ENDOCRINE BOARD REVIEW

David S. Cooper, MD, Program Chair
Professor of Medicine
Director, Thyroid Clinic
The Johns Hopkins University
School of Medicine

Richard J. Auchus, MD, PhD
Professor of Internal Medicine
Division of Metabolism,
Endocrinology & Diabetes
University of Michigan Medical School

Carolyn B. Becker, MD
Associate Professor of Medicine
and Master Clinician
Division of Endocrinology,
Diabetes and Hypertension
Brigham and Women's Hospital

Andrea D. Coviello, MD
Associate Professor of Medicine
Division of Endocrinology,
Metabolism, and Nutrition
Duke University School of Medicine

Frances J. Hayes, MD
Clinical Director
Endocrine Division
Massachusetts General Hospital

Serge A. Jabbour, MD
Professor and Division Director
Division of Endocrinology
Thomas Jefferson University
Sidney Kimmel Medical College

Michelle F. Magee, MD
Associate Professor of Medicine
Georgetown University
School of Medicine

Mark E. Molitch, MD
Professor of Medicine
Division of Endocrinology, Metabolism,
and Molecular Medicine
Northwestern University
Feinberg School of Medicine

Elizabeth N. Pearce, MD, MSc
Associate Professor
Endocrinology, Diabetes
& Nutrition Section
Boston University School of Medicine

Margaret E. Wierman, MD
Professor of Medicine
University of Colorado
School of Medicine

Abbie L. Young, MS, CGC, ELS(D)
Medical Editor

Endocrine Society
2055 L Street NW, Suite 600, Washington, DC 20036
1-888-ENDOCRINE • www.endocrine.org

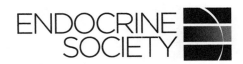
ENDOCRINE
SOCIETY

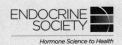

OVERVIEW

The Endocrine Board Review (EBR) is a board examination preparation course designed for endocrine fellows who have completed or are nearing completion of their fellowship, and are preparing to sit the board certification exam, as well as for practicing endocrinologists in search of a comprehensive self-assessment of endocrinology, either to prepare for recertification or to update their practice. EBR consists of 240 case-based, American Board of Internal Medicine (ABIM)–style, multiple-choice questions, presented in a mock exam format. Each section follows the ABIM Endocrinology, Diabetes, and Metabolism Certification Examination blueprint, covering the breadth and depth of the certification and recertification examinations. Each case is discussed in detail, with extensive answer explanations and references provided. A customized score report is provided to individuals participating in the live and online activities.

ACCREDITATION STATEMENT

The Endocrine Society is accredited by the Accreditation Council for Continuing Medical Education (ACCME) to provide continuing medical education (CME) for physicians. The Endocrine Society has achieved Accreditation with Commendation.

METHODS OF PARTICIPATION

This material is presented in 3 activities (1 live activity and 2 enduring activities), as follows:

- Endocrine Board Review 2017 (live activity in Chicago, IL, September 26-27, 2017)
- EBR Online 2017 (enduring online activity)
- Endocrine Board Review, 9th Edition (enduring book activity)

AMA PRA CATEGORY 1 CREDITS™ (CME) AND MAINTENANCE OF CERTIFICATION (MOC)

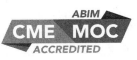

The Endocrine Society designates this activity for a maximum of 14.25 *AMA PRA Category 1 Credits*™. Physicians should claim only the credit commensurate with the extent of their participation in the activity.

Successful completion of this CME activity, which includes participation in the evaluation component, enables the participant to earn up to 14.25 MOC points and patient safety MOC credit in the ABIM Maintenance of Certification (MOC) program. Participants will earn MOC points equivalent to the amount of CME credits claimed for the activity. It is the CME activity provider's responsibility to submit participant completion information to the ACCME for the purpose of granting ABIM MOC credit.

To claim CME credit or MOC points, participants must complete the activity evaluation form online (accessible via the participant's Endocrine Society Center for Learning pending activities at *https://education.endocrine.org*).

CME or MOC points for the activities related to this material must be claimed by the following deadlines:

- Endocrine Board Review 2017 (live activity in Chicago, IL, September 26-27, 2017): October 31, 2017
- EBR Online 2017 (online activity): October 31, 2018
- Endocrine Board Review, 9th Edition (book activity): October 31, 2018

After completing the evaluation, you will be able to save or print a CME certificate. MOC points earned will be reported to the ABIM.

For questions about content or obtaining CME credit or MOC points, please contact the Endocrine Society at *https://education.endocrine.org/contact*.

LEARNING OBJECTIVES

Upon completion of this educational activity, learners will be able to demonstrate enhanced medical knowledge and clinical skills across all major areas of endocrinology; apply knowledge and skills in diagnosing, managing, and treating a wide spectrum of endocrine disorders; and successfully complete the board examination for certification or recertification in the subspecialty of endocrinology, diabetes, and metabolism.

TARGET AUDIENCE

This CME activity should be of substantial interest to endocrinologists, internists, and endocrine fellows preparing for the board examination or recertification or to endocrinologists and other health care practitioners seeking a review in endocrinology.

STATEMENT OF INDEPENDENCE

As a provider of CME accredited by the ACCME, the Endocrine Society has a policy of ensuring that the content and quality of this educational activity are balanced, independent, objective, and scientifically rigorous. The scientific content of this activity was developed under the supervision of the Endocrine Society's Endocrine Board Review Chair on the Clinical Endocrinology Update Steering Committee. The commercial supporters of this activity have no influence over the planning of this CME activity.

DISCLOSURE POLICY

The faculty, committee members, and staff who are in position to control the content of this activity are required to disclose to the Endocrine Society and to learners any relevant financial relationship(s) of the individual or spouse/partner that have occurred within the last 12 months with any commercial interest(s) whose products or services are related to the CME content. Financial relationships are defined by remuneration in any amount from the commercial interest(s) in the form of grants; research support; consulting fees; salary; ownership interest (eg, stocks, stock options, or ownership interest excluding diversified mutual funds); honoraria or other payments for participation in speakers' bureaus, advisory boards, or boards of directors; or other financial benefits. The intent of this disclosure is not to prevent CME planners with relevant financial relationships from planning or delivery of content, but rather to provide learners with information that allows them to make their own judgments of whether these financial relationships may have influenced the educational activity with regard to exposition or conclusion.

The Endocrine Society has reviewed all disclosures and resolved or managed all identified conflicts of interest, as applicable.

The faculty reported the following relevant financial relationship(s) during the content development process for this activity:

　Richard J. Auchus, MD, PhD: *Contracted Research*, Millendo Pharmaceuticals; *Contracted Research and Consultant*, Novartis Pharmaceuticals, Strongbridge Biopharma; *Consultant*, Alder Biopharmaceuticals, Corcept Pharmaceuticals, Diurnal Limited, Ipsen Pharmaceuticals, Janssen Pharmaceuticals, Spruce Biosciences

　Andrea D. Coviello, MD: *Consultant and Speaker*, Novo Nordisk Inc.

　Serge A. Jabbour, MD: *Consultant*, AstraZeneca, Eli Lilly & Co., Janssen Pharmaceuticals

　Mark E. Molitch, MD: *Consultant*, Pfizer Inc.; *Consultant and Primary Investigator*, Chiasma, Inc., Ipsen Pharmaceuticals, Novartis Pharmaceuticals

　Elizabeth N. Pearce, MD, MSc: *Primary Investigator*, Sociedad Química y Minera de Chile S.A.; *Speaker*, IBSA Institut Biochimique SA, Merck Serono

The following faculty reported no relevant financial relationships: Carolyn B. Becker, MD; David S. Cooper, MD; Frances J. Hayes, MD; Michelle F. Magee, MD; Margaret E. Wierman, MD

The medical editor for this activity reported no relevant financial relationships: Abbie L. Young, MS, CGC, ELS(D)

Endocrine Society staff associated with the development of content for this activity reported no relevant financial relationships.

DISCLAIMERS

The information presented in this activity represents the opinion of the faculty and is not necessarily the official position of the Endocrine Society.

USE OF PROFESSIONAL JUDGMENT:
The educational content in this activity relates to basic principles of diagnosis and therapy and does not substitute for individual patient assessment based on the health care provider's examination of the patient and consideration of laboratory data and other factors unique to the patient. Standards in medicine change as new data become available.

DRUGS AND DOSAGES:
When prescribing medications, the physician is advised to check the product information sheet accompanying each drug to verify conditions of use and to identify any changes in drug dosage schedule or contraindications.

POLICY ON UNLABELED/OFF-LABEL USE

The Endocrine Society has determined that disclosure of unlabeled/off-label or investigational use of commercial product(s) is informative for audiences and therefore requires this information to be disclosed to the learners at the beginning of the presentation. Uses of specific therapeutic agents, devices, and other products discussed in this educational activity may not be the same as those indicated in product labeling approved by the Food and Drug Administration (FDA). The Endocrine Society requires that any discussions of such "off-label" use be based on scientific research that conforms to generally accepted standards of experimental design, data collection, and data analysis. Before recommending or prescribing any therapeutic agent or device, learners should review the complete prescribing information, including indications, contraindications, warnings, precautions, and adverse events.

PRIVACY AND CONFIDENTIALITY STATEMENT

The Endocrine Society will record learner's personal information as provided on CME evaluations to allow for issuance and tracking of CME certificates. The Endocrine Society may also track aggregate responses to questions in activities and evaluations and use these data to inform the ongoing evaluation and improvement of its CME program. No individual performance data or any other personal information collected from evaluations will be shared with third parties.

ACKNOWLEDGMENT OF COMMERCIAL SUPPORT

The activity from which this material is produced was supported by an educational grant from Merck & Co., Inc.*

*As of August 16, 2017

Last Review: August 2017

Activity Release: September 2017

Activity Expiration Date (date after which this material is no longer certified for credit): see section titled "*AMA PRA Category 1 Credits*" (CME) and Maintenance of Certification (MOC)"

Contents

ENDOCRINE
BOARD
REVIEW

Diabetes Mellitus, Section 1 Board Review

Serge A. Jabbour, MD • Thomas Jefferson University

1 A 68-year-old man wants your opinion on how he can prevent diabetes in the future. He has a history of hypertension and dyslipidemia, both well controlled on ramipril and atorvastatin.

On physical examination, his BMI is 33 kg/m² and blood pressure is 120/60 mm Hg. He has 2+ edema in both lower extremities. Findings are otherwise unremarkable.

Recent laboratory test results:
    Plasma glucose (fasting) = 108 mg/dL
        (6.0 mmol/L)
    2-Hour postload glucose = 165 mg/dL
        (9.2 mmol/L)
    Hemoglobin A_{1c} = 5.9% (41 mmol/mol)
    Serum creatinine, normal
    Liver function tests, normal
    TSH, normal
    Estimated glomerular filtration rate = 76 mL/min
        per 1.73 m²

On the basis of available studies, which of the following is the best option?
    A. Once-weekly exenatide
    B. Dapagliflozin
    C. Metformin
    D. Lifestyle intervention
    E. Pioglitazone

2 A 25-year-old woman with a 10-year history of type 1 diabetes mellitus is seeing you for a follow-up visit. She has been stressed out at work for the past few months and reports having intermittent nausea for the last few days. She tells you that she feels unwell and attributes it to stress. She uses insulin pump therapy with insulin lispro at a basal rate of 1.4 units/h, an insulin-to-carbohydrate ratio of 1:10, and a sensitivity factor of 1:30. She has not been doing glucose fingerstick readings at home on a regular basis, but when she does the values range between 70 and 250 mg/dL (3.9 and 13.9 mmol/L) without a real pattern. A glucose fingerstick measurement in the office today is 385 mg/dL (21.4 mmol/L). Laboratory tests from 2 weeks ago show a hemoglobin A_{1c} value of 8.3% (67 mmol/mol) with normal basic metabolic panel, TSH, and complete blood cell count.

Which of the following is the best immediate next step?
    A. Basal rate testing
    B. Diabetes education
    C. Assessment for urine ketones
    D. Continuous glucose sensor
    E. Therapy for stress management

3 You are asked to see a 79-year-old man with a 30-year history of type 2 diabetes mellitus who is admitted to the hospital with severe hyperglycemia and change in mental status. The patient lives alone and was found by his neighbor in a confused state. It is unclear whether the patient has been taking his insulin and other medications.

On physical examination, the patient is lethargic and unable to answer any questions. His temperature is 100.5°F (38.1°C), blood pressure is 100/60 mm Hg, and pulse rate is 110 beats/min. His weight is 220 lb (100 kg), and BMI is 32 kg/m². Skin and mucous membranes are dry. There is no focal neurologic deficit.

Laboratory test results:
    Hemoglobin A_{1c} = 8.5% (69 mmol/mol)
    Plasma glucose = 1105 mg/dL (61.3 mmol/L)
    Serum sodium = 130 mEq/L (130 mmol/L)
    Serum potassium = 4.5 mEq/L (4.5 mmol/L)
    Serum bicarbonate = 21 mEq/L (21 mmol/L)
    Serum chloride = 106 mEq/L (106 mmol/L)
    Serum creatinine = 1.9 mg/dL (168.0 µmol/L)
    Arterial pH = 7.35

Serum β-hydroxybutyrate = 2.6 mg/dL
(249.8 μmol/L)
Effective serum osmolality = 312.3 mOsm/kg
(312.3 mmol/kg)

Which of the following is the best next step?

Answer	Fluids	Insulin
A.	1.5 L of 0.9% NaCl over the first hour	Intravenous insulin bolus of 10 units, then 10 units per hour
B.	1.5 L of 0.9% NaCl over the first hour	Intravenous insulin bolus of 10 units, then 2 units per hour
C.	1.5 L of 0.45% NaCl over the first hour	Intravenous insulin bolus of 10 units, then 10 units per hour
D.	1.5 L of 0.45% NaCl over the first hour	Intravenous insulin at the 10 units per hour
E.	1.5 L of 3% NaCl over the first hour	Intravenous insulin bolus of 10 units, then 10 units per hour

4 A 69-year-old man with type 2 diabetes mellitus is seeing you for a routine follow-up visit and is accompanied by his wife. His medical history is notable for hypertension and dyslipidemia. His main concern is fatigue, daytime sleepiness, and a 10-lb (4.5-kg) weight gain over the past few months. One of his friends told him he should have testing for "adrenal fatigue." His wife states that he has erectile dysfunction despite normal libido, as well as nighttime snoring. His medications include metformin, sitagliptin, rosuvastatin, ramipril, and baby aspirin.

On physical examination, his BMI is 36 kg/m² and blood pressure is 120/60 mm Hg.

Laboratory test results:
Hemoglobin A_{1c} = 6.8% (51 mmol/mol)
Serum sodium = 141 mEq/L (141 mmol/L)
Serum potassium = 4 mEq/L (4 mmol/L)
Serum creatinine = 0.6 mg/dL (53.0 μmol/L)
TSH = 3.8 mIU/L
Serum cortisol (8 AM) = 10 μg/dL (275.9 nmol/L)
Total testosterone = 250 ng/dL (8.7 nmol/L)
LH = 3.0 mIU/mL (3.0 IU/L)
FSH = 9.0 mIU/mL (9.0 IU/L)

Which of the following should you order next?
A. ACTH stimulation test
B. Pituitary MRI
C. Serum prolactin measurement
D. Polysomnography
E. Free T_4 measurement

5 You are evaluating a 48-year-old woman with new-onset type 2 diabetes mellitus. Nonalcoholic steatohepatitis was recently diagnosed after routine testing showed abnormal liver function. Subsequent workup, including a liver biopsy, revealed nonalcoholic steatohepatitis with pathologic evidence of steatosis, lobular inflammation, hepatocellular ballooning, and fibrosis. There was no evidence of cirrhosis.

Laboratory test results:
Hemoglobin A_{1c} = 8.0% (64 mmol/mol)
Creatinine = 0.8 mg/dL (70.7 μmol/L)
Alanine aminotransferase = 89 U/L (1.5 μkat/L)
TSH = 2.5 mIU/L

The hepatologist suggests that you prescribe an antidiabetes agent that would also improve her liver histology.

Which of the following would be the best choice?
A. Metformin
B. Dapagliflozin
C. Dulaglutide
D. Sitagliptin
E. Pioglitazone

6 A 26-year-old white woman with polycystic ovary syndrome is seeing you for the first time to establish care after her previous endocrinologist left the area. She has had irregular menses since menarche, facial hirsutism, and acne. She has had a good clinical response to hormonal contraception and spironolactone. She has no concerns at this time and has no pregnancy plans.

On physical examination, her BMI is 32 kg/m² and blood pressure is 110/60 mm Hg. A Ferriman-Gallwey score is 10 (normal <8). Otherwise, her examination findings are normal.

Her electrolytes, creatinine, and TSH are normal.

Which of the following is the most sensitive test to evaluate her risk for diabetes?
  - A. 2-Hour oral glucose tolerance test
  - B. Serum insulin measurement
  - C. Hemoglobin A_{1c} measurement
  - D. Fasting glucose measurement
  - E. Glucose-to-insulin ratio

7 An 18-year-old man is referred to you for management of type 1 diabetes mellitus, which was recently diagnosed during a hospital admission 6 weeks ago. After conversion from an intravenous insulin drip, he started basal and mealtime insulins. He is currently doing well with stable home blood glucose measurements and has no concerns. His mother asks whether he should be screened for other autoimmune conditions.

If tested, which of the following antibodies will he most likely have?
  - A. Tissue transglutaminase antibodies
  - B. Thyroid-stimulating immunoglobins
  - C. 21-Hydroxylase antibodies
  - D. Parathyroid gland antibodies
  - E. TPO antibodies

8 A 22-year-old woman who is a professional model has a 10-year history of type 1 diabetes mellitus. She is referred to you for management of poor glycemic control. She is on bedtime insulin glargine, 16 units, and mealtime insulin lispro at a dose of 1 unit for every 10 g of carbohydrates. Her glycemic control was initially acceptable with hemoglobin A_{1c} values around 7.0% (53 mmol/mol), but over the past few years, she has missed a few appointments and her hemoglobin A_{1c} has reached 9% to 10% (75-86 mmol/mol). She has had 3 episodes of diabetic ketoacidosis in the past 8 months. Recurrent hypoglycemic events have been occurring without a specific pattern. She always forgets to bring a record of her home glucose measurements or even her glucose meter to visits. She has no symptoms. She states she has lost 8 lb (3.6 kg) intentionally over the past year. Her menses are regular on hormonal contraception.

On physical examination, her blood pressure is 110/60 mm Hg. She refuses to be weighed. Her last BMI recorded in the chart was 22 kg/m² 2 years ago. Her examination findings are unremarkable.

Laboratory test results:
  Hemoglobin A_{1c} = 9.1% (76 mmol/mol)
  Estimated glomerular filtration rate = 75 mL/min
    per 1.73 m²
  Serum sodium = 141 mEq/L (141 mmol/L)
  Serum potassium = 3.6 mEq/L (3.6 mmol/L)
  Serum cortisol, not done due to laboratory error
  ACTH = 38 pg/mL (8.4 pmol/L)
  TSH = 2 mIU/L
  Tissue transglutaminase antibodies, negative

Which of the following is the best next step?
  - A. Initiation of insulin pump therapy
  - B. ACTH stimulation test
  - C. Gliadin antibody assessment
  - D. Psychological evaluation
  - E. Initiation of a tricyclic antidepressant

9 A 36-year-old Asian American man presents to his primary care physician for an annual visit. He feels well and has no concerns. He has no known medical conditions. His only medication is a daily multivitamin. He has no known family history of diabetes mellitus and does not smoke cigarettes or drink alcohol.

On physical examination, his blood pressure is 120/70 mm Hg and BMI is 24.0 kg/m². The rest of his examination findings are unremarkable.

In addition to lifestyle management counseling regarding diet and physical activity, when should screening be performed with respect to his prediabetes/diabetes risk?
  - A. Now
  - B. At age 45 years
  - C. When symptomatic
  - D. Only if BMI is greater than 25 kg/m²

10 A 42-year-old woman with an 8-year history of type 2 diabetes mellitus is referred for a second opinion regarding her unexplained high hemoglobin A_{1c} level. She has been on basal plus mealtime insulins for 3 years. She does self-monitoring of blood glucose 6 to 8 times daily, with values ranging between 75 and 120 mg/dL (4.2 and 6.7 mmol/L) before meals and between 110 and 130 mg/dL (6.1 and 7.2 mmol/L) 2 hours after meals. She reports rare hypoglycemic episodes.

Her review of systems is notable for recent fatigue and lightheadedness. She is scheduled for hysterectomy next month due to fibroids causing recurrent bleeding. Her medications include aspirin and ramipril. Her hemoglobin A_{1c} had been in the range of 6.5% to 6.9% (48 to 52 mmol/mol) for years, but 4 months ago it was 7.8% (62 mmol/mol) and a recent value was 8.5% (69 mmol/mol).

Laboratory test results:
Serum creatinine = 1.1 mg/dL (97.2 μmol/L)
Liver enzymes and TSH, normal
Urine albumin-to-creatinine ratio = 125 mg/g

Which of the following is the most likely cause of her high hemoglobin A_{1c}?
A. High nighttime blood glucose levels
B. Laboratory error
C. Hemolysis
D. Pregnancy
E. Iron deficiency

11 A 38-year-old man with sickle cell disease and a 20-year history of type 1 diabetes mellitus complicated by nephropathy and retinopathy is referred for help achieving better glycemic control. He is on insulin pump therapy at a basal rate of 1.1 units/h and an insulin-to-carbohydrate ratio of 1:12. Self-monitoring of blood glucose 4 times daily shows values ranging between 160 and 300 mg/dL (8.9 and 16.7 mmol/L). His hemoglobin A_{1c} level has been between 8.5% and 10% (69 and 86 mmol/mol). His medications include aspirin, ramipril, and atorvastatin.

Laboratory test results:
Hemoglobin A_{1c} = 9% (75 mmol/mol)
Serum creatinine = 2.2 mg/dL (194.5 μmol/L)
Urine albumin-to-creatinine ratio = 3886 mg/g
Liver function tests, normal
TSH = 7.5 mIU/L
Serum fructosamine = 210 μmol/L (reference range, 205-285 μmol/L)

The discrepancy between this patient's hemoglobin A_{1c} and fructosamine levels is most likely caused by which of the following?
A. Laboratory error
B. Sickle cell disease
C. Hemolysis
D. Hypothyroidism
E. Proteinuria

12 A 26-year-old man with type 1 diabetes mellitus who is on basal/mealtime insulins and resides in Louisiana went on a ski trip to Colorado. During his trip, he experienced frequent, unusually high fingerstick blood glucose readings not explained by food or activity changes.

Which of the following factor(s) can affect the accuracy of blood glucose meter readings?

Answer	Temperature	Altitude
A.	+	+
B.	−	−
C.	−	+
D.	+	−

13 A 33-year-old man with a 6-year history of type 1 diabetes mellitus returns for a follow-up visit frustrated by intermittent variation in glucose control despite use of an insulin pump and a continuous glucose sensor for the last 6 months. Recently, his blood glucose values have been more labile, with occasional unexplained highs above 350 mg/dL (>19.4 mmol/L). On further questioning, you learn there are also periods when his blood glucose levels are reasonably stable. His job requires some travel, often a week or two a month. He has occasional migraine headaches that can last 5 to 7 days. His medications include insulin lispro, a multivitamin, calcium, vitamin D, biotin, and acetaminophen as needed for headaches.

You review the data downloaded from his continuous glucose-monitoring device. Data from 2 consecutive weeks are shown (*see images*).

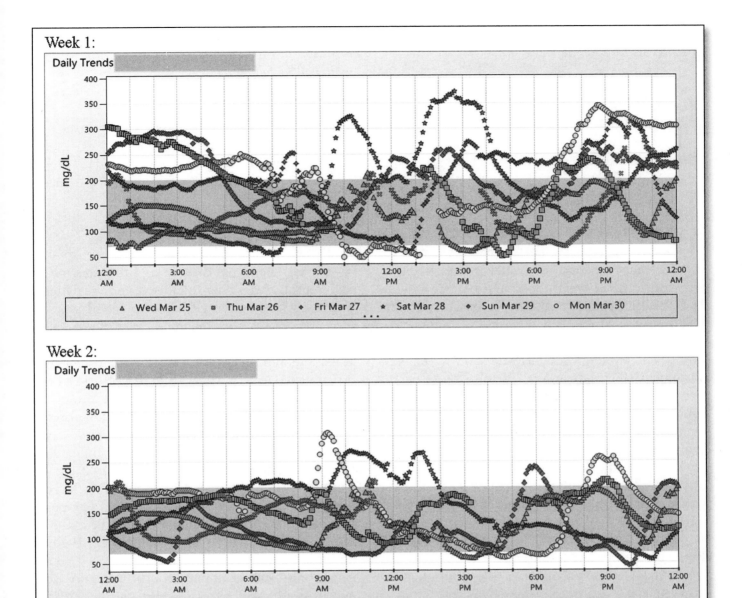

Week 1:

Daily Trends

| Wed Mar 25 | Thu Mar 26 | Fri Mar 27 | Sat Mar 28 | Sun Mar 29 | Mon Mar 30 |

Week 2:

Daily Trends

| Sat Mar 21 | Sun Mar 22 | Mon Mar 23 | Tue Mar 24 | Wed Mar 25 | Thu Mar 26 |

Besides variations in lifestyle management, which of the following do you hypothesize is causing his blood glucose spikes?

A. Biotin

B. Meal boluses that are low

C. Acetaminophen

D. Basal insulin rates that are low

14 A 32-year-old woman with a 12-year history of type 1 diabetes mellitus is seeing you for follow-up visit. She has had poor glycemic control for the past few years on insulin pump therapy and is reluctant to increase her pump settings as this could result in more weight gain. She has tried metformin and pramlintide in the past but she could not tolerate the gastrointestinal adverse effects. Her hemoglobin A_{1c} value is now 7.8% (62 mmol/mol), and her BMI is 27 kg/m^2.

Her basic metabolic panel, liver function, and TSH are normal. You suggest off-label use of empagliflozin to lower her hemoglobin A_{1c} and reduce her weight. She asks about potential adverse effects.

You tell her that empagliflozin could increase her risk of which of the following?

    A. Hip fracture
    B. Hyperkalemia
    C. Bladder tumor
    D. Hyponatremia
    E. Diabetic ketoacidosis

15 A 19-year-old woman with a 2-year history of type 1 diabetes mellitus comes to the emergency department after experiencing 1 week of polyuria, weight loss, and blurred vision. Her insulin regimen consists of basal/mealtime insulins, with a total daily insulin dose of approximately 0.5 units/kg per day. Before this, she was doing well, although she has gained 15 lb (6.8 kg) since her diabetes diagnosis. The only other pertinent history is treatment of depression with olanzapine for the past year, and she states that she is feeling stressed with preparation for college final exams next month.

On physical examination, her BMI is 24 kg/m². She has moderate midepigastric tenderness to palpation, but her examination findings are otherwise unremarkable.

Initial laboratory test results:
    Serum glucose = 436 mg/dL (24.2 mmol/L)
    Hemoglobin A_{1c} = 9.2% (77 mmol/mol)
    Bicarbonate = 14 mEq/L (14 mmol/L)
    Serum pH = 7.2
    Serum creatinine = 1.9 mg/dL (168.0 µmol/L)
    Serum potassium = 5.3 mEq/L (5.3 mmol/L)
    Urinalysis = 4+ glucose, large ketones, few white
      blood cells, no red blood cells, no blood
    Hematocrit = 51% (0.51)

After you consider what could have caused the deterioration in this patient's metabolic control, you do which of the following?

    A. Request a nephrology consult to evaluate her high creatinine
    B. Request a psychiatry consult to manage the discontinuation of olanzapine
    C. Review the electronic medical record to see when the prescriptions for insulin and syringes were last filled
    D. Increase her total daily insulin dose

16 A 17-year-old woman is referred to you for her recent diagnosis of diabetes mellitus. Her father has type 1 diabetes, and the patient, out of curiosity, checked her own blood glucose level with his glucose meter. She reported a value of 212 mg/dL (11.8 mmol/L) 2 hours after dinner. A hemoglobin A_{1c} measurement was subsequently documented to be 6.9% (52 mmol/mol) and a fasting glucose value was 91 mg/dL (5.1 mmol/L). Tests for islet-cell antibodies, insulin autoantibodies, and glutamic acid decarboxylase autoantibodies were negative. The patient began a low-carbohydrate diet and has been exercising regularly for 3 months, but her repeated hemoglobin A_{1c} level is now 7.4% (57 mmol/mol) and many of her postprandial glucose measurements are in the range of 200 to 250 mg/dL (11.1 to 13.9 mmol/L). She has no symptoms of hyperglycemia.

On physical examination, she has no skin tags or acanthosis nigricans. Her weight is 153 lb (69.5 kg) (BMI = 26 kg/m²). You wonder whether she has type 1 diabetes like her father.

Which of the following should you order next to help confirm the diagnosis of type 1 diabetes?

    A. Oral glucose tolerance testing
    B. Zinc transporter 8 (ZnT8) antibody testing
    C. Testing for *GCK* (glucokinase) gene mutations
    D. HLA haplotype determination

17 A 58-year-old man with no notable medical history presents to his primary care physician with a few months' history of an unintentional 5-lb (2.3-kg) weight loss and a 2-week history of polyuria and nocturia. His family history includes type 2 diabetes mellitus in a maternal aunt.

On physical examination, his blood pressure is 110/72 mm Hg, weight is 163 lb (74.1 kg), and BMI is 24 kg/m^2. His examination findings are unremarkable, with no localizing signs of infection.

Laboratory test results:
  Random serum glucose = 254 mg/dL
    (14.1 mmol/L)
  Hemoglobin A$_{1c}$ = 8.3% (67 mmol/mol)
  Creatinine = 0.7 mg/dL (61.9 μmol/L)
  Complete blood cell count and electrolytes, normal

He is referred to you 3 months later, while he is taking metformin, 1000 mg twice daily. You review the following laboratory test results:
  Random serum glucose = 233 mg/dL
    (12.9 mmol/L)
  Hemoglobin A$_{1c}$ = 8.4% (68 mmol/mol)
  C-peptide = 1.2 ng/mL (0.4 nmol/L) (reference range, 0.9-4.3 ng/mL [0.3-1.4 nmol/L])

Review of his twice-daily self-monitoring blood glucose log reveals most values in the range of the high 100s to low 200s (mg/dL) (5.6-11.1 mmol/L), with an average of 189 mg/dL (10.5 mmol/L).

Which of the following is the best next step to manage this patient's glycemia?
  A. Start insulin
  B. Add a sodium-glucose cotransporter 2 inhibitor
  C. Add a once-weekly glucagonlike peptide 1 receptor agonist
  D. Add a sulfonylurea

18 A 26-year-old man with a 6-year history of type 1 diabetes mellitus presents for follow-up. He has been on insulin glargine, 20 units at bedtime, and insulin aspart with meals. His insulin-to-carbohydrate ratio is 1 unit for every 8 g of carbohydrate, and his insulin sensitivity factor is 1 unit for every 30 mg/dL (1.7 mmol/L) above a blood glucose value of 100 mg/dL (5.6 mmol/L).

His fasting blood glucose values range from 80 to 130 mg/dL (4.4 to 7.2 mmol/L). His 2-hour postprandial blood glucose measurements are in the high 100s, low 200s. A recent hemoglobin A$_{1c}$ measurement was 7.6% (60 mmol/mol), down from 8.4% (68 mmol/mol) 4 months ago. He has had no recent hypoglycemic events.

His main concern is a 10-lb (4.5-kg) weight gain since his improved glycemic control over the past year and his inability to lose it. He refuses to switch to an insulin pump or to use a continuous glucose sensor. He refuses to increase his insulin requirements at meals because of fear of additional weight gain.

You recommend adding pramlintide injections immediately before each meal, starting at 15 mcg and titrating the dose as tolerated every 3 days to a maximal dose of 60 mcg.

Which of the following would you advise him to do upon starting pramlintide?
  A. Reduce insulin glargine to 10 units
  B. Change carbohydrate ratio to 1:16
  C. Continue same insulin regimen
  D. Change sensitivity factor to 1:60
  E. Reduce insulin glargine to 10 units and change carbohydrate ratios to 1:16

19 A 27-year-old man with type 1 diabetes mellitus who uses an insulin pump with good glycemic control started jogging for 1 to 2 hours several times weekly. He is concerned about the multiple hypoglycemic events he has been experiencing during exercise, sometimes followed by hyperglycemia hours later. He asks for advice on how to minimize this. His recent hemoglobin A$_{1c}$ level is 7.0% (53 mmol/mol).

In addition to monitoring blood glucose before, during, and after exercise, you advise that:

   A. He should consider a brief period of weightlifting before jogging to reduce the chance of hypoglycemia

   B. He should eat a big snack before and while jogging, as well as raise his basal rate for 2 hours when finished

   C. He should jog only if his blood glucose level is greater than 150 mg/dL (>8.3 mmol/L) before starting

   D. He should avoid aerobic activity

20 A 24-year-old woman without diabetes whose husband has type 1 diabetes mellitus is contemplating pregnancy and is inquiring about the risk of type 1 diabetes developing in her child. None of her family members have type 1 diabetes.

Which of the following characterizes the risk of type 1 diabetes developing in her offspring?

   A. 0.1%

   B. 0.4%

   C. 6.0%

   D. 20.0%

   E. 30.0%

21 A 67-year-old woman is referred by her primary care physician for a 9-year history of uncontrolled type 2 diabetes mellitus. Diet, exercise, and 3 agents (metformin, glimepiride, and canagliflozin) have been unsuccessful. One year ago, oral agents were discontinued and she was prescribed intensive insulin therapy with multiple daily injections. Currently, she is on 80 units of insulin glargine twice daily and 120 units daily of insulin aspart with meals. However, her hemoglobin A_{1c} levels have ranged from 9.4% to 10.7% (79 to 93 mmol/mol).

On physical examination, her BMI is 43.5 kg/m² and blood pressure is 130/79 mm Hg.

Her hemoglobin A_{1c} level is 9.8% (84 mmol/mol), and estimated glomerular filtration rate is 68 mL/min per 1.73m².

Which of the following is the best next step to improve this patient's glycemic control?

   A. Add metformin to current insulin therapy

   B. Convert multiple daily injections to insulin pump therapy

   C. Convert the insulin regimen to U500 insulin

   D. Switch insulin glargine to insulin degludec, 110 units in the morning and evening

22 A 71-year-old woman with a 17-year history of type 2 diabetes mellitus has developed episodes of confusion and disorientation over the past 4 weeks. Her current diabetes treatment regimen includes insulin glargine, 50 units at bedtime; metformin, 1000 mg twice daily; and repaglinide, 2 mg before meals. She measures her blood glucose levels 3 times daily, typically before meals. Over the past few weeks, she has had several blood glucose values less than 50 mg/dL (<2.8 mmol/L), but she has not felt any symptoms of hypoglycemia. Her hemoglobin A_{1c} level is 6.2% (44 mmol/mol). You diagnose hypoglycemia unawareness.

Blood chemistries, urinalysis, and liver function tests are within normal limits.

Which of the following is the best next step in her care?

Answer	Insulin Glargine	Repaglinide
A.	Decrease to 40 units at bedtime	Continue same dosage
B.	Decrease to 40 units at bedtime	Discontinue
C.	Replace with 50 units of insulin detemir	Discontinue
D.	Replace with 25 units of twice-daily NPH insulin	Discontinue

23 A 46-year-old man presents for advice on treatment of type 2 diabetes mellitus. He has been treated with metformin for 4 years. He has dyslipidemia and longstanding hypertension with chronic kidney disease. His only medications are metformin, rosuvastatin, and lisinopril.

On physical examination, his BMI is 33 kg/m² and blood pressure is 138/84 mm Hg.

His hemoglobin A_{1c} level is 7.8% (62 mmol/mol), and estimated glomerular filtration rate is 53 mL/min per 1.73 m².

You decide to add linagliptin. You explain to him that this drug, by increasing glucagonlike peptide 1 levels, will target the following pathogenetic defects:

A. Insulin resistance and β-cell dysfunction
B. Hepatic glucose output and gastric emptying
C. Renal glucose reabsorption and satiety
D. Glucagon secretion and gastric emptying
E. Hepatic glucose output and β-cell dysfunction

24 A 19-year-old man presents for continued management of type 1 diabetes, having "aged-out" of pediatric endocrine care. Diabetes was diagnosed at age 16 years when glycosuria and moderate hyperglycemia were found on a yearly checkup. Insulin therapy was started immediately. His current insulin dose is approximately 0.3 units/kg per day, administered as multiple daily injections, and his current hemoglobin A_{1c} level is 6.4% (46 mmol/mol) with occasional hypoglycemia. His family history is positive for type 1 diabetes in his mother, maternal grandfather, and an older sibling, all diagnosed at age 19 years or younger. His BMI is 23 kg/m².

Tests for glutamic acid decarboxylase antibodies, islet-cell antibodies, and insulinoma-associated protein 2 antibodies are negative; he did not have antibody testing at diagnosis. His serum C-peptide concentration is 1.1 ng/mL (0.4 nmol/L).

Which of the following is the optimal management of this patient's diabetes?

A. Insulin administration via a continuous subcutaneous insulin infusion pump
B. Discontinuation of insulin and initiation of empagliflozin
C. Discontinuation of insulin and initiation of metformin
D. Discontinuation of insulin and initiation of glimepiride

25 A 46-year-old Hispanic man presents for follow-up after he was admitted to an outside hospital 3 months ago with hyperglycemia. His hemoglobin A_{1c} level was 12.0% (108 mmol/mol). He was also told he had marked metabolic acidosis and ketonemia on admission. He was treated with intravenous insulin and discharged 3 days later on insulin glargine, 10 units at bedtime each day. He has not been monitoring his blood glucose values at home, but he reports feeling that his blood glucose is "low" in the morning. His medical history is otherwise unremarkable, and his family history is notable only for type 2 diabetes diagnosed in his father at age 65 years.

On physical examination, his blood pressure is 122/73 mm Hg. The rest of his examination findings are unremarkable.

You obtain the outside hospital records, which confirm his history in addition to revealing marked metabolic acidosis and ketonemia on admission.

Which of the following measurements would most accurately guide this patient's long-term insulin management?

A. BMI, glutamic acid decarboxylase antibodies, and insulinoma-associated protein 2 antibodies
B. Glutamic acid decarboxylase antibodies, hemoglobin A_{1c}, and insulinoma-associated protein 2 antibodies
C. BMI, C-peptide, and hemoglobin A_{1c}
D. C-peptide, glutamic acid decarboxylase antibodies, and insulinoma-associated protein 2 antibodies

26 A 54-year-old woman with end-stage renal disease from polycystic kidney disease undergoes a renal transplant. She comes to see you 2 months later for management of new-onset diabetes. She is on tacrolimus and glucocorticoids. Her only concern is shortness of breath on exertion. She has a family history of type 2 diabetes mellitus. Her home fasting blood glucose measurements are between 150 and 210 mg/dL (8.3 and 11.7 mmol/L) despite a few weeks of lifestyle modifications with the help of a dietician.

On physical examination, her BMI is 32 kg/m². She has 2+ edema in her lower extremities.

Her hemoglobin A_{1c} level is 8.0% (64 mmol/mol), and estimated glomerular filtration rate is 52 mL/min per 1.73 m².

Which of the following is the most appropriate medication for the management of her condition?

A. Repaglinide
B. Pioglitazone
C. Dapagliflozin
D. Insulin glargine

27 A 20-year-old woman with cystic fibrosis affecting her lungs and liver is seeing you for the first time after a hemoglobin A_{1c} level of 6.2% (44 mmol/mol) was documented and oral glucose tolerance testing showed a 2-hour plasma glucose level of 245 mg/dL (13.6 mmol/L). Three months later, her hemoglobin A_{1c} level is 6.1% (43 mmol/mol) and the 2-hour plasma glucose level is 260 mg/dL (14.4 mmol/L). She has no family history of diabetes. Her BMI is 23 kg/m^2.

Which of the following medications should be started as the next step?
- A. Metformin
- B. Glimepiride
- C. Dulaglutide
- D. Insulin

28 A 28-year-old man is referred to you for new-onset diabetes discovered on routine testing. He has had low libido and erectile dysfunction for 1 year. His family history is notable for diabetes and liver disease of uncertain etiology in several relatives.

On physical examination, his BMI is 26 kg/m^2 and blood pressure is 110/60 mm Hg. He has no cushingoid features. He has a mildly enlarged, nontender liver.

Laboratory test results:
Hemoglobin A_{1c} = 6.9% (52 mmol/mol)
Creatinine = 0.8 mg/dL (70.7 μmol/L)
Alanine aminotransferase = 142 U/L (2.4 μkat/L)
Total testosterone = 220 ng/dL (7.6 nmol/L)

Which of the following tests is the best next step?
- A. Glutamic acid decarboxylase antibody titers
- B. Total iron-binding capacity and serum ferritin measurements
- C. Pancreatic CT
- D. Pituitary MRI

29 A 29-year-old woman is referred to you for weight management. She has schizophrenia that has been treated with olanzapine for the past 2 years. The patient reports a 15-lb (6.8-kg) weight gain since starting treatment.

On physical examination, her blood pressure is 130/70 mm Hg and BMI is 32 kg/m^2.

Laboratory test results:
Hemoglobin A_{1c} = 6.3% (45 mmol/mol)
Total cholesterol = 215 mg/dL (5.57 mmol/L)
Triglycerides = 310 mg/dL (3.50 mmol/L)
LDL cholesterol = 125 mg/dL (3.24 mmol/L)
HDL cholesterol = 36 mg/dL (0.93 mmol/L)
Creatinine = 0.9 mg/dL (79.6 μmol/L)
TSH = 1.6 mIU/L

You should suggest that her psychiatrist change her regimen from olanzapine to:
- A. Clozapine
- B. Aripiprazole
- C. Quetiapine
- D. Risperidone

30 A 32-year-old woman with a 20-year history of type 1 diabetes mellitus is referred to you to establish care. She has no diabetes complications and is not planning pregnancy. Her treatment regimen consists of insulins degludec and aspart.

On physical examination, her blood pressure is 120/70 mm Hg and BMI is 27 kg/m^2.

Laboratory test results:
Hemoglobin A_{1c} = 7.2% (55 mmol/mol)
Total cholesterol = 216 mg/dL (5.59 mmol/L)
LDL cholesterol = 136 mg/dL (3.52 mmol/L)
HDL cholesterol = 40 mg/dL (1.04 mmol/L)
Triglycerides = 210 mg/dL (2.37 mmol/L)
Serum creatinine = 0.86 mg/dL (76.0 μmol/L)
Urinary albumin-to-creatinine ratio = 19 mg/g

How should you advise the patient regarding the best course of action to reduce her risk for cardiovascular disease?
- A. Intensify her treatment regimen to attain a target hemoglobin A_{1c} level less than 7.0% (<53 mmol/mol)
- B. Start treatment with a statin
- C. Start treatment with an ACE inhibitor
- D. Refer to a nutritionist

Adrenal Board Review

Richard J. Auchus, MD, PhD • University of Michigan

1 A 43-year-old man is referred for evaluation of resistant hypertension and hypokalemia. His blood pressure while taking amlodipine, carvedilol, lisinopril, metformin, and potassium chloride was 148/96 mm Hg in his primary care physician's office 4 weeks ago. His primary care physician ordered measurement of aldosterone and plasma renin activity, then started spironolactone, 25 mg daily. The patient started the spironolactone, but did not have his blood drawn until 3 weeks later.

At his appointment today, his blood pressure is 133/86 mm Hg, and he feels well with no adverse effects from his medications.

Laboratory test results:
Sodium = 142 mEq/L (142 mmol/L)
Potassium = 3.6 mEq/L (3.6 mmol/L)
Serum aldosterone = 35 ng/dL (971 pmol/L)
Plasma renin activity = <0.6 ng/mL per h

Which of the following is the best next step in this patient's evaluation?
 A. Stop spironolactone for 6 weeks and measure aldosterone and renin activity again
 B. Stop carvedilol and lisinopril for 2 weeks and measure aldosterone and renin activity again
 C. Perform CT with fine cuts of the adrenals
 D. Perform adrenal MRI
 E. Substitute eplerenone for spironolactone

2 A 27-year-old woman was diagnosed at birth with classic 21-hydroxylase deficiency and has been treated with hydrocortisone and fludrocortisone acetate her entire life. She had vaginal reconstruction as an infant. For the last 18 months, she has been sexually active and wants to conceive, but this effort has been unsuccessful despite optimally timed intercourse. She currently takes hydrocortisone, 10 mg 3 times daily with each meal, and fludrocortisone acetate, 0.2 mg with the morning meal. She has regular monthly menses and shaves her upper lip and chin once a month.

On physical examination, she has mild moon facies, no striae or facial plethora, no acne, and a trace of shaved stubble.

Which of the following is the key laboratory parameter to monitor when adjusting her glucocorticoid therapy?
 A. Follicular-phase androstenedione
 B. Follicular-phase progesterone
 C. Premorning-dose 17-hydroxyprogesterone
 D. Periovulatory testosterone
 E. Luteal-phase 17-hydroxyprogesterone

3 A 45-year-old woman presents with resistant hypertension that has been more difficult to control in the past few years. She has also gained 22 lb (10 kg) over the last 2 years and now has diet-controlled diabetes mellitus. She developed hypokalemia while taking amlodipine and hydrochlorothiazide. Lisinopril and potassium chloride supplements were added, with resolution of the hypokalemia but without normalization of blood pressure.

On physical examination, she has subtle facial plethora and dermal atrophy. Proximal muscle strength is normal. She has no dorsocervical fat pad or striae.

Laboratory test results:
Sodium = 138 mEq/L (138 mmol/L)
Potassium = 3.7 mEq/L (3.7 mmol/L)
Chloride = 103 mEq/L (103 mmol/L)
Bicarbonate = 23 mEq/L (23 mmol/L)
Fasting glucose = 157 mg/dL (8.7 mmol/L)
Serum aldosterone = 16 ng/dL (444 pmol/L)
Plasma renin activity = <0.6 ng/mL per h
Serum urea nitrogen = 32 mg/dL (11.4 mmol/L)
Creatinine = 0.6 mg/dL (53.0 µmol/L)

Abdominal CT with contrast demonstrates a 3.8-cm left adrenal mass and an atrophic right adrenal gland (*see image, arrows*).

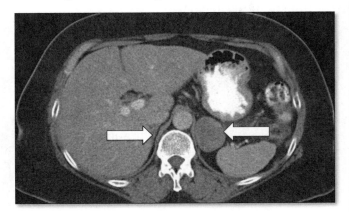

The patient is referred to you for further evaluation and recommendations.

Which of the following is the best next step?
   A. Prescribe spironolactone, 50 mg daily
   B. Measure plasma metanephrines and perform a 1-mg overnight dexamethasone suppression test
   C. Schedule adrenal venous sampling to measure aldosterone and cortisol
   D. Perform left adrenalectomy
   E. Perform a saline infusion test measuring aldosterone after administration of 2 L normal saline

4 A 54-year-old man with a 3-month history of weight gain, bruising, and facial changes is referred for possible Cushing syndrome. He has longstanding HIV infection and has a suppressed viral load while taking tenofovir, ritonavir, and didanosine. His symptoms started 2 weeks after starting salmeterol/fluticasone twice daily for worsening asthma due to the high spring pollen count.

On physical examination, he has facial plethora and moon facies, bruising, and central obesity. His primary care physician ordered a brain MRI, which shows an 8-mm hypoenhancing mass in the pituitary.

Which of the following sets of laboratory values do you predict?

Answer	Plasma ACTH	Serum DHEA-S	Cortisol After Dexamethasone
A.	High	High	High
B.	Low	Low	High
C.	Normal	Normal	Low
D.	Low	Low	Low
E.	Low	Normal	Low

5 You are asked to evaluate a 34-year-old man for bilateral adrenal masses. He was born in rural Laos and recently moved to the United States. He developed a viral gastroenteritis 2 weeks previously and remained bedridden for a week while other affected family members recovered in 2 days. He reports that all his life, he has had difficulty recovering from ordinary viral infections.

On physical examination, his height is 59 in (150 cm) and he is muscular. His blood pressure is 102/66 mm Hg, and pulse rate is 102 beats/min.

Laboratory test results:
   Sodium = 128 mEq/L (128 mmol/L)
   Potassium = 5.2 mEq/L (5.2 mmol/L)

Due to persistent abdominal pain, a CT scan is performed, which reveals bilateral, heterogeneous masses with macroscopic fat diagnostic of myelolipomas (*see image*).

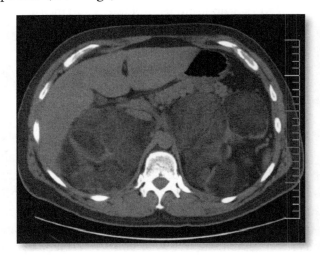

Which of the following additional laboratory tests will reveal the diagnosis?
  A. Serum DHEA-S measurement
  B. Plasma metanephrines measurement
  C. Serum 17-hydroxyprogesterone measurement
  D. Late-night salivary cortisol measurement
  E. Purified protein derivative skin test

6 You are evaluating a 34-year-old woman with weight gain, depression, hirsutism, irregular menses, and hypertension. Her symptoms began 2 years ago and are gradually progressive. Her medications are an oral contraceptive (ethinylestradiol and drospirenone); sertraline, 100 mg daily; and omeprazole, 20 mg daily.

On physical examination, she has facial plethora, disproportionate supraclavicular fat pads, 1- to 2-cm nonblanching purple striae on the abdomen and upper arms, central obesity, and proximal muscle weakness.

Laboratory test results:
  Serum cortisol after 1 mg dexamethasone =
    25 μg/dL (690 nmol/L)
  Plasma ACTH = 188 pg/mL (41.4 pmol/L)
  Late-night salivary cortisol = 0.42 μg/dL
    (11.6 nmol/L)
  Repeat late-night salivary cortisol = 0.48 ng/dL
    (13.2 nmol/L)
  Serum glucose = 85 mg/dL (4.7 mmol/L)

MRI of the sella without and with contrast shows an irregular 2-mm area of delayed contrast enhancement on the right side of the pituitary gland found only on the dynamic scans, which the radiology report describes as "consistent with pituitary adenoma."

Which of the following is the best next step in this patient's management?
  A. Stop the contraceptive for 6 weeks and repeat the dexamethasone suppression test
  B. Refer for pituitary surgery
  C. Measure 24-hour urinary free cortisol excretion
  D. Start mifepristone, 600 mg daily
  E. Refer for inferior petrosal sinus sampling

7 A 46-year-old woman with no notable medical history has developed hypertension with paroxysmal sweating and palpitations over the past 6 months. During one such episode, she went to the emergency department and was subsequently hospitalized for a blood pressure of 205/140 mm Hg. An evaluation for a suspected pheochromocytoma is in progress, and the patient has not yet received adrenergic blockade.

Which of the following agents can be safely administered without concern for causing catecholamine crisis?
  A. Metoclopramide
  B. Intravenous low-osmolar iodinated contrast
  C. Intravenous glucocorticoids
  D. Glucagon
  E. Inhalational anesthetics

8 You are asked to provide consultation for a 28-year-old man with possible adrenal insufficiency. He was hospitalized 2 weeks ago for unexplained hypotension following a party, and an etiology was not identified. He recovered with fluid resuscitation and a single dose of methylprednisolone, 40 mg intravenously. He received no further glucocorticoids and takes no medication or nutritional supplements. Since discharge, he has had some malaise and fatigue but no hypotension, and his appetite is normal. He is about to be discharged, and you come to his bedside at 4:00 PM (1600 h).

Which laboratory test result obtained at this time will conclusively exclude adrenal insufficiency?
  A. Serum cortisol concentration of 8.0 μg/dL (220.7 nmol/L) (reference range, 4.0-11.0 μg/dL [110.3-303.5 nmol/L])
  B. Salivary cortisol concentration of 0.1 μg/dL (2.8 nmol/L) (reference range, 0.01-0.2 μg/dL [0.3-5.5 nmol/L])
  C. Plasma ACTH concentration of 10 pg/mL (2.2 pmol/L) (reference range, 6-48 pg/mL [1.3-10.6 pmol/L])
  D. Serum DHEA-S concentration of 120 μg/dL (3.3 μmol/L) (reference range, 38-523 μg/dL [1.0-14.2 μmol/L])
  E. Adrenal insufficiency cannot be excluded without dynamic testing

9 A 16-year-old girl presents with a 1-year history of progressive weight gain, muscle weakness, and easy bruising. Her menses have been irregular and ceased 3 months ago. She has no vision loss or diarrhea.

On physical examination, she has central obesity, dermal atrophy, and moon facies. Closer examination of the face reveals the finding shown in the photograph (*see image*).

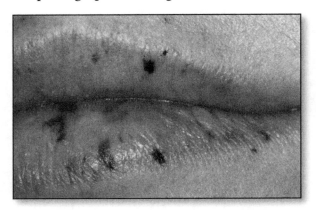

Screening laboratory test results:
Sodium = 138 mEq/L (138 mmol/L)
Potassium = 3.8 mEq/L (3.8 mmol/L)
Serum DHEA-S = 30 µg/dL (0.8 µmol/L)
   (reference range, 35-535 µg/dL
   [0.9-14.5 µmol/L])
Plasma ACTH = <5 pg/mL (<1.1 pmol/L)
Urinary free cortisol = 435 µg/24 h
   (1200.6 nmol/d)
Serum aldosterone = 3 ng/dL (83.2 pmol/L)
Plasma renin activity = 0.8 ng/mL per h
Serum testosterone = 60 ng/dL (2.1 nmol/L)
Serum cortisol = 23 µg/dL (634.5 nmol/L)

The serum cortisol concentration is 25 µg/dL (689.7 nmol/L) after 1 mg of dexamethasone the night before.

CT scan shows normal-sized but irregular adrenals (*see image, arrows*).

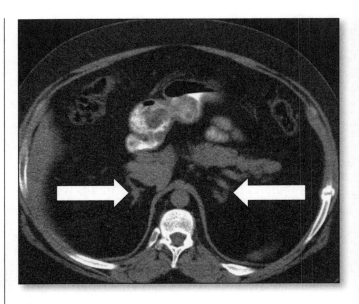

What other endocrinopathy is this patient at risk for developing?
   A. Paraganglioma
   B. Primary hyperparathyroidism
   C. Gastrinoma
   D. Primary aldosteronism
   E. Acromegaly

10 A 57-year-old woman was diagnosed with a pancreatic gastrinoma 10 years ago, when she presented with duodenal ulcers and abdominal pain. At the time of the resection, CT scan demonstrated a 1.3-cm pancreatic primary tumor and a single 4-cm hepatic metastasis. She underwent resection of the primary tumor and liver metastasis and was treated with depot octreotide, 30 mg monthly. Pathology showed a well-differentiated neuroendocrine tumor with a Ki-67 index (reflecting mitotic rate) of 1%. She remained well, but serial imaging demonstrated gradual appearance of multiple liver metastases (all smaller than 1.5 cm) with slight interval growth each year. In the 3 months since her last CT, she abruptly developed hypertension and hypokalemia, diabetes mellitus, poor sleep, muscle weakness, and depression.

On physical examination, her blood pressure is 167/96 mm Hg. She has a flat affect with slow response to commands, 2+ bilateral pedal edema, and muscle weakness.

Laboratory test results:

Serum potassium = 2.8 mEq/L (2.8 mmol/L)

Serum cortisol = 120 µg/dL (3310.6 nmol/L)

Plasma ACTH = 750 pg/mL (165 pmol/L)

Fasting serum gastrin = 95 pg/mL (95 ng/L)
(reference range, <100 pg/mL [<100 ng/L])

Serum albumin = 4.1 g/dL (41 g/L)

Hemoglobin A_{1c} = 10.0% (86 mmol/mol)

On repeated CT, the liver metastases are not measurably changed from the scan 3 months ago. The adrenal glands are thickened but show no tumors.

Which of the following is the most appropriate next step in this patient's management?

A. Biopsy a liver metastasis

B. Perform bilateral adrenalectomy

C. Increase the depot octreotide dosage to 60 mg monthly

D. Refer to oncology for anthracycline-based chemotherapy

E. Perform liver MRI with gadolinium contrast

11 A 40-year-old woman presents with rapidly progressive hirsutism, secondary amenorrhea, balding, voice deepening, and hypertension over the last 6 months. Her primary care physician obtained some initial laboratory tests:

Sodium = 143 mEq/L (143 mmol/L)

Potassium = 3.1 mEq/L (3.1 mmol/L)

Serum aldosterone = <2 ng/dL (<55.5 pmol/L)

Plasma renin activity = <0.6 ng/mL per h

Plasma ACTH = 11 pg/mL (2.4 pmol/L)

Serum cortisol = 14 µg/dL (386.2 nmol/L)

Serum DHEA-S = 2833 µg/dL (76.8 µmol/L)
(reference range, 44-352 µg/dL [1.2-9.5 µmol/L])

Serum total testosterone = 310 ng/dL
(10.8 nmol/L)

Sex hormone–binding globulin = 1.0 µg/mL
(8.9 nmol/L) (reference range, 12-120 µg/mL
[106.7-1067.5 nmol/L])

Which of the following is the most likely diagnosis?

A. Macronodular adrenocortical hyperplasia

B. Nonclassic 11β-hydroxylase deficiency

C. Adrenocortical carcinoma

D. Licorice ingestion

E. Anabolic steroid abuse

12 A 52-year-old man with hypertension and hypokalemia is completing evaluation for primary aldosteronism.

Screening laboratory test results:

Sodium = 147 mEq/L (147 mmol/L)

Potassium = 3.2 mEq/L (3.2 mmol/L)

Serum aldosterone = 24 ng/dL (666 pmol/L)
(repeated measurement = 26 ng/dL
[721 pmol/L])

Plasma renin activity = <0.6 ng/mL per h (repeated measurement = <0.6 ng/mL per h)

CT with fine cuts of the adrenals demonstrates normal-appearing glands.

He undergoes adrenal venous sampling with continuous infusion of cosyntropin at 50 mcg per hour. The results are shown (*see table*).

Measurement	Right Adrenal Vein	Left Adrenal Vein	Inferior Vena Cava
Aldosterone	3000 ng/dL (83,220 pmol/L)	900 ng/dL (24,966 pmol/L)	30 ng/dL (832 pmol/L)
Cortisol	2750 µg/dL (75,867 nmol/L)	200 µg/dL (5518 nmol/L)	25 µg/dL (690 nmol/L)
Aldosterone-to-Cortisol Ratio	1.1	4.5	1.2

How do you interpret the results of the adrenal venous sampling study?

A. Unsuccessful study: unable to localize

B. Successful study: left adrenal gland is the source (left adenoma)

C. Successful study: both adrenal glands are sources (bilateral idiopathic hyperaldosteronism)

D. Unsuccessful study: however, there is enough information to localize the source to the right adrenal (right adenoma)

E. Insufficient information to interpret whether the study was successful

13 A 54-year-old man has a 2.2-cm mass in the left adrenal gland incidentally noted on a CT performed to evaluate hematuria. The mass is homogeneous, 30 Hounsfield units before contrast, with 30% washout at 15 minutes. His blood pressure is 122/78 mm Hg, and he reports no symptoms of sweating, palpitations, or headache. He takes no medications, but he has a positive family history of hypertension developing after age 50 years.

Screening laboratory test results:
Plasma metanephrine = 670 pg/mL (3400 pmol/L) (reference range, <57 pg/mL [<289 pmol/L])
Plasma normetanephrine = 641 pg/mL (3500 pmol/L) (reference range, <148 pg/mL [<808 pmol/L])
Serum cortisol after 1 mg dexamethasone = 0.5 µg/dL (13.8 nmol/L)

The CT image before contrast is shown (*see image*).

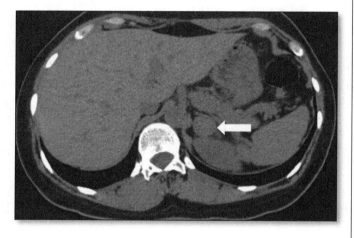

Which of the following is the most appropriate next step in this patient's management?
A. Prescribe α-adrenergic blockade and refer for left adrenalectomy
B. Measure plasma renin activity and serum aldosterone
C. Perform adrenal MRI
D. Repeat the CT in 12 months
E. Perform adrenal biopsy

14 A 20-year-old woman is sent for evaluation of unwanted facial hair, acne, and irregular menses. She developed pubic hair and body odor at age 5 years and was the tallest girl in her class until she stopped growing at age 11 years. She developed acne and facial hair at age 12 years (before menarche at age 14 years). Her menses have always been irregular, and she has not menstruated for 6 months.

On physical examination, the patient has coarse terminal hairs and shaved stubble on her chin, upper lip, and sides of her face, and acne on her forehead. Findings on pelvic examination, including external genitalia, are normal. She has no moon facies, dermal atrophy, myopathy, striae, or acanthosis nigricans. Her blood pressure is 120/80 mm Hg, and BMI is 23 kg/m².

Screening laboratory test results at 10:00 AM:
Serum cortisol = 12 µg/dL (331 nmol/L)
Serum DHEA-S = 680 µg/dL (18.4 µmol/L) (reference range, 62-615 µg/dL [1.7-16.7 µmol/L])
Serum 17-hydroxyprogesterone = 300 ng/dL (9.1 nmol/L)
Serum total testosterone = 75 ng/dL (2.6 nmol/L)
Sex hormone–binding globulin = 1.0 µg/mL (8.9 nmol/L)

Which of the following is the most appropriate next step in this patient's evaluation?
A. Cosyntropin stimulation test measuring 17-hydroxyprogesterone
B. Cosyntropin stimulation test measuring 17-hydroxypregnenolone
C. Adrenal-directed CT
D. Plasma ACTH measurement
E. No further testing

15 A 47-year-old woman presents for evaluation of Cushing syndrome. She describes a 6-month history of increased waist circumference, poor sleep, easy bruising, and worsening hypertension.

On physical examination, her blood pressure is 140/92 mm Hg. She has mild supraclavicular fullness, a few small bruises, slight dermal atrophy, mild central obesity, no purple striae, and no dorsocervical fat pad.

Laboratory test results:
Plasma ACTH = 5 pg/mL (1.1 pmol/L)
Serum DHEA-S = 93 µg/dL (2.5 µmol/L) (reference range, 44-352 µg/dL [1.2-9.5 µmol/L])
Serum cortisol after 1 mg dexamethasone = 7.2 µg/dL (199 nmol/L)
Urinary free cortisol = 81 µg/24 h (223 nmol/d)

CT of the adrenal glands shows multiple adrenal nodules, the largest being 4-cm on the right side and 2-cm on the left side (*see image*).

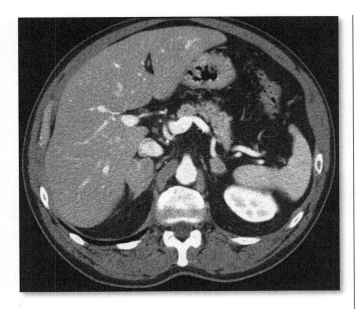

Which of the following interventions do you recommend?
- A. Right adrenalectomy
- B. Bilateral adrenalectomy
- C. Pasireotide, 600 mcg twice daily
- D. Cabergoline, 1 mg twice weekly
- E. Spironolactone, 100 mg daily

16 You are asked to evaluate a 67-year-old man with an incidentally discovered right adrenal mass on a CT scan performed as follow-up for colon cancer. He underwent partial colectomy and chemotherapy 2 years ago, and his adrenal glands were normal on CT imaging 1 year ago. The adrenal mass measures 3.2 cm in maximal diameter with a precontrast attenuation value of 27 Hounsfield units and 35% contrast washout at 15 minutes. His blood pressure is normal, and he has normal glucose, potassium, and plasma metanephrine measurements. The serum cortisol concentration after 1 mg of dexamethasone the previous night is 0.8 µg/dL (22.1 nmol/L).

Which of the following is the best next step?
- A. Refer for laparoscopic right adrenalectomy
- B. Perform MRI of the adrenal mass with in-phase and out-of-phase images
- C. Perform an ^{18}F-fluorodeoxyglucose (FDG)-PET scan
- D. Perform another CT in 1 year
- E. Measure serum aldosterone and plasma renin activity

17 A 38-year-old man is sent for evaluation of severe hypertension and adrenal masses. He has new-onset hypertension and mild hyperglycemia. His mother and a maternal uncle also developed severe hypertension in their 30s. The uncle died of a myocardial infarction, and the patient's mother underwent adrenalectomies for bilateral pheochromocytoma.

Laboratory test results:
- Sodium = 138 mEq/L (138 mmol/L)
- Potassium = 3.8 mEq/L (3.8 mmol/L)
- Plasma normetanephrine = 1502 pg/mL (8200 pmol/L)
- Plasma metanephrine = 60 pg/mL (304 pmol/L)
- Serum aldosterone = 3 ng/dL (83.2 pmol/L)
- Plasma renin activity = 0.8 ng/mL per h

CT scan after intravenous contrast is shown (*see image*).

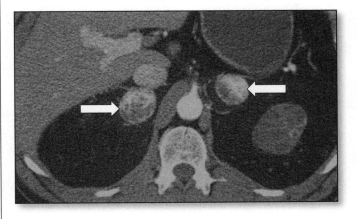

A mutation in which of the following genes is most likely responsible for the pheochromocytoma in this kindred?
- A. *RET*
- B. *MEN1*
- C. *VHL*
- D. *SDHD*
- E. *TMEM127*

18 A 55-year-old woman is referred to you for evaluation of a right adrenal mass that was incidentally discovered during an evaluation performed for a transient episode of flank pain. She is normotensive and has no signs or symptoms of adrenal gland dysfunction. Her only medication is a bisphosphonate for the treatment of osteoporosis.

The mass measures 3.4 cm in diameter, precontrast attenuation is –5 Hounsfield units, and there is more than 60% contrast medium washout 15 minutes after contrast administration. The left adrenal gland has no nodularity.

On physical examination, she has normal blood pressure and no facial plethora, dermal atrophy, bruising, or supraclavicular fat pads.

Laboratory test results:
Sodium = 143 mEq/L (143 mmol/L)
Potassium = 3.8 mEq/L (3.8 mmol/L)
Plasma ACTH (8 AM) = 7 pg/mL (1.5 pmol/L); repeated measurement = 8 pg/mL (1.8 pmol/L)
Serum DHEA-S = <15 µg/dL (<0.41 µmol/L)
Serum cortisol after 1 mg dexamethasone = 4 µg/dL (110.4 nmol/L); repeated measurement is the same
Urinary free cortisol = 22 µg/24 h (60.7 nmol/d)
Plasma normetanephrine = 120 pg/mL (655 pmol/L)
Plasma metanephrine = 40 pg/mL (203 pmol/L)

How should you counsel this patient about the adrenal mass and test results?
A. She should not consider surgery unless the urinary free cortisol is elevated
B. This degree of cortisol excess has no clinical consequences
C. The risk of developing increasing cortisol excess is less than 5%
D. Her osteoporosis is unrelated to the adrenal tumor
E. The adrenal tumor increases her risk of cardiovascular events

19 A 78-year-old woman is hospitalized for acute liver injury after unintentionally overdosing on acetaminophen-oxycodone for chronic pain. One year ago, an unclassified connective tissue disease was diagnosed that manifests as myositis and arthritis, and she has since been treated with prednisone, 20 mg daily. She increased the amount of pain medication she was taking over the last week due to worsening joint and muscle pain. On hospital admission, she was hypotensive with abdominal pain and nausea, and you are consulted about her corticosteroid regimen.

On physical examination, she is jaundiced and lethargic with dermal atrophy, bruising, muscle weakness, and prominent supraclavicular fat pads. Her blood pressure is 94/68 mm Hg, and pulse rate is 100 beats/min.

Laboratory test results:
Sodium = 128 mEq/L (128 mmol/L)
Potassium = 3.8 mEq/L (3.8 mmol/L)
Serum DHEA-S = <15 µg/dL (<0.41 µmol/L)
Plasma ACTH = <2 pg/mL (<0.4 pmol/L)
Serum aldosterone = 16 ng/dL (444 pmol/L)
Plasma renin activity = 8 ng/mL per h
Serum cortisol (8 AM) = <0.5 µg/dL (<13.8 nmol/L)
Serum alanine aminotransferase = 2680 U/L (44.8 µkat/L)

In addition to fluid resuscitation, which of the following do you recommend?
A. Perform a cosyntropin stimulation test
B. Add fludrocortisone, 0.1 mg twice daily
C. Increase prednisone to 20 mg twice daily
D. Substitute prednisolone, 20 mg daily, for prednisone
E. Perform adrenal CT

20 A 66-year-old woman presents to her local physician with hypertension of 20 years' duration, which has been poorly controlled for the past 6 years. The patient does not use tobacco or alcohol. She takes amlodipine, 10 mg daily; losartan, 100 mg daily; and hydrochlorothiazide, 12.5 mg daily. Her blood pressure is 155/93 mm Hg.

She is referred to you after the following laboratory values are obtained:
Sodium = 140 mEq/L (140 mmol/L)
Potassium = 3.6 mEq/L (3.6 mmol/L)
Serum creatinine = 1.1 mg/dL (97.2 µmol/L)
Serum aldosterone = 14 ng/dL (388.4 pmol/L)
Plasma renin activity = <0.6 ng/mL per h

Which of the following should you order first?
- A. 24-Hour urinary aldosterone and sodium measurement on the third day of a high-salt diet
- B. MR-angiogram of the renal arteries
- C. Adrenal-directed CT
- D. 1-mg overnight dexamethasone suppression test measuring cortisol and aldosterone
- E. Adrenal venous sampling

21 A 62-year-old man is status post left open adrenalectomy for a 6-cm adrenocortical carcinoma with Cushing syndrome. The pathology specimen showed high-grade tumor extending to the margin of the resection, and 4 of 10 lymph nodes were positive for tumor. Postoperatively, he was treated with hydrocortisone, 20 mg on arising and 10 mg in the afternoon, and he recovered well with some resolution of his cushingoid features. After 4 weeks, mitotane was added for residual disease and titrated up to 1 g 4 times daily. At a clinic visit 6 weeks later, his serum mitotane value is at therapeutic goal, but he reports nausea, anorexia, and fatigue.

Laboratory test results:
  Serum mitotane = 16.4 mg/L (therapeutic goal >14 mg/L)
  Serum potassium = 4.2 mEq/L (4.2 mmol/L)
  Plasma ACTH = <2 pg/mL (<0.4 pmol/L)
  Serum testosterone = 320 ng/dL (11.1 nmol/L)
  Sex hormone–binding globulin = 11.5 µg/mL (102.3 nmol/L)

Which of the following is the best next step in this patient's management?
- A. Add fludrocortisone, 0.1 mg daily
- B. Reduce the mitotane dosage to 0.5 g 4 times daily
- C. Change the hydrocortisone regimen to 20 mg 3 times daily
- D. Add testosterone enanthate, 100 mg weekly
- E. Add anastrozole, 1 mg daily

22 A 32-year-old woman with a history of Cushing disease status post surgery, diabetes mellitus, and hypertension has noted weight gain, poor sleep, irregular menses, and worsening glycemia for the past 6 months. Her medications include amlodipine, 10 mg daily, and metformin, 1500 mg daily.

On physical examination, her blood pressure is 135/85 mm Hg and she has facial plethora.

Laboratory test results:
  Fasting glucose = 205 mg/dL (11.4 mmol/L)
  Potassium = 3.1 mEq/L (3.1 mmol/L)
  Serum cortisol = 18 µg/dL (496.6 nmol/L)
  Hemoglobin A_{1c} = 8.5% (69 mmol/mol)
  Plasma ACTH = 65 pg/mL (14.3 pmol/L)
  Late-night salivary cortisol = 0.32 µg/dL (8.8 nmol/L)
  Urinary free cortisol = 360 µg/24 h (993.6 nmol/d)
  Urinary pregnancy test = negative

Pituitary MRI shows only postoperative changes. After a discussion of treatment options, you plan to begin mifepristone, 300 mg daily.

Before starting mifepristone, you should first treat her to achieve which of the following?
- A. Adequate contraception
- B. Normal blood pressure
- C. Normal fasting glucose
- D. Normal serum potassium
- E. No additional treatment is required

23 A 68-year-old man is diagnosed with primary aldosteronism after having difficult-to-control hypertension with intermittent hypokalemia for at least 10 years and microalbuminuria for the last 2 years. Adrenal venous sampling demonstrates bilateral hyperaldosteronism, and you begin medical therapy with eplerenone, 50 mg daily, added to amlodipine, 10 mg daily. Over 6 weeks, his blood pressure falls from 158/96 mm Hg to 135/88 mm Hg, and you increase the eplerenone dosage to 50 mg twice daily. After another 8 weeks, his blood pressure is 125/82 mm Hg.

Laboratory test results (baseline before eplerenone):
    Serum potassium = 3.1 mEq/L (3.1 mmol/L)
    Serum creatinine = 1.4 mg/dL (124 μmol/L)
    Serum aldosterone = 28 ng/dL (777 pmol/L)
    Plasma renin activity = <0.6 ng/mL per h

Laboratory test results (after 8 weeks taking eplerenone, 50 mg twice daily):
    Serum potassium = 4.4 mEq/L (4.4 mmol/L)
    Serum creatinine = 1.8 mg/dL (159 μmol/L)
    Serum aldosterone = 33 ng/dL (915 pmol/L)
    Plasma renin activity = 1.3 ng/mL per h

Repeated testing 2 weeks later shows equivalent results.

On the basis of these results, which of the following changes would you make to his blood pressure therapy?
    A. Reduce the eplerenone dosage to 50 mg daily
    B. Change eplerenone to spironolactone, 100 mg daily
    C. Discontinue amlodipine
    D. Discontinue eplerenone and add atenolol, 50 mg daily
    E. No changes

24 A 29-year-old woman with a history of systemic lupus erythematosus presents to the emergency department for evaluation of a 2-day history of vomiting and orthostasis. She received a 12-week course of prednisone for nephritis 1 year ago with subsequent improvement. She was well until 4 weeks ago, when she developed a deep vein thrombosis in her left leg, and she was found to have the antiphospholipid syndrome. Warfarin was added and titrated to achieve an international normalized ratio (INR) in the target range. She became acutely ill 2 days ago with flank pain but no fever or dysuria.

Laboratory test results:
    Sodium = 121 mEq/L (121 mmol/L)
    Potassium = 6.4 mEq/L (6.4 mmol/L)
    Plasma ACTH = 1330 pg/mL (293 pmol/L)
    Serum aldosterone = <2 ng/dL (<55.5 pmol/L)
    Plasma renin activity = 27 ng/mL per h
    Serum cortisol = <0.5 μg/dL (<13.8 nmol/L)

Which of the following tests will reveal the cause of her adrenal insufficiency?
    A. Serum DHEA-S measurement
    B. Pituitary MRI
    C. Urine synthetic glucocorticoid screen
    D. Serum 21-hydroxylase antibody assessment
    E. Adrenal CT

25 A 48-year-old man with a history of stage IV small cell lung cancer is referred for rapid onset of cushingoid features, hypertension, and hypokalemia.

Laboratory test results:
    Serum cortisol = 80 μg/dL (2207 nmol/L)
    Plasma ACTH = 580 pg/mL (128 pmol/L)
    Serum glucose = 402 mg/dL (22.3 mmol/L)

Eplerenone, 100 mg twice daily, is started to control the hypokalemia and hypertension, with good response. Ketoconazole is initiated and advanced to the dosage of 200 mg 3 times daily. He is tolerating this regimen well, and you note improvements in glucose and cortisol levels.

Which of the following changes should you anticipate as a result of ketoconazole therapy?
    A. Increase in 11-deoxycortisol
    B. Increase in ACTH
    C. Increase in estradiol
    D. Decrease in testosterone
    E. Decrease in corticosteroid-binding globulin

Calcium and Bone Board Review

Carolyn B. Becker, MD ● Brigham & Women's Hospital

1 A 40-year-old woman is found to have a serum calcium level that is mildly but consistently elevated over several months of observation (ranging from 10.3 to 10.9 mg/dL [2.6-2.7 mmol/L]). Her PTH level ranges from 67 to 78 pg/mL (67-78 ng/L) (reference range, 10-65 pg/mL [10-65 ng/L]) over multiple measurements and her serum 25-hydroxyvitamin D level is 33 ng/mL (82.4 nmol/L). A 24-hour urine collection reveals the calculated calcium-to-creatinine clearance ratio to be 0.01. Her parents are deceased and she has no siblings or children. No previous laboratory results are available. She feels well.

Which of the following is the best next step in this patient's management?
   A. Referral to a surgeon for 4-gland parathyroid exploration
   B. Bone mineral densitometry (DXA) testing
   C. Genetic testing for a calcium-sensing receptor (*CASR*) mutation
   D. Sestamibi parathyroid scan
   E. Continued annual monitoring

2 You are evaluating an 80-year-old man who presents with 2 days of acute back pain after lifting a heavy package. He is status post pelvic irradiation and androgen deprivation therapy for prostate cancer 5 years ago. He is otherwise in good health.

On physical examination, he is tender over his lower spine. Radiographs of the spine show an anterior wedge compression fracture at L1 and significant degenerative arthritic changes. Four years ago, following his treatment for prostate cancer, a DXA scan revealed T scores of −2.0 at the lumbar spine and −1.5 at the femoral neck with FRAX scores that did not meet treatment thresholds.

Current laboratory test results, including complete blood cell count, routine chemistries, alkaline phosphatase, prostate-specific antigen, 25-hydroxyvitamin D, serum/urine protein electrophoresis, and PTH, are all normal. Serum testosterone on a morning specimen is 270 ng/dL (9.4 nmol/L) (reference range, 300-900 ng/dL [10.4-31.2 nmol/L]). Sex hormone–binding globulin is within the reference range.

Which of the following is the best next step in this patient's care?
   A. Begin alendronate
   B. Begin testosterone and finasteride
   C. Begin teriparatide
   D. Refer for bone biopsy and possible kyphoplasty at L1
   E. Obtain another DXA

3 A 60-year-old man with end-stage renal disease due to type 2 diabetes mellitus has been receiving hemodialysis for 10 years. He comes to you because of multiple vertebral fractures, a pelvic fracture, and a femoral neck T score of −3.8 on DXA. Long-term medications include calcitriol, 0.5 mcg twice daily, and cinacalcet, 90 mg twice daily.

Laboratory test results:
   Serum calcium = 8.1 mg/dL (2.0 mmol/L) (reference range, 8.2-10.2 mg/dL [2.1-2.6 mmol/L])
   Phosphate = 5.2 mg/dL (1.7 mmol/L) (reference range, 2.3-4.7 mg/dL [0.7-1.5 mmol/L])
   25-Hydroxyvitamin D = 24 ng/mL (59.9 nmol/L) (reference range [optimal], 25-80 ng/mL [62.4-199.7 nmol/L])
   PTH = 78 pg/mL (78 ng/L) (reference range, 10-65 pg/mL [10-65 ng/L])
   Total alkaline phosphatase = 48 U/L (0.80 μkat/L) (reference range, 50-120 U/L [0.84-2.00 μkat/L])

An iliac crest biopsy is done after double-tetracycline labeling.

While awaiting bone biopsy results, which of the following changes in management should be made immediately?
    A. Increase the calcitriol dosage
    B. Decrease the calcitriol dosage
    C. Begin teriparatide
    D. Begin denosumab
    E. Decrease the cinacalcet dosage

4 You are evaluating a 68-year-old woman who has had several serum calcium measurements in the range of 10.6 to 11.0 mg/dL (2.7-2.8 mmol/L) (reference range, 8.2-10.2 mg/dL [2.1-2.6 mmol/L]). She feels well.

Laboratory test results:
    Serum albumin, normal
    Estimated glomerular filtration rate = 40 mL/min per 1.73 m^2 (reference range, >60 mL/min per 1.73 m^2)
    Serum PTH = 110 pg/mL (110 ng/L) (reference range, 10-65 [pg/mL [10-65 ng/L])
    Urinary calcium = 188 mg/24 h (4.7 mmol/d) (reference range, 100-300 mg/24 h [2.5-7.5 mmol/d])
    25-Hydroxyvitamin D = 32 ng/mL (74.9 nmol/L) (reference range [optimal], 25-80 ng/mL [62.4-199.7 nmol/L])

Which of the following is the best next step?
    A. Measurement of 1,25-dihydroxyvitamin D
    B. Parathyroidectomy with identification of all parathyroid glands
    C. Sestamibi scan
    D. Renal ultrasonography
    E. Repeated measurement of serum calcium, creatinine, and PTH in 6 months

5 A 45-year-old woman undergoes total thyroidectomy for papillary carcinoma of the thyroid and is left with permanent surgical hypoparathyroidism. She takes 1200 mg of elemental calcium 3 times per day with meals; calcitriol, 0.5 mcg twice daily; and levothyroxine, 150 mcg daily. She feels well.

On physical examination, she has a well-healed thyroidectomy scar and negative Chvostek and Trousseau signs.

Laboratory test results 6 months after surgery:
    Serum calcium = 10.0 mg/dL (2.5 mmol/L) (reference range, 8.2-10.2 mg/dL [2.1-2.6 mmol/L])
    Albumin = 4.0 g/dL (40 g/L) (reference range, 3.5-5.0 g/dL [35-50 g/L])
    Phosphate = 4.9 mg/dL (1.6 mmol/L) (reference range, 2.3-4.7 mg/dL [0.7-1.5 mmol/L])
    Urinary calcium = 380 mg/24 h (9.5 mmol/d) (reference range, 100-300 mg/24 h [2.5-7.5 mmol/d])

Which of the following would you recommend now?
    A. Continue current regimen
    B. Decrease calcium supplementation
    C. Add sevelamer (oral phosphate binder)
    D. Add recombinant human PTH(1-84)
    E. Add hydrochlorothiazide

6 A 25-year-old woman presents with fatigue, and primary hyperparathyroidism is diagnosed.

Laboratory test results:
    Serum calcium = 11.9 mg/dL (3.0 mmol/L) (reference range, 8.2-10.2 mg/dL [2.1-2.6 mmol/L])
    Serum PTH = 120 pg/mL (120 ng/L) (reference range, 10-65 pg/mL [10-65 ng/L])
    Urinary calcium excretion = 400 mg/24 h (10 mmol/d) (reference range, 100-300 mg/24 h [2.5-7.5 mmol/d])

Her family history is positive for recurrent hyperparathyroidism and chronic diarrhea in her father, as well as kidney stones and peptic ulcers in 1 of her 3 siblings.

Which of the following is the most likely diagnosis in this case?
    A. Familial "idiopathic" hyperparathyroidism (*CDC73* gene)
    B. Hereditary "renal leak" hypercalciuria (*TRPV5* gene)
    C. Hereditary activation of the calcium sensing receptor (*CASR* gene)
    D. Multiple endocrine neoplasia type 1 (*MEN1* gene)
    E. Hyperparathyroidism–jaw tumor syndrome (*CDC73* gene)

7 A 40-year-old transgender woman is admitted to the hospital with symptomatic hypercalcemia. She is status post bilateral orchiectomy and her only medication is oral estradiol. She reports no recent use of alcohol, tobacco, or illicit drugs.

On physical examination, she is afebrile, lethargic, and dehydrated. She has bilateral breast implants and multiple firm, nontender nodules over both buttocks and hips.

Chest x-ray is negative.

Laboratory test results:
  Calcium = 14.5 mg/dL (3.6 mmol/L) (reference range, 8.2-10.2 mg/dL [2.1-2.6 mmol/L])
  Albumin = 4.1 g/dL (41 g/L) (reference range, 3.5-5.0 g/dL [35-50 g/L])
  Creatinine = 2.0 mg/dL (176.8 μmol/L) (reference range, 0.6-1.1 mg/dL [53.0-97.2 μmol/L])
  Phosphate = 4.9 mg/dL (1.6 mmol/L) (reference range, 2.3-4.7 mg/dL [0.7-1.5 mmol/L])
  PTH = <10 pg/mL (<10 ng/L) (reference range, 10-65 pg/mL [10-65 ng/L])
  25-Hydroxyvitamin D = 15 ng/mL (37.4 nmol/L) (reference range [optimal], 25-80 ng/mL [62.4-199.7 nmol/L])
  1,25-Dihydroxyvitamin D = 82 pg/mL (213.2 pmol/L) (reference range, 16-65 pg/mL [41.6-169.0 pmol/L])

In addition to vigorous intravenous hydration, which of the following is the best next step?
  A. Serum PTHrP measurement
  B. CT of the chest, abdomen, and pelvis
  C. Bone marrow aspiration and biopsy
  D. Octreotide scan
  E. Biopsy of one of the nodules

8 A 55-year-old woman has her third episode of renal colic. Analysis of the stone shows calcium oxalate. Her workup reveals normal serum calcium and PTH levels, with a 24-hour urinary calcium excretion of 335 mg/24 h (8.4 mmol/d) (reference range, 100-300 mg/24 h [2.5-7.5 mmol/d]), but normal 24-hour urinary oxalate, uric acid, sodium, and citrate levels. Her urine volume is 2600 mL/24 h. Her daily diet contains about 1000 mg of elemental calcium.

Which of the following recommendations would provide the greatest reduction in her risk of future calcium oxalate stone disease?
  A. Begin hydrochlorothiazide
  B. Begin allopurinol
  C. Reduce dietary oxalate
  D. Reduce dietary calcium
  E. Increase fluid intake

9 A 78-year-old man with type 2 diabetes mellitus, congestive heart failure, and chronic kidney disease is admitted for exacerbation of congestive heart failure and new-onset atrial fibrillation.

Laboratory test results:
  Serum calcium = 12.0 mg/dL (3.0 mmol/L) (reference range, 8.2-10.2 mg/dL [2.1-2.6 mmol/L])
  Serum creatinine = 1.8 mg/dL (159.1 μmol/L)
  PTH = 176 pg/mL (176 ng/L) (reference range, 10-65 pg/mL [10-65 ng/L])

Which of the following is the most appropriate management for his hypercalcemia?
  A. Perform urgent exploratory parathyroid surgery
  B. Start cinacalcet
  C. Start alendronate
  D. Start amiloride
  E. Start nasal calcitonin

10 A 20-year-old man comes to you for follow-up of hypoparathyroidism. He presented at age 5 years with a seizure from severe hypocalcemia and has been maintained on calcium and calcitriol ever since. Over the past several months, he has noted anorexia, 10-lb (4.5-kg) weight loss, weakness, and dizziness.

Physical examination reveals a supine blood pressure of 80/60 mm Hg, pulse rate of 120 beats/min, and dystrophic fingernails and toenails.

Which of the following laboratory measurements is key to the diagnosis?
  A. Serum ceruloplasmin
  B. Serum ferritin, iron, and total iron-binding capacity
  C. Serum calcium and magnesium
  D. Serum electrolytes, cortisol, and ACTH

11 A 65-year-old healthy woman is noted to have an elevated serum PTH level of 92 pg/mL (92 ng/L) (reference range, 10-65 pg/mL [10-65 ng/L]) as part of an evaluation for osteopenia. Her DXA reveals T scores of –1.8 at the spine, –1.6 at the total hip, and –2.0 at the femoral neck. Serum total and ionized calcium levels have been consistently normal. A repeated PTH measurement is 80 pg/mL (80 ng/L). She has no history of kidney stones, fractures, or loss of height and no relevant family history. Physical examination findings are unremarkable.

Additional laboratory test results:
Urinary calcium = 180 mg/24 h (4.5 mmol/d) (reference range, 100-300 mg/24 h [2.5-7.5 mmol/d])
Serum creatinine = 0.8 mg/dL (70.7 µmol/L) (reference range, 0.6-1.1 mg/dL [53.0-97.2 µmol/L])
Phosphate = 2.6 mg/dL (0.8 mmol/L) (reference range, 2.3-4.7 mg/dL [0.7-1.5 mmol/L])
25-Hydroxyvitamin D = 48 ng/mL (119.8 nmol/L)

Which of the following is the most appropriate next step?
A. DXA of the one-third distal radius
B. Sestamibi scan
C. Spinal radiographs
D. Renal ultrasonography
E. Bone turnover markers

12 A 74-year-old woman with severe osteoporosis (femoral neck T score of –3.2, compression fractures of T8 and T9 after minimal or no trauma) has been self-injecting teriparatide, 20 mcg daily, for the past 3 months every morning. She has been on hydrochlorothiazide/triamterene, 25/37.5 mg daily, for hypertension for many years. She gets 600 mg of calcium from food sources daily and takes a calcium supplement, 600 mg once daily with food. Before starting teriparatide, her baseline serum calcium level was normal.

On the day of her visit, she skips her morning teriparatide injection and comes to see you in the late afternoon. She feels well. Her blood pressure is 138/90 mm Hg.

Laboratory test results 36 hours after her last teriparatide injection:
Serum calcium = 10.6 mg/dL (2.7 mmol/L) (reference range, 8.2-10.2 mg/dL [2.1-2.6 mmol/L])
Albumin = 3.9 g/dL (39 g/L)
Serum urea nitrogen = 12 mg/dL (4.3 mmol/L)
Creatinine = 0.9 mg/dL (79.6 µmol/L)

In addition to rechecking laboratory values within 1 to 2 weeks, which of the following should you advise?
A. Stop hydrochlorothiazide
B. Decrease the hydrochlorothiazide dosage to 12.5 mg daily
C. Stop the calcium supplement
D. Stop teriparatide
E. No changes needed

13 An 18-year-old female refugee from a war-torn country presents with a history of bone pain, joint deformities, and severe dental problems since childhood. On physical examination, she has short stature, severe genu varum (bow-leggedness), and very poor dentition, but no abnormal skin pigmentation. Family history is unavailable because she was separated from her family as an infant and grew up in an orphanage.

Laboratory blood tests results:
Calcium = 8.8 mg/dL (2.2 mmol/L) (reference range, 8.2-10.2 mg/dL [2.1-2.6 mmol/L])
Albumin = 4.0 g/dL (40 g/L) (reference range, 3.5-5.0 g/dL [35-50 g/L])
Phosphate = 1.3 mg/dL (0.4 mmol/L) (reference range, 2.3-4.7 mg/dL [0.7-1.5 mmol/L])
25-Hydroxyvitamin D = 24 ng/mL (59.9 nmol/L) (reference range [optimal], 25-80 ng/mL [62.4-199.7 nmol/L])
1,25-Dihydroxyvitamin D = 30 pg/mL (78 pmol/L) (reference range, 16-65 pg/mL [41.6-169.0 pmol/L])
Intact PTH = 110 pg/mL (110 ng/L) (reference range, 10-65 pg/mL [10-65 ng/L])

Which of the following is the most likely diagnosis?
   A. Vitamin D–resistant rickets
   B. Oncogenic osteomalacia (tumor induced osteomalacia)
   C. McCune-Albright syndrome
   D. X-linked hypophosphatemic rickets
   E. Vitamin D–deficient rickets

14 A 63-year-old postmenopausal woman with osteoporosis and rheumatoid arthritis affecting her hands has been on prednisone, 5 mg daily, and alendronate, 70 mg weekly, for the past 2 years. Recently, temporal arteritis was diagnosed and her prednisone dosage was increased to 20 mg daily. One month later, she sustained a painful vertebral fracture during yoga class. She is very adherent to her treatment regimen of alendronate, calcium, and vitamin D, and a workup for secondary causes of vertebral fracture is negative. DXA documents T scores of –2.6, –1.8, and –1.4 at the lumbar spine, total hip, and femoral neck, respectively. Bone mineral density at the spine has improved 4% over the past 2 years.

Which of the following would you recommend now?
   A. Continue alendronate
   B. Switch to teriparatide
   C. Switch to zoledronic acid
   D. Switch to denosumab
   E. Add teriparatide to alendronate

15 You are evaluating an 82-year-old woman with osteoporosis who has been on oral alendronate, 70 mg weekly, for 5 years. She has no known history of fracture. Her current DXA shows T scores of –1.5 at the lumbar spine, –2.8 at the femoral neck, and –2.6 at the total hip. Her bone mineral density increased dramatically during the first 2 years on alendronate and then stabilized at the current level.

On physical examination, she appears frail but has no kyphosis or tenderness; her gait is slow and she is unable to balance on 1 foot or rise from a chair without using her arms. She has had 3 falls since her visit 6 months ago.

Laboratory testing documents normal serum calcium, phosphate, creatinine, and 25-hydroxyvitamin D levels.

She asks whether she can go on a "drug holiday."

Which of the following should be the next step in this patient's management?
   A. Discontinue alendronate and reassess in 1 to 2 years
   B. Switch to zoledronic acid
   C. Switch to teriparatide
   D. Switch to denosumab

16 A 55-year-old woman with osteoporosis has been on risedronate, 35 mg orally weekly, for the past 2 years. Her diet provides more than 1000 mg of elemental calcium each day, and she takes 1000 IU of cholecalciferol daily. Her last menstrual period occurred 3 years ago and she has never taken hormone therapy. A follow-up DXA on the same machine now shows significant declines in bone mineral density at both the spine (6% decline) and hip (5% decline) compared with values obtained 2 years ago. On review of systems, she feels well and has no new symptoms. Physical examination findings are unchanged.

Laboratory test results, including serum calcium, albumin, creatinine, intact PTH, 25-hydroxyvitamin D, and 24-hour urinary calcium excretion, are normal.

Which of the following is the most likely reason for her poor response to therapy?
   A. Nonadherence to treatment
   B. Malabsorption
   C. An undiagnosed underlying disorder
   D. Positioning error by the DXA technician
   E. Lack of potency of risedronate to stop rapid postmenopausal bone loss

17 You are called to see a 40-year-old man with hypercalcemia. He comes to the emergency department following 24 hours of nausea, vomiting, and abdominal pain. His medical history is notable for heavy alcohol use and severe gastroesophageal reflux disease. He takes no prescription medications but does take several over-the-counter therapies "for his stomach."

On physical examination, he is afebrile and lethargic with very dry mucous membranes and epigastric tenderness. Chest x-ray and abdominal CT are normal.

Initial laboratory test results:

Potassium = 3.0 mEq/L (3.0 mmol/L) (reference range, 3.5-5.0 mEq/L [3.5-5.0 mmol/L])

Bicarbonate = 39 mEq/L (39 mmol/L) (reference range, 21-28 mEq/L [21-28 mmol/L])

Calcium = 16.8 mg/dL (4.2 mmol/L) (reference range, 8.2-10.2 mg/dL [2.1-2.6 mmol/L])

Phosphate = 3.5 mg/dL (1.1 mmol/L)

Serum urea nitrogen = 50 mg/dL (17.9 mmol/L) (reference range, 8-23 mg/dL [2.9-8.2 mmol/L])

Creatinine = 3.5 mg/dL (309.4 µmol/L) (reference range, 0.7-1.3 mg/dL [61.9-114.9 µmol/L])

Intact PTH = <10 pg/mL (<10 ng/L) (reference range, 10-65 pg/mL [10-65 ng/L])

The patient receives vigorous intravenous saline hydration along with potassium supplementation. By the next morning, he is alert and oriented, and laboratory values are greatly improved. Two days after hospital admission, his creatinine normalizes and his serum calcium level is 8.0 mg/dL (2.0 mmol/L).

Which of the following best explains this patient's clinical presentation?

A. Acute pancreatitis
B. Dehydration
C. Milk-alkali syndrome
D. Vitamin D intoxication
E. Malignancy

18 A 28-year-old woman with a history of nephrotic syndrome is found to have a low serum calcium level.

Laboratory test results:

Serum calcium = 7.9 mg/dL (2.0 mmol/L) (reference range, 8.2-10.2 mg/dL [2.1-2.6 mmol/L])

Serum creatinine = 0.9 mg/dL (79.6 µmol/L)

Phosphate = 2.7 mg/dL (0.9 mmol/L) (reference range, 2.3-4.7 mg/dL [0.7-1.5 mmol/L])

She reports no paresthesias or muscle cramps. On physical examination, she has 2+ pitting pretibial edema, but negative Trousseau and Chvostek signs.

Serum measurement of which of the following would be the most useful to determine the etiology of her hypocalcemia?

A. Intact PTH
B. 25-Hydroxyvitamin D
C. 1,25-Dihydroxyvitamin D
D. Magnesium
E. Albumin

19 A 55-year-old white woman is referred to you after results of a screening DXA. Her last menstrual period was 3 years ago and she has no menopausal symptoms. Her BMI is 20 kg/m². She is generally healthy, but she fractured 2 toes last year after missing a step. She does not smoke cigarettes, she drinks 1 glass of wine nightly, and she takes no medications. Her daily intake provides 1200 mg of calcium and 1000 IU of vitamin D. Her mother fractured a hip.

The patient's DXA documented the following:

Site	BMD, g/cm²	T Score
Total hip	0.698	−1.5
Femoral neck	0.658	−1.7
L1-L4	0.983	−0.3

Vertebral fracture assessment is negative for spinal compression fractures. Her FRAX 10-year risk is 12% for any major osteoporotic fracture and 0.7% for hip fracture.

Which of the following is the correct management plan?

A. Start alendronate and repeat DXA in 1 year
B. Continue calcium and vitamin D and repeat DXA in 2 years
C. Start raloxifene and perform DXA in 1 year
D. Start estrogen replacement therapy
E. Start nasal calcitonin therapy

20 A 35-year-old man is referred to you for evaluation of muscle and bone pain, fatigue, weakness, spontaneous fractures, and difficulty walking. Physical examination reveals diffuse bony tenderness, proximal muscle weakness, and ataxic gait. DXA documents T scores of −3 to −4 at all sites.

Laboratory test results:

Chemistry panel, normal

Serum 25-hydroxyvitamin D = 28 ng/mL (69.9 nmol/L)

Serum 1,25-dihydroxyvitamin D = 12 pg/mL (31.2 pmol/L)

PTH = 98 pg/mL (98 ng/L) (reference range, 10-65 pg/mL [10-65 ng/L])

Serum phosphate = 1.1 to 1.3 mg/dL (0.36 to 0.42 mmol/L) (reference range, 2.3-4.7 mg/dL [0.74-1.52 mmol/L])

Maximum tubular phosphate reabsorption (phosphorus tubule maximum/glomerular filtration rate) = low

Which of the following is the key diagnostic test to order next?

A. Serum and urine protein electrophoresis

B. Sestamibi scan

C. 24,25-Dihydroxyvitamin D measurement

D. Fibroblast growth factor 23 measurement

E. 24-Hour urine collection for calcium, electrolytes, amino acids, glucose, and creatinine

21 A 72-year-old man with chronic left hip pain was recently diagnosed with Paget disease of bone. Radiographs show Paget disease in his left hemipelvis and femoral head, as well as moderate degenerative arthritis in the left hip. His alkaline phosphatase level is 250 mg/dL (4.2 μkat/L) (reference range, 40-120 mg/dL [0.7-2.0 μkat/L]), and his gamma-glutamyltranspeptidase level is normal. Bone scan shows intense increased uptake in the left ilium, acetabulum, and femoral head. You advise treatment of his Paget disease with zoledronic acid. He wonders what to expect in the next few years.

Which of the following is most likely to occur?

A. Spread of Paget disesase to the right hip

B. Hearing loss due to Paget disease

C. Worsening arthritis in the hip

D. Total resolution of all hip pain

E. Osteonecrosis of the femoral neck

22 A 25-year-old woman is referred because of low bone density. Her risk factors include a family history of osteoporosis and a personal history of secondary amenorrhea due to anorexia nervosa (from which she recovered). After getting help for her eating disorder and regaining weight, regular menses resumed and have been normal for the past 2 years. She does not smoke cigarettes and is otherwise in excellent health. She has never fractured. Her current DXA reveals Z scores of −2.7 at the spine and −1.5 at the femoral neck. A workup for secondary causes of low bone density is negative.

In addition to optimal calcium, vitamin D, and exercise, which of the following would you recommend for this patient?

A. Teriparatide

B. Denosumab

C. Risedronate

D. Oral contraceptive pill

E. Monitoring only

23 A 26-year-old man presents for evaluation of fragility fractures and low bone density. He had normal childhood and pubertal development but has sustained multiple fractures since adolescence with minimal or no trauma. He notes that he continues to get taller.

On physical examination, his height is 80 in (203 cm), and he is eunuchoid in appearance. He is well virilized with normal male external genitalia and no gynecomastia.

DXA shows Z scores of −4.4 at the spine and −3.2 at the hip. Bone age is greatly reduced with unfused epiphyses.

Laboratory test results:

Total testosterone = 1700 ng/dL (59.0 nmol/L) (reference range, 300-900 ng/dL [10.4-31.2 nmol/L])

Sex hormone–binding globulin = 1.2 μg/mL (10.7 nmol/L) (reference range, 1.1-6.7 μg/mL [10-60 nmol/L])

LH = 35.0 mIU/mL (35.0 IU/L) (reference range, 1.0-9.0 mIU/mL [1.0-9.0 IU/L])

Which of the following additional tests is the key to the diagnosis?

    A. Pituitary-directed MRI

    B. Karyotype analysis

    C. Sequencing of the gene encoding the androgen receptor

    D. Serum estradiol measurement

    E. Free testosterone measurement by equilibrium dialysis

24 A 40-year-old man is referred to you for management of osteogenesis imperfecta. This condition was diagnosed in childhood after he sustained multiple fractures, and he was treated with intermittent intravenous pamidronate until his late teenage years. His main concern is worsening bone pain and several recent extremity fractures with minor trauma. Current DXA reveals T scores of –3.0 at the spine, –3.2 at the femoral neck, and –3.5 at the total hip.

On physical examination, he has short stature with a height of 60 in (152 cm). Sclerae are blue. He has multiple joint deformities and dentinogenesis imperfecta. He wears bilateral hearing aids.

You decide to restart bisphosphonate therapy.

Which of the following benefits is most likely to occur with bisphosphonate therapy in this patient?

    A. Increased bone mineral density

    B. Decreased bone pain

    C. Improved dentition

    D. More rapid fracture healing

    E. Decreased fracture risk

25 A 52-year-old postmenopausal woman with type 1 diabetes mellitus and chronic kidney disease trips while stepping off a curb and fractures her right hip. DXA reveals T scores of –2.8 at the lumbar spine and –3.0 at the left total hip.

Laboratory test results:

    Serum calcium = 8.6 mg/dL (2.2 mmol/L) (reference range, 8.2-10.2 mg/dL [2.1-2.6 mmol/L])

    Albumin = 4.0 g/dL (40 g/L) (reference range, 3.5-5.0 g/dL [35-50 g/L])

    Creatinine = 3.8 mg/dL (335.9 μmol/L) (reference range, 0.6-1.1 mg/dL [53.0-97.2 μmol/L])

25-Hydroxyvitamin D = 32 ng/mL (79.9 nmol/L) (reference range [optimal], 25-80 ng/mL [62.4-199.7 nmol/L])

One month after surgical repair of the hip fracture, you treat her with denosumab, 60 mg subcutaneously.

In this patient, which of the following is the most likely adverse effect of this therapy?

    A. Worsening renal function

    B. Symptomatic hypocalcemia

    C. Osteonecrosis of the jaw

    D. A severe flulike syndrome

    E. Impaired fracture healing

26 A 65-year-old woman is referred to you because of vitamin D deficiency and secondary hyperparathyroidism. Her medical history is positive for morbid obesity and type 2 diabetes mellitus. Long-term medications include metformin and lisinopril. Her internist prescribed cholecalciferol, 1000 IU daily, 3 months ago. She has no bone pain, proximal muscle weakness, or fractures. Her BMI is 42 kg/m², blood pressure is 120/70 mm Hg, and physical examination findings are otherwise normal.

Laboratory test results (baseline):

    Serum calcium = 8.9 mg/dL (2.2 mmol/L) (reference range, 8.2-10.2 mg/dL [2.1-2.6 mmol/L])

    Albumin = 4.0 g/dL (40 g/L) (reference range, 3.5-5.0 g/dL [35-50 g/L])

    Intact PTH = 88 pg/mL (88 ng/L) (reference range, 10-65 pg/mL [10-65 ng/L])

    25-Hydroxyvitamin D = 15 ng/mL (37.4 nmol/L) (reference range [optimal], 25-80 ng/mL [62.4-199.7 nmol/L])

    Urinary calcium excretion = 110 mg/24 h (2.8 mmol/d) (reference range, 100-300 mg/24 h [2.5-7.5 mmol/d])

    Hemoglobin A_{1c} = 6.3% (45 mmol/mol)

    Complete blood cell count, normal

    Vitamin B_{12}, normal

    Iron and total iron-binding capacity, normal

Laboratory test results (3 months after starting cholecalciferol):

> Serum calcium, unchanged
> Intact PTH = 82 pg/mL (82 ng/L) (reference range, 10-65 pg/mL [10-65 ng/L])
> 25-Hydroxyvitamin D = 18 ng/mL (44.9 nmol/L)

Which of the following is the most likely cause for this patient's blunted response to cholecalciferol supplementation?

    A. Malabsorption
    B. Low vitamin D–binding protein
    C. Obesity
    D. Activating mutation in the gene encoding the 24,25-hydroxylase enzyme
    E. Treatment nonadherence

27 An 88-year-old man is admitted to the hospital after several weeks of progressive muscle twitching and multiple falls. His history is notable for congestive heart failure. Last year he was hospitalized with bleeding gastric ulcers due to heavy use of nonsteroidal anti-inflammatory drugs and was started on omeprazole, 40 mg 3 times daily. Current medications include furosemide, 40 mg daily, and omeprazole, 40 mg twice daily.

On physical examination, he is a thin, elderly man with markedly positive Chvostek and Trousseau signs.

Laboratory test results:

> Serum calcium = 6.8 mg/dL (1.7 mmol/L) (reference range, 8.2-10.2 mg/dL [2.1-2.6 mmol/L])
> Ionized calcium = 3.00 mg/dL (0.75 mmol/L) (reference range, 4.60-5.08 mg/dL [1.2-1.3 mmol/L])
> Phosphate = 4.7 mg/dL (1.5 mmol/L) (reference range, 2.3-4.7 mg/dL [0.7-1.5 mmol/L])
> Creatinine = 0.9 mg/dL (79.6 µmol/L) (reference range, 0.7-1.3 mg/dL [61.9-114.9 µmol/L])
> Intact PTH = 30 pg/mL (30 ng/L) (reference range, 10-65 pg/mL [10-65 ng/L])

Measurement of which of the following is most likely to explain this patient's presentation?

    A. 25-Hydroxyvitamin D
    B. 1,25-Dihydroxyvitamin D
    C. Tissue transglutaminase antibodies
    D. 24-Hour urinary calcium excretion
    E. Serum magnesium

28 A 73-year-old woman comes to see you for an opinion regarding her skeletal health. She is currently due for her sixth annual infusion of zoledronic acid for treatment of osteopenia. She did not tolerate oral bisphosphonates. She has never fractured but her mother died of complications of a hip fracture. On further questioning, she notes aching in her left thigh and groin bilaterally which she attributes to increased weight-bearing exercise. A radiograph of the left femur is shown (*see image*).

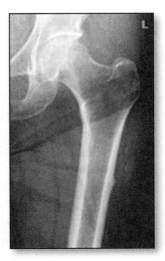

Which of the following would be the most helpful diagnostic test to do next?

    A. Radionuclide bone scan
    B. Serum CTX measurement
    C. Radiograph of the right femur
    D. Bone mineral density test
    E. Iliac crest bone biopsy after double-tetracycline labeling

29 A 58-year-old man presents with nausea, vomiting, and mental confusion. On physical examination, the patient is lethargic and disoriented with a 3-cm firm mass on the left side of his neck.

Laboratory test results:
  Serum calcium = 16 mg/dL (4.0 mmol/L)
    (reference range, 8.2-10.2 mg/dL
    [2.1-2.6 mmol/L])
  Intact PTH = 750 pg/mL (750 ng/L) (reference
    range, 10-65 pg/mL [10-65 ng/L])
  Creatinine = 2.2 mg/dL (194.5 µmol/L) (reference
    range, 0.7-1.3 mg/dL [61.9-114.9 µmol/L])

He is treated with vigorous intravenous hydration followed by zoledronic acid and has marked clinical and biochemical improvement. Family history is noncontributory. A CT scan of the neck reveals a 3.5-cm left-sided neck mass but no other worrisome features.

Which of the following is the best next step?
  A. Sestamibi scan
  B. FNAB of the neck mass
  C. *RET* proto-oncogene genetic testing
  D. Referral for wide surgical resection
  E. Serum parafibromin measurement

30 A 68-year-old woman has been taking alendronate, 70 mg weekly, for the past 2 years. She says that she has taken it correctly (except for missing a few doses) and that she has not had any adverse effects. She had a repeated bone density test at the same center as her initial study. The report indicates a significant loss of bone mineral density in the spine and increases in bone mineral density in the femoral neck and total hip. The DXA images and numeric results are shown (*see images and table*).

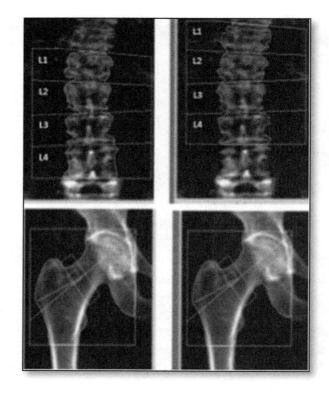

Site	Baseline Bone Mineral Density	Follow-up Bone Mineral Density
L1	0.451	0.423
L2	0.548	0.449
L3	0.593	0.549
L4	0.617	0.591
Total L1-L4	0.557	0.507
Femoral neck	0.480	0.532
Total hip	0.590	0.595

Which of the following is your conclusion?
  A. She is not taking alendronate correctly
  B. She is not responding to alendronate
  C. She has an underlying cause of secondary
     osteoporosis
  D. Her hip bone mineral density was measured
     incorrectly
  E. Her spine bone mineral density was measured
     incorrectly

Obesity/Lipids Board Review

Andrea D. Coviello, MD ● Duke University

1 A 36-year-old woman comes to you for help with weight management. Her height is 65 in (165 cm), and weight is 250 lb (113.5 kg) (BMI = 41.6 kg/m²). She uses a smartphone app to track her caloric intake and has been faithfully following a 1500-calorie a day diet composed of 50% carbohydrates, 30% monounsaturated and polyunsaturated fats, and 20% protein. She exercises 5 days a week at her gym, with 40 minutes of aerobic exercise and 20 minutes of weight training. She thinks her appetite is under control.

She is interested in starting a weight-loss medication that is not directed at appetite suppression.

Which of the following US FDA-approved medications should you recommend?
   A. Phentermine
   B. Orlistat
   C. Phentermine/topiramate
   D. Lorcaserin
   E. Naltrexone/bupropion

2 This patient also states she is interested in the medication associated with the most weight loss.

Which of the following medications should you recommend that is approved for long-term weight loss?
   A. Phentermine/topiramate titrated to 15 mg/92 mg daily
   B. Lorcaserin, 10 mg twice daily
   C. Naltrexone/bupropion ER titrated to 16 mg/180 mg twice daily
   D. Liraglutide titrated to 3.0 mg daily

3 A 36-year-old woman with a BMI of 36 kg/m² presents to you for weight loss. She is otherwise healthy and takes no medications. She would like to lose 20 lb (9.1 kg) before her upcoming wedding. She exercises regularly. She does not want to take weight-loss medications. You prescribe a very low-calorie diet. When you see her back in 3 months, she has lost 18 lb (8.2 kg) or 10% of her body weight (BMI = 32.5 kg/m²). She is pleased, but tells you it is a struggle to maintain her weight. She feels hungry all the time.

This patient's degree of weight loss is expected to result in which of the following changes in gut hormones that regulate appetite?

Answer	Ghrelin	Glucagonlike Peptide 1	Peptide YY	Cholecystokinin
A.	↑	↑	↓	↓
B.	↓	↓	↓	↓
C.	↑	↓	↓	↓
D.	↑	↑	↑	↑

4 A 42-year-old woman with polycystic ovary syndrome is referred to you for weight management. Polycystic ovary syndrome was diagnosed at age 15 years. She gained weight through college and while she worked at her first job, which was sedentary. She had a baby at age 36 years with the assistance of clomiphene but had difficulty losing weight after delivery. She has lost 18 lb (8.2 kg) by participating in a commercial weight-loss program and exercising regularly for the last 6 months, but her weight has plateaued. She has prediabetes, depression, and chronic migraines for which she takes metformin, a selective serotonin reuptake inhibitor, and sumatriptan. She also has fatty liver disease and gallstones, which were documented on ultrasonography 6 months ago. Her BMI is 38 kg/m².

Which of the following should you recommend for continued weight loss?

    A. Naltrexone/bupropion

    B. Lorcaserin

    C. Liraglutide, 3.0 mg daily

    D. Phentermine/topiramate

5 The mother of an 18-year-old girl is concerned about her daughter's weight and long-term health risks. She tells you that her daughter was always the tallest kid in her class. She gained weight quickly as an infant and toddler and her weight was greater than the 95th percentile by the age of 2 years. She was hungry all the time as a child and struggled with obesity despite being very physically active and playing sports. Academically she performed well and had many friends. She went through puberty at age 11 years and has always had regular menses. Her BMI is 36 kg/m².

Which of the following is the most likely genetic cause of obesity in this young woman?

    A. Melanocortin 4 receptor (*MC4R*) mutation

    B. Leptin (*LEP*) mutation

    C. Leptin receptor (*LEPR*) mutation

    D. Proopiomelanocortin (*POMC*) mutation

6 A 45-year-old man with a BMI of 41 kg/m² is interested in weight loss. He tells you that he was not overwegiht as a child and was very physically active. He played football in college but steadily gained weight after graduating. Both of his parents and 3 siblings are obese and struggle with their weight. He is wondering whether his family carries a genetic mutation for obesity.

You tell the patient that a mutation in which of the following genes is the most common genetic variant associated with obesity?

    A. *FTO*

    B. *IRS1*

    C. *TLR4*

    D. *MC4R*

    E. *HHIP*

7 A 53-year-old man presents to your clinic for help with weight loss. His BMI is 44 kg/m² (class III obesity). He has hypertension, hyperlipidemia, and type 2 diabetes mellitus. His hemoglobin A_{1c} level increased to 8.2% (66 mmol/mol) 6 months ago, and sitagliptin was added to a regimen of metformin and glipizide. His most recent hemoglobin A_{1c} value was 7.6% (60 mmol/mol). After starting him on a diet and exercise regimen, you recommend initiating liraglutide, 3.0 mg daily (a glucagonlike peptide 1 receptor agonist) for weight loss.

Current medications include metformin, 500 mg twice daily with meals; glipizide, 5 mg twice daily with meals; sitagliptin, 100 mg once daily; lisinopril, 20 mg daily; and atorvastatin, 40 mg daily.

Before starting liraglutide, you stop his sitagliptin and do which of the following?

    A. Increase the metformin dosage

    B. Increase the glipizide dosage

    C. Decrease the glipizide dosage

    D. Increase the atorvastatin dosage

    E. Decrease the atorvastatin dosage

8 A 64-year-old man whom you follow for type 2 diabetes mellitus asks your advice on weight-loss surgery, which he has been considering to address his severe obesity. His height is 70 in (178 cm), and weight is 365 lb (166 kg) (BMI = 52.4 kg/m²). He also has hypertension, hyperlipidemia, coronary artery disease, and osteoarthritis in his knees. He needs bilateral knee replacements, but his surgeon told him that he must weight less than 300 lb (<136.5 kg) (>20% weight loss) before surgery.

Which bariatric procedure will most likely result in the greatest weight loss for this patient?

    A. Sleeve gastrectomy

    B. Roux-en-Y gastric bypass

    C. Laparoscopic banding procedure

    D. Endoscopically placed duodenal sleeve

9 A 38-year-old woman presents for help with weight loss. She has polycystic ovary syndrome and prediabetes. She has always struggled with her weight. She follows a low-fat, low-glycemic index diet, exercises daily, and takes metformin, 500 mg twice daily. She is very concerned about her risk for progressing to type 2 diabetes. Her current hemoglobin A_{1c} level is 6.3% (45 mmol/mol).

On physical examination, her height is 64 in (162.5 cm), and weight is 210 lb (95.5 kg) (BMI = 36 kg/m²).

Given her insulin resistance, you prescribe liraglutide, 3 mg daily. You tell her that with weight loss of ≥5% (≥10 lb), her risk of progressing to type 2 diabetes will be reduced by:

    A. 10%
    B. 20%
    C. 50%
    D. 80%
    E. 100%

10 A 51-year-old man with type 2 diabetes mellitus is considering having gastric bypass surgery with a sleeve gastrectomy. He has had diabetes for 8 years and is currently treated with metformin, glipizide, and sitagliptin. His hemoglobin A_{1c} level is 9.2%. He has been resistant to starting insulin due to fear of further weight gain. He has heard that although gastric bypass surgery can result in diabetes remission, the remission only lasts a year or two.

You tell this patient that the rate of diabetes remission (defined as a hemoglobin A_{1c} level <6.0% on no glucose-lowering medications 5 years after sleeve gastrectomy) is approximately:

    A. 0%
    B. 10%
    C. 20%
    D. 50%
    E. 75%

11 A 57-year-old man is referred to you for weight loss. His medical history is notable for hypertension, type 2 diabetes mellitus, hyperlipidemia, and coronary artery disease. He had a non-ST–elevation myocardial infarction 6 months ago complicated by tachyarrhythmias initially but with preserved cardiac function according to transthoracic echocardiography. He just completed a cardiac rehabilitation program. His cardiologist referred him to you for weight loss to help reduce his risk of a second cardiovascular event.

On physical examination, his blood pressure is 138/76 mm Hg, pulse rate is 108 beats/min, respiratory rate is 18 breaths/min, and BMI is 63 kg/m². Lungs are clear to auscultation, with no rales. On cardiovascular exam, he has an increased heart rate, regular rhythm, and no murmurs. Findings on abdominal exam are normal. He has ankle edema bilaterally and venous stasis changes.

In addition to a diet and exercise program, which of the following medications would you recommend?

    A. Lorcaserin
    B. Phentermine extended release
    C. Phentermine/topiramate
    D. Liraglutide, 3.0 mg daily
    E. Diethylpropion

12 A 36-year-old woman with polycystic ovary syndrome comes to see you for help with weight loss. Her weight is 268 lb (122 kg) (BMI = 37 kg/m²). She and her husband have been trying to have a child for years and recently went to a fertility specialist who recommended weight loss of 25 lb (11.5 kg) (~8%-9% weight loss) to improve her chances of conceiving a child. She wants to lose the weight as soon as possible and is interested in a very low-calorie diet program. She also has type 2 diabetes mellitus, depression, fatty liver, and cholelithiasis. She is currently taking metformin, 1000 mg twice daily. Her hemoglobin A_{1c} level is 9.0% (75 mmol/mol).

Given her overall clinical picture, you are hesitant to prescribe a very low-calorie diet due to which of the following:

    A. Fatty liver disease
    B. Dyslipidemia
    C. Cholelithiasis
    D. Depression
    E. Type 2 diabetes mellitus

13 A 28-year-old woman presents for help with weight loss. Her height is 65 in (165 cm) and weight is 197 lb (89.5 kg) (BMI = 32.8 kg/m²). You take a weight history and learn that her weight after high school was 132 lb (60 kg) (BMI = 22 kg/m²). She gained 10 lb (4.5 kg) during college. Her first job was very sedentary and she gained another 15 lb (6.8 kg) over 2 years (BMI

= 26 kg/m^2). She began eating a more healthful diet and exercising 3 times a week and her weight plateaued. However, she reports gaining 40 lb (18.2 kg) over the last year. Her current medications are paroxetine (which she started 18 months ago for depression), a multivitamin, and ethinyl estradiol/norethindrone.

You suggest that she stop paroxetine and replace it with which of the following?
   A. Amitriptyline
   B. Mirtazapine
   C. Venlafaxine
   D. Sertraline
   E. Fluoxetine

14 A 54-year-old postmenopausal women presents to your clinic for medically supervised weight loss with a meal replacement program. Her height is 66 in (167.5 cm), and weight is 188 lb (85.5 kg) (BMI = 30.3 kg/m^2). She has seasonal allergies, asthma, hypertension, type 2 diabetes mellitus, and hyperlipidemia. Physical examination findings are notable for central adiposity. You review her current medications and are surprised she is on multiple weight-promoting medications.

Of the patient's medications, which of the following is considered weight neutral?
   A. Atenolol
   B. Glipizide
   C. Cetirizine
   D. Atorvastatin
   E. Fluticasone

15 A 57-year-old woman had a laparoscopic gastric banding procedure done in another state 4 years ago. One year after surgery, she had lost 71 lb (32.3 kg) from a peak lifetime weight of 290 lb (131.8 kg) to a weight nadir of 219 lb (99.5 kg). However, she has regained weight over the last 6 months and currently weighs 282 lb (128.2 kg). Over the last 10 days, she has noted increasing abdominal pain and bloating associated with redness and tenderness over her injection port. On physical examination, she has moderate abdominal tenderness and decreased bowel sounds.

Which of the following is the most likely diagnosis?
   A. Surreptitious manipulation of the injection port
   B. Staple line dehiscence
   C. Gastric band erosion
   D. Anastomotic leak
   E. Food impaction in the band

16 You are referred a 34-year-old man with hyperlipidemia but no known coronary disease. He tells you that he has a strong family history of hypercholesterolemia and early-onset cardiovascular disease with multiple first-degree male relatives who had a myocardial infarction in their 40s. He does not have diabetes mellitus and there is no family history of type 2 diabetes. His 8-year-old daughter reportedly has high cholesterol. His primary care physician has recommended that he start statin therapy, but the patient is hesitant to initiate such a medication at his age.

Laboratory test results:
   Total cholesterol = 617 mg/dL (15.98 mmol/L)
   LDL cholesterol = 538 mg/dL (13.93 mmol/L)
   HDL cholesterol = 49 mg/dL (1.37 mmol/L)
   Triglycerides = 149 mg/dL (1.68 mmol/L)

On physical examination, you note arcus cornealis bilaterally and look specifically for which of the following?
   A. Lipemia retinalis
   B. Achilles tendon xanthomas
   C. Eruptive xanthomas
   D. Palmar xanthoma
   E. Orange tonsils

17 A 56-year-old man is referred to you for treatment of persistently high cholesterol. He also has hypertension and type 2 diabetes mellitus. He had his first heart attack at age 54 years. He also tells you he has a significant family history of cardiovascular disease in his father who had his first heart attack at age 52 years followed by another at age 58 and finally a fatal myocardial infarction at age 63. The patient has been taking atorvastatin, 80 mg daily, for the last 8 years since diabetes was diagnosed. However, he is concerned because he had anginal symptoms 3 months ago, which prompted a left heart catheterization with the placement of 2 stents. His last LDL-cholesterol measurement was 68 mg/dL (1.76 mmol/L). He wants to know what he can do to decrease his risk of another cardiovascular event.

Which of the following is the best management strategy?
   A. No further treatment (his LDL cholesterol is already <70 mg/dL [<1.81 mmol/L])
   B. Add ezetimibe
   C. Add niacin
   D. Add evolocumab
   E. Perform lipopheresis

18 A 45-year-old woman with polycystic ovary syndrome, obesity, and type 2 diabetes mellitus is referred to you after an episode of pancreatitis. She was first told she had high cholesterol and high triglycerides (2386 mg/dL [26.96 mmol/L]) at a health fair screening in college. She had started oral contraceptive pills a few months before her blood was drawn. She stopped the oral contraceptive and her triglycerides dropped to 356 mg/dL (4.02 mmol/L). Last year, type 2 diabetes was diagnosed and the following laboratory values were documented:
   Hemoglobin A_{1c} = 7.0% (53 mmol/mol)
   Total cholesterol = 152 mg/dL (3.94 mmol/L)
   Triglycerides = 330 mg/dL (3.73 mmol/L)

She started metformin and rosuvastatin. She did well initially, but one month ago she was admitted to the hospital with pancreatitis (triglycerides, 1197 mg/dL [13.53 mmol/L]; hemoglobin A_{1c}, 12.9% [117 mmol/mol]). Her father has type 2 diabetes and high cholesterol treated with a statin and fish oil, but he has never had pancreatitis.

Laboratory test results (on rosuvastatin):
   Total cholesterol = 158 mg/dL (4.09 mmol/L)
   LDL cholesterol (direct measure) = 56 mg/dL (1.45 mmol/L)
   HDL cholesterol = 41 mg/dL (1.06 mmol/L)
   Triglycerides = 425 mg/dL (4.80 mmol/L)
   TSH = 2.29 mIU/L
   Free T_4 = 0.75 ng/dL (9.6 pmol/L) (reference range, 0.8-1.8 ng/dL [10.30-23.17 pmol/L])

Which of the following is the most likely primary cause of her hypertriglyceridemia?
   A. Familial hypertriglceridemia
   B. Polycystic ovary syndrome
   C. Lipoprotein lipase deficiency
   D. Apolipoprotein C1 deficiency

19 A 24-year-old graduate student from Japan comes to see you for a high cholesterol level identified by screening at the student health clinic. He is healthy and takes a multivitamin but no other medications. He drinks a couple beers 2 or 3 times a week but does not binge drink.

Fasting lipid levels:
   Total cholesterol = 220 mg/dL (5.70 mmol/L)
   HDL cholesterol = 115 mg/dL (2.98 mmol/L)
   Triglycerides = 78 mg/dL (0.88 mmol/L)
   LDL cholesterol = 89 mg/dL (2.31 mmol/L)

Which of the following is the most likely explanation for his lipid levels?
   A. Alcohol use
   B. Cholesteryl ester transfer protein deficiency
   C. Interference with lipid assays
   D. Apolipoprotein A1 deficiency
   E. Lipoprotein lipase deficiency

20 A 54-year-old man with hyperlipidemia is referred to you for further evaluation and decision about treatment. He has no other medical problems and takes only an oral multivitamin. He is physically fit and is an avid runner. His father and brother both have hyperlipidemia and take statins. Despite statin therapy, his father had a myocardial infarction at age 56 years. The patient is leery of taking a statin due to possible myalgias or myopathy.

On physical examination, his blood pressure is 126/76 mm Hg, pulse rate is 64 beats/min, and BMI is 24 kg/m². There are no stigmata of hyperlipidemia.

Lipid profile:
   Total cholesterol = 262 mg/dL (6.79 mmol/L)
   HDL cholesterol = 46 mg/dL (1.19 mmol/L)
   Triglycerides = 135 mg/dL (1.53 mmol/L)
   LDL cholesterol = 187 mg/dL (4.84 mmol/L)

You calculate his American Heart Association 10-year risk of having a heart attack or stroke, which is 7.4%. You are concerned that his risk of cardiovascular disease is underestimated given his LDL-cholesterol level and family history of cardiovascular disease.

Which of the following should you recommend?
   A. Measure apolipoprotein B
   B. Measure lipoprotein (a)
   C. Measure high-sensitivity C-reactive protein
   D. No further testing

21 A 59-year-old man has type 2 diabetes mellitus, hypertension, and hyperlipidemia with an LDL-cholesterol level of 180 mg/dL (4.66 mmol/L). His doctor advised him to start a statin for primary prevention of cardiovascular disease. After starting atorvastatin, 80 mg daily, his LDL-cholesterol level decreased to 95 mg/dL (2.46 mmol/L). However, he developed pain in his lower extremities and his creatine kinase level rose to twice the upper normal limit. He stopped the atorvastatin and the pain resolved. His TSH level is normal.

Which of the following medications should be started now?
   A. Low-dosage rosuvastatin
   B. Fenofibrate
   C. Ezetimibe
   D. Evolocumab
   E. Niacin

22 A 56-year-old man is referred to you for treatment of high cholesterol. He also has hypertension treated with lisinopril and type 2 diabetes mellitus treated with metformin and glipizide. He has never had a myocardial infarction, but he does have coronary disease and a stent was placed 6 months ago. He has been intolerant to high-intensity statins (both rosuvastatin and atorvastatin) due to myalgias, although his creatine phosphokinase level has always been normal. He currently takes simvastatin, 40 mg daily, and is tolerating it without myalgias.

Laboratory test results (on current medications):
   Hemoglobin A_{1c} = 8.2% (66 mmol/mol)
   Total cholesterol = 160 mg/dL (4.14 mmol/L)
   HDL cholesterol = 38 mg/dL (0.98 mmol/L)
   LDL cholesterol = 100 mg/dL (2.59 mmol/L)
   Triglycerides = 110 mg/dL (1.24 mmol/L)

Which of the following is the best next step in this patient's management?
   A. Add niacin
   B. Add ezetimibe
   C. Add fenofibrate
   D. Change simvastatin to pitavastatin
   E. No change, his LDL cholesterol is at goal

23 A 27-year-old woman with a history of hypertriglyceridemia and pancreatitis has controlled her hypertriglyceridemia reasonably well with diet and fenofibrate. Her triglyceride levels on this program have ranged from 595 to 880 mg/dL (6.72-9.94 mmol/L). She has 2 children, aged 4 and 7 years, and she developed gestational diabetes during her last pregnancy. She was not prescribed oral contraceptive pills because of her hypertriglyceridemia. She now returns 8 months after her last visit and tells you that she is 12 weeks pregnant and still taking fenofibrate.

Laboratory test results:
   Total cholesterol = 300 mg/dL (7.77 mmol/L)
   Triglycerides = 815 mg/dL (9.21 mmol/L)
   HDL cholesterol = 31 mg/dL (0.80 mmol/L)
   Fasting glucose = 105 mg/dL (5.8 mmol/L)
   Hemoglobin A_{1c} = 7.0% (53 mmol/mol)

Which of the following is the most reasonable strategy now?
   A. Continue fenofibrate
   B. Substitute atorvastatin for fenofibrate
   C. Substitute nicotinic acid for fenofibrate
   D. Substitute omega-3 fatty acids for fenofibrate

24 A 50-year-old man with type 2 diabetes mellitus has a hemoglobin A_{1c} level of 7.8% (62 mmol/mol) and is currently treated with rosuvastatin, 40 mg daily. His other risk factor for cardiovascular disease is hypertension.

Which of the following cholesterol-reducing therapies also might assist with his glucose control?
- A. Niacin
- B. Colesevelam
- C. Pitavastatin
- D. Ezetimibe
- E. Anacetrapib

25 A 24-year-old man is referred to you for management of high triglycerides. Two weeks ago, he was hospitalized with acute pancreatitis after attending a party. He notes that he had only "a few beers" and normally does not drink alcohol at all. His peak triglyceride level was 4800 mg/dL (54.24 mmol/L).

On physical examination, he has a rash of small eruptive xanthomas (*see image*) and lipemia retinalis on fundoscopic exam. He relates that as a teenager and in college he had episodes of severe abdominal pain after eating too many cheeseburgers and fries.

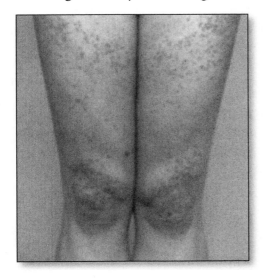

Which of the following is the most likely etiology of his hypertriglyceridemia?
- A. Apolipoprotein B elevation
- B. Adipose triglyceride lipase deficiency
- C. Hepatic lipase deficiency
- D. Lipoprotein lipase deficiency
- E. Pancreatic lipase deficiency

26 A 17-year-old man is referred to you for abnormal cholesterol levels. His parents noticed clouding of his corneas and took him to an ophthalmologist who ordered a fasting cholesterol panel. He tells you that he has been very tired and can no longer play basketball.

On physical examination, he is a thin, ill-appearing young man. His tonsils are of normal color and size and he has no tendinous or eruptive xanthomas.

Laboratory test results (fasting):
    HDL cholesterol = 6 mg/dL (0.16 mmol/L)
    LDL cholesterol = 190 mg/dL (4.92 mmol/L)
    Triglycerides = 290 mg/dL (3.28 mmol/L)
    Creatinine = 2.8 mg/dL (247.5 μmol/L)
    Urinanalysis = 3+ proteinuria

Which of the following is this patient's most likely diagnosis?
- A. ABCA1 deficiency (Tangier disease)
- B. Lecithin-cholesterol acyltransferase (LCAT) deficiency
- C. Defective apolipoprotein B
- D. Lipoprotein lipase deficiency
- E. Surreptitious anabolic steroid use

27 You are referred a 53-year-old woman for high cholesterol after her physician ordered a lipid panel. She has been in good health and has no personal or family history of vascular disease. After menopause, she gained 20 lb (9.1 kg), and during the past year she has attempted to reduce her weight with a high-fat, low-carbohydrate diet. On this diet, her BMI has decreased from 35 to 29 kg/m². She was unaware that she had a cholesterol problem. Her total cholesterol concentration is greater than 600 mg/dL (>15.54 mmol/L) with an equal increase in triglycerides (>600 mg/dL [>6.78 mmol/L]). Thyroid function is normal.

A picture of her palm is shown (*see image*).

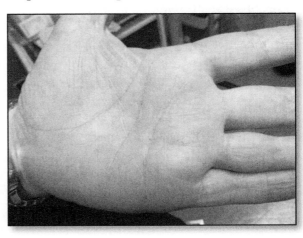

To make the definitive diagnosis of this patient's disorder, you should order which of the following tests?
- A. Apolipoprotein AI measurement by radioimmunoassay
- B. Assessment of LDL particle size
- C. Apolipoprotein E genotyping
- D. Lipoprotein (a) gene analysis

28 A 38-year-old woman is referred to you from the liver transplant service for severe hyperlipidemia. She is undergoing evaluation for liver transplant due to primary biliary cirrhosis. She is currently taking ursodiol, 300 mg 3 times daily. She has polymyositis, which was diagnosed 9 years ago, for which she takes prednisone. She does not smoke cigarettes or drink alcohol. She does not have diabetes mellitus or heart disease and has no family history of premature cardiovascular disease.

On physical examination, her BMI is 23.8 kg/m², she has mild icterus, and fundoscopic exam is negative for lipemia retinalis. She has no xanthelasma or tendon xanthomata.

Laboratory test results:
- Total cholesterol = 608 mg/dL (15.75 mmol/L)
- LDL cholesterol = 426 mg/dL (11.03 mmol/L)
- HDL cholesterol = 63 mg/dL (1.63 mmol/L)
- Triglycerides = 190 mg/dL (2.15 mmol/L)
- Alanine aminotransferase = 150 U/L (2.51 µkat/L) (reference range, 10-40 U/L [0.17-0.67 µkat/L])
- Aspartate aminotransferase = 145 U/L (2.42 µkat/L) (reference range, 20-48 U/L [0.33-0.80 µkat/L])
- Total bilirubin = 2.2 mg/dL (37.6 µmol/L) (reference range, 0.3-1.2 mg/dL [5.1-20.5 µmol/L])
- Alkaline phosphatase = 816 U/L (13.6 µkat/L) (reference range, 50-120 U/L [0.84-2.00 µkat/L])
- Hepatitis B and C serology, negative

Which of the following is the most likely explanation for her lipid values?
- A. Accumulation of lipoprotein (a)
- B. A complication of ursodeoxycholic acid treatment
- C. Lecithin-cholesterol acyltransferase (LCAT) deficiency
- D. Liver disease causing increased apolipoprotein B production
- E. Accumulation of lipoprotein X

29 A 58-year-old man recently presented with anginal symptoms and a positive exercise stress test. He reports no history of hypertension, diabetes mellitus, or cigarette smoking. His father died of a myocardial infarction at age 55 years and his brother underwent a revascularization procedure at age 56 years. Both his father and brother had lipid profiles characterized by high triglycerides, low HDL cholesterol, and high LDL cholesterol. His physical examination findings are unremarkable.

Fasting lipid levels:
- Triglycerides = 300 mg/dL (3.39 mmol/L)
- HDL cholesterol = 30 mg/dL (0.78 mmol/L)
- LDL cholesterol = 175 mg/dL (4.53 mmol/L)

Which of the following best explains his lipid profile?
- A. Familial hypercholesterolemia
- B. Lipoprotein lipase deficiency
- C. Familial defective apolipoprotein B
- D. Familial combined hyperlipidemia
- E. Apolipoprotein A1 deficiency

30 A 32-year-old woman is referred to you because of "low" blood cholesterol levels. She had a bout of abdominal pain several weeks ago and her physician ordered right upper-quadrant ultrasonography, which revealed a fatty liver. She was previously healthy and takes no medications. Her BMI is 25 kg/m². Her physical examination findings are unremarkable. Given her fatty liver disease, her physician ordered a cholesterol panel and a hemoglobin A_{1c} measurement.

Laboratory test results:
- Hemoglobin A_{1c} = 5.5% (37 mmol/mol)
- Total cholesterol = 56 mg/dL (1.45 mmol/L)
- HDL cholesterol = 24 mg/dL (0.62 mmol/L)
- LDL cholesterol = 24 mg/dL (0.62 mmol/L)
- Triglycerides = 38 mg/dL (0.43 mmol/L)
- Hepatic profile, within normal limits

Which of the following is the most likely diagnosis?
- A. Hypobetalipoproteinemia
- B. Abetalipoproteinemia
- C. Dysbetalipoproteinemia
- D. Hypoalphalipoproteinemia

Pituitary Board Review

Mark E. Molitch, MD • Northwestern University

1 A 51-year-old man presents with new-onset atrial fibrillation and a 10-lb (4.5-kg) weight loss. In retrospect, he has noticed some fatigue, a mild tremor, and heat intolerance for several months. His sister has hypothyroidism.

On physical examination, his blood pressure is 139/67 mm Hg, pulse rate is 92 beats/min (irregular), and BMI is 24.1 kg/m². He has no proptosis but does have slight lid-lag. His thyroid gland is about 2-fold diffusely enlarged and is soft. He has brisk reflexes and a fine tremor of his outstretched hands.

Laboratory test results:
Free T_4 = 4.5 ng/dL (57.9 pmol/L) (reference range, 0.8-1.8 ng/dL [10.30-23.17 pmol/L])
Total T_3 = 482 ng/dL (7.4 nmol/L) (reference range, 70-200 ng/dL [1.08-3.08 nmol/L])
TSH = 9.47 mIU/L

Results from repeated tests are similar. Thyroid-stimulating immunoglobulin index is 1.4 (normal <1.3). MRI of the pituitary gland is normal.

Which of the following tests would be the most helpful in determining the etiology of his hyperthyroidism?
  A. Measurement of β-subunit
  B. T_3 suppression test
  C. Measurement of HAMA (human anti-mouse antibodies)
  D. Petrosal sinus sampling for TSH measurements

2 A 32-year-old woman is referred by her gynecologist because of amenorrhea of 1.5 years' duration, galactorrhea, and a prolactin level of 39.3 ng/mL (1.7 nmol/L).

Her examination findings are normal except for bilateral expressible galactorrhea. There is no clinical evidence of Cushing syndrome or acromegaly.

MRI shows a 1.4-cm pituitary adenoma with minimal suprasellar extension.

Laboratory test results:
Prolactin = 41.3 ng/mL (1.8 nmol/L)
LH = 2.3 mIU/mL (2.3 IU/L)
FSH = 1.7 mIU/mL (1.7 IU/L)
Cortisol (8 AM) = 17.3 μg/dL (477.3 nmol/L)
IGF-1 = 469 ng/mL (61.4 nmol/L) (reference range, 113-297 ng/mL [14.8-38.9 nmol/L])

Which of the following should be the next step in this patient's management?
  A. Measure GH during an oral glucose tolerance test
  B. Remeasure prolactin levels after 1:100 dilution
  C. Start cabergoline, 0.5 mg twice weekly
  D. Start octreotide LAR, 20 mg monthly

3 A 37-year-old woman is found to have a prolactin level of 1012 ng/mL (44.0 nmol/L) when evaluated for amenorrhea and galactorrhea. She also has decreased energy levels and headaches.

Laboratory test results:
Free T_4 = 0.6 ng/mL (7.7 pmol/L)
TSH = 0.62 mIU/L
Cortisol = 4.7 μg/dL (129.7 nmol/L)
LH = 2.1 mIU/mL (2.1 IU/L)
FSH = 2.9 mIU/mL (2.9 IU/L)
IGF-1 = 142 ng/mL (18.6 nmol/L) (reference range, 160-360 ng/mL [21.0-47.2 nmol/L])

MRI shows a 2.5-cm macroadenoma that extends laterally into the cavernous sinus on the left side and inferiorly into the sphenoid sinus. After replacement with hydrocortisone and levothyroxine, cabergoline is initiated and the dosage is gradually increased to 1 mg twice weekly. Over the next 3 months, her prolactin level normalizes, her menses resume, her energy improves, and her headaches resolve. However, over the past 2 weeks, she has noticed profuse, watery rhinorrhea.

Which of the following should be the next step in this patient's management?
  A. Perform pituitary MRI
  B. Increase the cabergoline dosage
  C. Reduce the cabergoline dosage
  D. Add pseudoephedrine
  E. Measure β2-transferrin in the nasal discharge

4 A 37-year-old man has had recurrence of his Cushing disease 5 years after what appeared to be a curative resection of a pituitary adenoma. A late-night salivary cortisol measurement was elevated on his annual screening, and he subsequently began to develop facial rounding, erythema, and increased abdominal fat. He again became hyperglycemic with a hemoglobin A_{1c} level of 6.8% (51 mmol/mol).

Laboratory test results:
  Urinary free cortisol = 110 µg/24 h (303.6 nmol/d)
  Cortisol (AM) = 21.3 µg/dL (587.6 nmol/L)
  ACTH = 83 pg/mL (18.3 pmol/L)

However, MRI shows no evidence of tumor regrowth. After discussion of therapeutic options, he begins taking mifepristone, 300 mg daily, increasing to 600 mg daily. Over the next several months, his symptoms resolve and he feels back to normal. However, the following laboratory test results are documented:

  Urinary free cortisol = 230 µg/24 h (634.8 nmol/d)
  Cortisol (AM) = 35.1 µg/dL (968.3 nmol/L)
  ACTH = 253 pg/mL (55.7 pmol/L)

Which of the following should be the next step in this patient's management?
  A. Increase the mifepristone dosage to 900 mg daily
  B. Continue the mifepristone dosage at 600 mg daily
  C. Decrease the mifepristone dosage to 300 mg daily
  D. Add pasireotide LAR, 20 mg every 4 weeks
  E. Refer for gamma-knife radiotherapy

5 A 45-year-old woman is referred after a 2.2 × 1.8-cm hypodense right adrenal nodule is found during a staging CT scan for recently diagnosed breast cancer. She is asymptomatic and has no clinical signs of Cushing syndrome.

Laboratory test results:
  DHEA-S, normal
  Androstenedione, normal
  Testosterone, normal
  Urinary free cortisol, normal
  Cortisol (AM) = 13.1 µg/dL (361.4 nmol/L)
    (fails to suppress with dexamethasone)

With a diagnosis of an incidental adenoma causing subclinical Cushing syndrome rather than an adrenal metastasis, she undergoes surgery and irradiation for breast cancer. Four months after completion of these treatments, she reports some facial rounding and erythema, peripheral edema, and worsening hirsutism. On physical examination, she has increased hair growth and appears mildly cushingoid.

Urinary free cortisol excretion is 228 µg/24 h (629.3 nmol/d).

Which of the following should be the next step in this patient's management?
  A. Perform an ACTH stimulation test with measurement of 17-hydroxyprogesterone
  B. Refer for laparoscopic right adrenalectomy
  C. Perform petrosal sinus sampling for ACTH
  D. Perform bilateral adrenal venous sampling for cortisol
  E. Measure 8-AM cortisol and ACTH levels

6 A 37-year-old woman is being evaluated for persistent fatigue. Ten years ago, she had partial resection of TSH-secreting pituitary tumor with subsequent radiotherapy for the residual tumor. Last year, she underwent resection via a craniotomy of a sarcoma arising from the dorsum sella thought to be related to the prior radiotherapy. Her current medications include levothyroxine, 137 mcg daily; hydrocortisone, 10 mg in the morning and 5 mg in the afternoon; and a low-dosage oral contraceptive. She read on the Internet that GH treatment might improve her energy levels.

On physical examination, she is a well-appearing woman with a blood pressure of 124/78 mm Hg, pulse rate of 76 beats/min, and BMI of 24.1 kg/m^2.

Laboratory test results:
Free T$_4$ = 1.2 ng/dL (15.4 pmol/L) (reference range, 0.8-1.8 ng/dL [10.30-23.17 pmol/L])
Prolactin = 7.6 ng/mL (0.3 nmol/L)
LH = 1.7 mIU/mL (1.7 IU/L)
FSH = 1.4 mIU/mL (1.4 IU/L)
IGF-1 = 97 ng/dL (12.7 nmol/L) (reference range, 55-360 ng/dL [7.2-47.2 nmol/L])
Comprehensive chemistry panel, normal
Complete blood cell count, normal

Which of the following should be the next step in evaluating for GH deficiency?
A. Perform an insulin tolerance test to assess GH levels
B. Perform a glucagon stimulation test to assess GH levels
C. Measure IGF-1 again
D. No assessment for GH deficiency is indicated as she is not a candidate for GH therapy

7 A 71-year-old woman with metastatic melanoma being treated with chemotherapy is admitted to the hospital with weight loss, lethargy, and orthostatic hypotension. She has taken levothyroxine for hypothyroidism due to Hashimoto thyroiditis for many years.

Laboratory test results:
Random cortisol = 1.5 µg/dL (41.4 nmol/L)
ACTH = 9 pg/mL (2.0 pmol/L)
LH = 0.3 mIU/mL (0.3 IU/L)
FSH = 2.0 mIU/mL (2.0 IU/L)
IGF-1 = 35 ng/mL (4.6 nmol/L) (reference range, 41-279 ng/mL [5.4-36.5 nmol/L])
Prolactin = 1.8 ng/mL (0.08 nmol/L)
TSH = 0.2 mIU/L

MRI shows homogeneous enlargement of the pituitary and stalk, which was not present on MRI 2 months ago.

Which of the following medications is the most likely cause of these pituitary abnormalities?
A. Bevacizumab
B. Ipilimumab
C. Temozolomide
D. Sunitinib

8 A 46-year-old man presents with loss of libido and erectile dysfunction. His primary care physician documented his testosterone level to be 180 ng/dL (6.3 nmol/L) and referred him for further evaluation.

Laboratory test results:
Repeated testosterone = 171 ng/dL (5.9 nmol/L)
LH = 0.9 mIU/mL (0.9 IU/L)
FSH = 1.1 mIU/mL (1.1 IU/L)
Prolactin = 2513 ng/mL (109.3 nmol/L)
TSH, normal
Cortisol, normal

MRI shows a 1.7-cm adenoma with substantial extension into the left cavernous sinus.

At a cabergoline dosage of 1.0 mg twice weekly, his prolactin level normalizes, his tumor is greatly reduced in size, his testosterone level increases to 497 ng/dL (17.2 nmol/L), and his erectile function returns. However, his wife complains that he has become obsessed with playing online poker and has lost about $5000 over the past 3 months.

Which of the following is the most likely explanation for his current behavior?
A. Restoring testosterone to normal has unmasked previously suppressed obsessive behavior
B. Hypothalamic damage from the tumor
C. An adverse effect of cabergoline
D. Behavior change unrelated to his tumor or treatment

9 A 31-year-old woman presents with galactorrhea and amenorrhea and is found to have a prolactin level of 3230 ng/mL (140.4 nmol/L) and a 14-mm pituitary adenoma. With cabergoline treatment, 0.5 mg twice weekly, her prolactin normalizes, her galactorrhea and amenorrhea resolve, and her tumor decreases in size to 5 mm. She stops cabergoline when she learns she is pregnant. Now, 7 months later, she reports increasing headaches that are quite severe. Findings on formal visual field testing are normal.

Which of the following is the best step in this patient's management?
- A. Restart cabergoline now
- B. Start bromocriptine
- C. Proceed with transsphenoidal surgical tumor removal
- D. Deliver the baby
- E. Perform pituitary-directed MRI

10 A 57-year-old woman with acromegaly still has elevations of GH and IGF-1 after transsphenoidal surgery. As one of the complications of acromegaly, she has difficult-to-control diabetes mellitus (hemoglobin A_{1c}, 8.4% [68 mmol/mol]). She is very concerned about the type of adjunctive medical therapy she should have.

Which of the following medications is most likely to worsen her diabetes control?
- A. Octreotide LAR
- B. Lanreotide depot
- C. Pegvisomant
- D. Cabergoline
- E. Pasireotide

11 A 33-year-old woman has developed Cushing syndrome during her second month of pregnancy. She has hypertension, diabetes mellitus, hirsutism, and wide, purple striae on her abdomen.

Laboratory test results:
Serum cortisol (8 AM) = 37 µg/dL (1020.8 nmol/L)
ACTH = 129 pg/mL (28.4 pmol/L) (reference range, 10-60 pg/mL [2.2-13.2 pmol/L])
Urinary free cortisol = 475 µg/24 h (1311 nmol/d) (reference range, 4-50 µg/24 h [11-138 nmol/d])

MRI shows a 6-mm pituitary adenoma.

Which of the following treatment options is absolutely contraindicated?
- A. Ketoconazole
- B. Mifepristone
- C. Transsphenoidal surgery
- D. Pasireotide
- E. Cabergoline

12 A 28-year-old woman has had amenorrhea and non-bothersome galactorrhea for 4 years and is found to have a serum prolactin level of 48.3 ng/mL (2.1 nmol/L). Evaluation documents normal thyroid, renal, and hepatic function and a negative pregnancy test. MRI reveals a 4-mm hypointense area in the pituitary compatible with a microadenoma. Although she is sexually active, she is not planning to try for pregnancy for at least 4 to 5 years. Her health insurance is minimal and she is concerned about her health care costs over the next 4 years.

Which of the following is the best treatment plan for this woman?
- A. Transsphenoidal surgery
- B. Bromocriptine
- C. Cabergoline
- D. Oral contraceptives
- E. Reassurance

13 Cushing disease is diagnosed in a 45-year-old man. Forty-eight hours after transsphenoidal surgery for a 4-mm microadenoma, his morning cortisol level is 11 µg/dL (303.5 nmol/L) and he is discharged home. Two days later, urinary free cortisol excretion is 37 µg/24 h (102.1 nmol/d) (reference range, 4-50 µg/24 h [11-138 nmol/d]).

Which of the following should you tell this patient?
- A. He may need another transsphenoidal operation performed by an experienced pituitary surgeon in the next few years
- B. He will need to take maintenance hydrocortisone daily, as well as stress dosing for close to a year
- C. He should be started on medical therapy for persistent Cushing disease
- D. He should be referred for gamma-knife stereotactic radiotherapy
- E. He should have petrosal sinus sampling to determine the location of any residual tumor

14 A 26-year-old woman is found to have sarcoidosis involving her hypothalamus after she presents with polyuria and polydipsia. On further evaluation, panhypopituitarism, complete diabetes insipidus, and a markedly impaired thirst mechanism are diagnosed. While on anterior pituitary hormone replacement and twice-daily DDAVP, a serum sodium concentration of 116 mEq/L (116 mmol/L) is documented. Her blood pressure is 124/68 mm Hg, her pulse rate is 76 beats/min, her skin is "doughy," and she is very confused.

In addition to holding the DDAVP, which of the following is the best treatment plan?
   A. Restrict fluid intake to 1000 mL/day and check serum sodium in 12 hours
   B. Restrict fluid intake to 1000 mL/day and check serum sodium every 2 to 4 hours
   C. Give hypertonic saline to raise the serum sodium by 6 mEq/L (6 mmol/L) over 6 hours
   D. Give normal saline at 250 mL/h plus furosemide, 40 mg intravenously
   E. Give conivaptan

15 A 28-year-old woman who is 29 weeks' pregnant has been told by her mother-in-law that her facial features seem to be coarsening. After documenting an elevated IGF-1 level, her obstetrician refers her for evaluation of possible acromegaly.

Which of the following should be the next step?
   A. Deferral of further workup until after delivery
   B. Another measurement of IGF-1
   C. Measurement of GH response during an oral glucose tolerance test
   D. Pituitary-directed MRI
   E. Use of octreotide long-acting release until after delivery

16 A 49-year-old man is treated for a 2.6-cm prolactinoma. He responds well to cabergoline, 1.0 mg twice weekly, with an initial normalization of his prolactin level and shrinkage of his tumor to about 7 mm in height. However, now, 2 years later, his prolactin concentration has increased to 312 ng/mL (13.6 nmol/L). On MRI, his tumor has grown to 1.4 cm despite taking his medication regularly. His cabergoline dosage is gradually increased to 2 mg daily over the next year. However, his prolactin level continues to rise to 4513 ng/mL (196.2 nmol/L) and his tumor is now 3.2 cm. He subsequently undergoes a 2-stage transsphenoidal/transcranial near-total resection.

However, the tumor regrows rapidly even on cabergoline, and he undergoes gamma-knife radiotherapy. Over the next 2 years, the tumor continues to grow.

Which of the following treatments is the best choice now?
   A. Conventional radiotherapy
   B. Repeat craniotomy
   C. Lanreotide
   D. Ipilimumab
   E. Temozolomide

17 A 19-year-old man had acute lymphocytic leukemia treated with chemotherapy and cranial irradiation at ages 4 to 6 years with resultant panhypopituitarism. He has been treated with levothyroxine, hydrocortisone, GH, and testosterone. Over the past year, he has grown only 1 cm and his height is now 65 in (165.1 cm). A recent hand and wrist x-ray shows complete epiphyseal closure. After 1 month off GH therapy, his IGF-1 concentration is −2.7 standard deviations. Following testing, he restarts his GH therapy. However, he is now off to college and wants to know whether he should continue GH treatment.

If he continues GH treatment, which of the following outcomes is most likely?
   A. Further growth of 2 to 3 inches
   B. Increased peak bone mass
   C. Decreased mortality rate
   D. Improvement in recent memory
   E. Increased libido

18 A 34-year-old woman reports that she has decreased libido and mild depression, and her primary care physician subsequently documents a prolactin level of 37 ng/mL (1.6 nmol/L). Her physician re-measures prolactin (which is 45 ng/mL [2.0 nmol/L]) and orders further laboratory tests. The patient has a normal chemistry metabolic profile and a TSH level of 1.1 mIU/L. Her menses have been regular, and she has not noticed any galactorrhea. She was able to conceive without problems about 18 months ago and the pregnancy and delivery were without incident. She breast-fed the baby for 2 to 3 months and did not have persistent galactorrhea. She is otherwise well. Her examination findings are normal, with no goiter or expressible galactorrhea.

Which of the following tests should now be done?
A. Pituitary-directed MRI
B. LH and FSH measurement
C. Assessment for macroprolactin
D. Prolactin measurement at 1:100 dilution
E. Estradiol measurement

19 An 18-year-old woman is referred for gigantism. She also has primary amenorrhea. Her height is 76 in (193 cm), and weight is 217 lb (98.6 kg). Her hands and feet are enlarged, and she has frontal bossing and prognathism. She has a bitemporal visual field defect. A maternal aunt was thought to have had a pituitary adenoma of uncertain type. There is no known family history of calcium disorders or kidney stones.

Laboratory test results:
GH = 90 ng/mL (90 µg/L) (does not suppress adequately during an oral glucose tolerance test)
Serum IGF-1 = 1233 ng/mL (161.5 nmol/L) (reference range, 147-527 ng/mL [19.3-69.0 nmol/L])
Serum calcium, normal

MRI of the brain shows a 4.3 × 3.2 × 2.8-cm pituitary adenoma with suprasellar extension. Following transsphenoidal surgery, her GH and IGF-1 levels remain elevated and poorly responsive to octreotide LAR and pasireotide.

A germline mutation in which of the following genes is most likely responsible for the findings in this patient?
A. *GNAS* (GNAS complex locus)
B. *TBX19* (T-box 19) (previously *TPIT*)
C. *PROP1* (PROP paired-like homeobox 1)
D. *AIP* (aryl hydrocarbon receptor interacting protein)
E. *MEN1* (menin)

20 A 78-year-old man is referred because a head CT performed after he fell and struck his head showed a pituitary mass. On MRI, this appears to be a 1.2-cm pituitary adenoma with minimal left parasellar extension. He has been feeling well, but in general he thinks he has been slowing down. He has no headaches or vision symptoms. He had a myocardial infarction 10 years ago and currently takes a statin, lisinopril for hypertension, and a baby aspirin.

On physical examination, his blood pressure is 136/70 mm Hg and pulse rate is 74 beats/min. His skin has normal texture, and his reflexes are normal.

Laboratory test results:
Testosterone = 218 ng/dL (7.6 nmol/L)
LH = 2.3 mIU/mL (2.3 IU/L)
FSH = 1.4 mIU/mL (1.4 IU/L)
Cortisol (8 AM) = 15.7 µg/dL (433.1 nmol/L)
Prolactin = 5.7 ng/mL (0.2 nmol/L)
Free T$_4$ = 1.2 ng/dL (15.4 pmol/L) (reference range, 0.8-1.8 ng/dL [10.3-23.2 pmol/L])

Which of the following is the most appropriate management for this patient?
A. Another MRI in 6 to 12 months
B. Referral to an experienced pituitary surgeon
C. Visual field testing
D. Gamma-knife radiotherapy
E. Conventional radiotherapy

21 A 28-year-old woman developed headaches, nausea, vomiting, and fatigue during her 33rd week of pregnancy. She had been previously well and was able to become pregnant within 2 months of trying. Her pregnancy course had been smooth until then. Her symptoms have continued to worsen, and she now presents at 35 weeks' gestation. Her physical examination findings are normal for 35 weeks' gestation. Because of the progressive nature of her headaches, her obstetrician persuades the radiologist to perform a noncontrast MRI of her head, and the patient is found to have a diffusely enlarged pituitary, measuring 16 mm in height, without abutment of the optic chiasm.

Laboratory test results:

Free T$_4$ = 1.2 ng/dL (15.4 pmol/L) (reference range, 0.8-1.8 ng/dL [10.3-23.2 pmol/L])

TSH = 1.3 mIU/L

Cortisol (8 AM) = 6.0 μg/dL (165.5 nmol/L)

Prolactin = 137 ng/mL (6.0 nmol/L)

Which of the following is indicated now?
  A. Bromocriptine
  B. Cabergoline
  C. Transsphenoidal decompression
  D. Hydrocortisone replacement
  E. Urgent cesarean delivery

22 A 68-year-old woman reports fatigue, weight gain, and decreased libido. She has been well all her life until these symptoms started. Menopause was at age 52 years and she never took hormone replacement therapy. She attributes her symptoms to aging, but her husband has urged her to be evaluated. Although she recently retired, she has not changed her lifelong pattern of little exercise.

On physical examination, no abnormalities are noted except that she is overweight. The thyroid is not enlarged, and there are no cushingoid features. Her blood pressure is 130/92 mm Hg, pulse rate is 60 beats/min, and BMI is 28.2 kg/m^2.

Laboratory test results:

Complete blood cell count, normal

Blood chemistries, normal

TSH = 0.5 mIU/L

Free T$_4$ = 0.5 ng/dL (6.4 pmol/L) (reference range, 0.8-1.8 ng/dL [10.3-23.2 pmol/L])

Cortisol (8 AM) = 10 μg/dL (275.9 nmol/L)

LH = 2.1 mIU/mL (2.1 IU/L)

FSH = 1.7 mIU/mL (1.7 IU/L)

Which of the following tests is the most important next step?
  A. Pituitary-directed MRI
  B. Serum estradiol measurement
  C. Ferritin measurement
  D. α-Subunit measurement

23 A 63-year-old man with severe ascites due to cirrhosis from hepatitis C is admitted to the hospital with altered mental status.

On physical examination, he is mildly confused. He has massive ascites, pulmonary congestion, and 4+ peripheral edema.

Laboratory test results:

Serum sodium = 121 mEq/L (121 mmol/L)

Urinary sodium = 14 mEq/L

Urine osmolality = 373 mOsm/kg (373 mmol/kg)

Serum alanine aminotransferase = 342 U/L (5.7 μkat/L)

Bilirubin = 4.7 mg/dL (80.4 μmol/L)

Which of the following treatments is appropriate?
  A. Restrict free water intake to less than 1500 mL/24 h
  B. Administer 3% saline at a rate of 0.1 mL/kg per h
  C. Start demeclocycline
  D. Start conivaptan
  E. Start a furosemide intravenous drip

24 You are asked to see a 24-year-old man who was recently discharged from a rehabilitation hospital. He had been there for 3 months after falling from a roof. He had suffered extensive head injuries, including a basal skull fracture, and had been recovering from brain/cranial surgery. He seemed to be regaining his strength more slowly than expected. However, he was eating and drinking from a tray without assistance. Over the past week, he seemed to get weaker, and when he saw his primary care physician, laboratory testing showed the following:

Serum sodium = 129 mEq/L (129 mmol/L)

Serum urea nitrogen = 6 mg/dL (2.1 mmol/L)

Creatinine = 0.5 mg/dL (44.2 μmol/L)

Which of the following is the most likely cause of his hyponatremia?
  A. Hypopituitarism
  B. Syndrome of inappropriate antidiuretic hormone secretion
  C. Excessive diuretic use to prevent brain swelling
  D. Cerebral salt wasting
  E. Iatrogenic water intoxication

25 A 68-year-old man is found to have a 2.3-cm mass abutting the optic chiasm after his ophthalmologist identified a left eye visual field defect. MRI shows a relatively normal-sized sella with a large mass extending in a suprasellar fashion. In retrospect, he has had poor energy, frequent urination, increased thirst, and a 46-lb (20.9-kg) weight gain over the past 2 years. Testing reveals a prolactin concentration of 42.7 ng/mL (1.9 nmol/L) (similar on dilution), panhypopituitarism, and diabetes insipidus.

Which of the following is the most likely diagnosis?
   A. Gonadotroph adenoma
   B. Prolactinoma
   C. Craniopharyngioma
   D. Silent corticotroph adenoma
   E. Sarcoidosis

Diabetes Mellitus, Section 2 Board Review

Michelle F. Magee, MD • Georgetown University

31 A 49-year-old woman with type 2 diabetes mellitus presents to the emergency department with symptomatic hyperglycemia. Since starting insulin 2 months ago, she has been measuring blood glucose by fingerstick 4 times daily and calling her endocrinologist every 2 weeks for insulin dosage titration. Glucose readings have been in the range of 300 to 400 mg/dL (16.7 to 22.2 mmol/L). She is now taking 95 units of insulin glargine twice daily and 30 units of insulin aspart with each meal (total daily insulin dose = 288 units). Her BMI is 25 kg/m^2.

Laboratory test results:
Random blood glucose = 466 mg/dL
(25.9 mmol/L)
Hemoglobin A$_{1c}$ = >13% (>119 mmol/mol)
(upper limit of the device range)

She receives intravenous hydration and insulin aspart per emergency department protocol, and her blood glucose decreases to less than 240 mg/dL (<13.2 mmol/L) over 4 to 6 hours.

How should you advise the emergency department team to manage her uncontrolled type 2 diabetes?
A. Admit her to the hospital for management of uncontrolled hyperglycemia
B. Stop both insulin glargine and insulin aspart and begin U500 regular insulin
C. Ask her to show you how she self-administers insulin injections
D. Increase the doses of insulin glargine and insulin aspart by 20% each

32 An 82-year-old woman with a 32-year history of type 2 diabetes mellitus and hypertension is referred for glycemic management following an emergency department visit for severe hypoglycemia with an unconscious reaction.

Emergency medical technicians report that her initial blood glucose value was 27 mg/dL (1.5 mmol/L). Her current at-home diabetes treatment regimen consists of 25 units of insulin detemir at bedtime, 9 units of rapid-acting insulin with each meal, and correction doses for blood glucose values greater than 180 mg/dL (>10.0 mmol/L).

Since her insulin doses were last increased, her blood glucose measurements are as follows:

- Fasting values mostly in the upper 100s mg/dL (~5.6 mmol/L), with an occasional low value (68-75 mg/dL [3.8-4.2 mmol/L]) or high value (211-274 mg/dL [11.7-15.2 mmol/L])
- Prelunch and predinner values in the upper 100s mg/dL (~5.6 mmol/L), unless lunch is late when values are 90 mg/dL (5.0 mmol/L) to low 100s mg/dL (~5.6 mmol/L)
- Bedtime values of 150 mg/dL (8.3 mmol/L) to low 200s mg/dL (~11.1 mmol/L), except for an occasional reading in the range of 110-130 mg/dL (6.1-7.2 mmol/L)

She often does not record the insulin doses she has taken. She asks you to review how and when to take correction insulin doses.

On physical examination, her BMI is 19 kg/m^2 and blood pressure is 142/78 mm Hg. She has markedly reduced sensation in both feet. Her mood and affect are normal and her memory appears to be sharp.

Laboratory test results:
Hemoglobin A$_{1c}$ = 8.7% (72 mmol/mol)
(corresponds with an estimated average glucose value of 203 mg/dL [11.3 mmol/L])
Estimated glomerular filtration rate = 52 mL/min per 1.73 m^2
C-peptide = 3.6 ng/mL (1.2 nmol/L)

Which of the following would you recommend to reduce the risk for further episodes of severe hypoglycemia in this older woman?

    A. Refer to a diabetes educator to help her better understand how to take insulin

    B. Reduce basal insulin to 20 units and keep meal boluses at 9 units

    C. Change basal insulin to 20 units in the morning, stop the mealtime insulin, and start an oral agent

    D. Advise that she live with a family member or move to an assisted living situation

33 A 73-year-old woman has type 1 diabetes mellitus, which was diagnosed at age 15 years. She is referred to you for evaluation of erratic glycemic control. She takes multiple daily insulin injections. She eats consistent meals and takes her insulin as prescribed. She has no gastrointestinal bloating, nausea, or constipation. Her blood glucose values vary widely from 36 to 350 mg/dL (2.0 to 19.4 mmol/L). She senses that something is wrong when her blood glucose is low and treats most instances of hypoglycemia appropriately.

When she stands up to put on a gown, it looks as if she has a ball in her jacket pocket. Palpation reveals a firm mass that is the size of one-half of a tennis ball on her left upper abdomen (*see image, arrow*). She tells you that she has been injecting insulin into this site for many years and that she reuses her needles until they feel blunt.

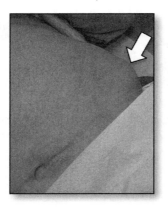

Which of the following is the most likely etiology of her erratic glycemic control?

    A. Gastrointestinal autonomic neuropathy

    B. Adrenal insufficiency

    C. Tight glycemic control

    D. Lipohypertrophy

34 A 35-year-old woman with an 18-year history of type 1 diabetes mellitus presents for a follow-up visit. She receives her insulin via continuous subcutaneous insulin infusion with an insulin pump. She has had consistently good glycemic control (hemoglobin A_{1c} 6.5%-7.0% [48-53 mmol/mol]) without evidence of microvascular complications. At a follow-up visit, she tells you that she has been having hypoglycemia and more erratic blood glucose measurements than usual, particularly when her pump is on the right side of her abdomen. She rotates pump insertion sites between the right and left sides of her abdomen.

When you examine her insertion sites, you notice an area on the right lower abdominal wall about 3 cm in diameter where the skin is slightly "indented" when you run your fingers across it. There is no associated erythema and the skin in the area otherwise looks normal.

Antiinsulin antibody (IAA) levels are high (49.6%; reference range, <8.5%).

Which of the following management strategies would you initially recommend?

    A. Rotate the pump insertion sites more widely

    B. Switch to a different insulin preparation

    C. Prescribe prednisone, 10 mg daily, for 2 weeks

    D. Switch to a different insertion set

35 A 52-year-old woman with type 2 diabetes mellitus is taking metformin and sitagliptin, and her hemoglobin A_{1c} level is 9.2% (77 mmol/mol). Her BMI is 36 kg/m². You suggest that she start taking a glucagonlike peptide 1 receptor agonist plus basal insulin combination injection.

She is reluctant to initiate a glucagonlike peptide 1 receptor agonist, as one of her friends experienced marked nausea and vomiting and had to stop taking the medication.

When you discuss risks and benefits of glucagonlike peptide 1 analogues as part of a shared decision-making process, which of the following injectable medications will you tell her had the lowest risk of nausea in clinical trials?

A. Liraglutide
B. Insulin degludec/liraglutide combination injectable
C. Lixisenatide
D. Insulin glargine/lixisenatide combination injectable

36 A 28-year-old woman with a 20-year history of type 1 diabetes mellitus is considering an isolated pancreas transplant. Her blood glucose values have been labile. Her hemoglobin A_{1c} level has ranged from 8% to 10% (64 to 86 mmol/mol), and she has hypoglycemic unawareness despite being on a sensor-augmented insulin pump. She has early nephropathy, proliferative retinopathy, gastroparesis, and peripheral neuropathy.

Laboratory test results:
Hemoglobin A_{1c} = 8.8% (73 mmol/mol)
Creatinine = 1.9 mg/dL (168 μmol/L)
Urinary albumin-to-creatinine ratio = 98 mg/g creat

Which of the following outcomes can this patient expect within 5 years after a successful pancreas transplant?

A. Regression of retinopathy
B. Recovery of peripheral sensation
C. Regression of gastroparesis
D. Reduced albuminuria

37 A 23-year-old woman was treated for gestational diabetes during a previous pregnancy and maintained her hemoglobin A_{1c} level less than 6.5% (<48 mmol/mol). After delivery, she did not have follow-up glycemic testing. Now, 10 months later, she has a positive pregnancy test 6 weeks after her last menstrual period. She has no symptoms of diabetes at this time. Her blood glucose value is 143 mg/dL (7.9 mmol/L) about 90 minutes after breakfast. You order further testing.

Laboratory test results:
Hemoglobin A_{1c} = 5.7% (39 mmol/mol)
2-Hour plasma glucose (75-g oral glucose tolerance test) = 210 mg/dL (11.7 mmol/L)

Which of the following is the best assessment of this woman's current glycemic status?

A. Gestational diabetes mellitus
B. Type 2 diabetes mellitus
C. Prediabetes
D. Indeterminate

38 A 29-year-old woman with type 2 diabetes mellitus is 8 weeks' pregnant. She is being treated with medical nutrition therapy and takes insulin levemir, 14 units in the morning, and insulin aspart, 4 units with each meal. She shows you her blood glucose log (fingerstick measurements) for the past 3 days following her visit with the diabetes educator.

Day	Before Breakfast	2 Hours After Breakfast	2 Hours After Lunch	2 Hours After Dinner	Comments
1	97 mg/dL (5.4 mmol/L)	119 mg/dL (6.6 mmol/L)	115 mg/dL (6.4 mmol/L)	145 mg/dL (8.0 mmol/L)	Pizza for dinner
2	101 mg/dL (5.6 mmol/L)	54 mg/dL (3.0 mmol/L)	153 mg/dL (8.5 mmol/L)	118 mg/dL (6.5 mmol/L)	Walk after breakfast
3	96 mg/dL (5.3 mmol/L)	93 mg/dL (5.2 mmol/L)	119 mg/dL (6.6 mmol/L)	95 mg/dL (5.3 mmol/L)	…

Which of the following recommendations would you make for adjusting her insulin dosages based on the blood glucose patterns over the last 3 days?

A. Reduce her prebreakfast insulin aspart to 3 units
B. Increase her basal insulin to 15 units in the morning
C. Increase her predinner insulin aspart to 5 units
D. Reduce her basal insulin to 13 units in the morning

39 A 56-year-old man with type 2 diabetes mellitus (hemoglobin A_{1c} of 10.6% [92 mmol/mol]) has been on a regimen of metformin and basal-bolus insulin consisting of 52 units of basal insulin split as 26 units with breakfast and at bedtime, plus 14 units of rapid-acting insulin analogue with each meal. He misses the bedtime dose of insulin at least 3 or 4 days a week, as he falls asleep not long after dinner. He is switched to a disposable patch pump insulin delivery device.

Which of the following is the most likely outcome of insulin delivery using this device?
   A. A 25% reduction in the total daily dose insulin requirement
   B. Reduction in hemoglobin A_{1c} of about 3% points
   C. Reduced incidence of hypoglycemia
   D. Significant increase in direct pharmacy costs

40 A 39-year-old man with a 19-year history of type 1 diabetes mellitus reports that his ophthalmologist recently informed him that he has signs of early nonproliferative diabetic retinopathy. He is concerned about progression and losing his sight and asks you what he can do to help prevent this complication.

In addressing his concern, you explain that the amount of vision loss due to diabetic retinopathy that can be prevented at this early stage with appropriate care is:
   A. Less than 10%
   B. 20%-30%
   C. 50%
   D. 75%
   E. More than 90%

41 A 52-year-old woman has had poorly controlled type 2 diabetes mellitus for 21 years. She has not seen an ophthalmologist for several years. She is experiencing decreased visual acuity. You perform funduscopic examination and note the findings shown (*see image*).

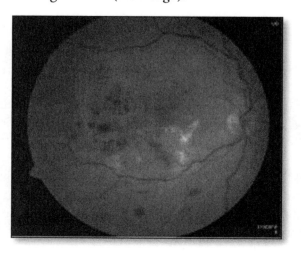

Which of the following should she undergo next?
   A. Ranibizumab injections
   B. Focal laser photocoagulation
   C. Stereo views of the retina
   D. Panretinal laser photocoagulation

42 At an annual dilated ophthalmologic examination, a 53-year-old woman with longstanding type 1 diabetes mellitus is told that she has new-onset macular edema.

Which of the following is the optimal treatment for her condition?
   A. Follow-up ophthalmologic examination in 6 months
   B. Focal laser therapy to the affected area now and again in 1 month
   C. Panretinal photocoagulation
   D. Intravitreal anti-VEGF (vascular endothelial growth factor) agent injections once each month for the first year

43 A 22-year-old man has a 5-year history of type 1 diabetes mellitus and is concerned about his risk for developing long-term complications, particularly nephropathy, because his father died of end-stage diabetic kidney disease. He is normotensive and has a hemoglobin A_{1c} level of 6.9% (52 mmol/mol), normal urine albumin excretion, no retinopathy, and a normal LDL-cholesterol level but a low HDL-cholesterol level.

Which of the following can you tell him with confidence?
   A. The development of microalbuminuria begins 15 to 20 years after the onset of diabetes and increases over time
   B. Microalbuminuria represents a stage of diabetic nephropathy during which treatment is often successful in preventing progression to macroalbuminuria
   C. ACE inhibitors and angiotensin-receptor blockers effectively prevent microalbuminuria in normotensive patients
   D. Low HDL cholesterol is associated with the development of microalbuminuria
   E. Risk for nephropathy is not associated with risk for retinopathy

44 A 54-year-old man who has had type 2 diabetes mellitus and hypertension for 19 years sees you for his annual diabetes examination. He is troubled by erectile dysfunction that has developed over the last 2 to 3 years. He has retinopathy and has had coronary artery bypass surgery. Medications include lisinopril, atorvastatin, metformin, insulin glargine, and metoprolol.

On physical examination, his BMI is 31.3 kg/m^2. Seated, his pulse rate is 92 beats/min and blood pressure is 140/92 mm Hg. Standing for 2 minutes, his pulse rate is 92 beats/min and blood pressure is 119/72 mm Hg. He has absent sensation to a 10-g monofilament to the mid-shin. Electrocardiography shows sinus rhythm, with a fixed R-R interval and evidence of a previous myocardial infarction.

Recent laboratory test results:
Hemoglobin A$_{1c}$ = 8.6% (70 mmol/mol)
Estimated glomerular filtration rate = 55 mL/min per 1.73 m^2
Testosterone = 220 ng/dL (7.6 nmol/L)

Which of the following is the best initial management of his erectile dysfunction?
  A. Refer to urology for penile prosthesis implantation
  B. Improve glycemic control
  C. Begin intracavernosal alprostadil injections
  D. Begin sildenafil

45 A 51-year-old woman with poorly controlled type 2 diabetes mellitus presents to the emergency department because she is worried she is having a stroke. She has noticed drooping on the left side of her face and some trouble speaking. There is some pain in the area. She has no other symptoms. She has a history of retinopathy and distal somatosensory neuropathy.

On physical examination, she has right facial droop with minimal tenderness in the affected area. There is no rash present. Her ear canal and tympanic membrane look normal. The rest of her neurologic examination findings are normal, except for reduced sensation in the lower extremities to the mid-shin.

Laboratory test results:
Hemoglobin A$_{1c}$ = 8.3% (67 mmol/mol)
Complete blood cell count and chemistries, normal

Head CT without contrast is negative for cerebrovascular accident.

Which of the following is the most likely cause of her facial palsy?
  A. Diabetic radiculopathy
  B. Diabetic autonomic neuropathy
  C. Herpes zoster
  D. Otitis media
  E. Stroke

46 A 68-year-old man with type 2 diabetes mellitus describes tingling in his hands and legs over the last 6 months. These sensations are different from his longstanding foot numbness. He also feels unsteady when he gets up at night to void. He eats a well-balanced diet. He has taken metformin since diabetes was diagnosed 11 years ago.

On physical examination, his blood pressure is 126/74 mm Hg and BMI is 28 kg/m^2. Cranial nerves II through XII are intact, muscle bulk and strength are normal, and coordination in the upper and lower extremities is normal. He has reduced sharp sensation to the knee, decreased vibratory sense in the great toes, and loss of patellar and Achilles reflexes.

Laboratory test results:
Hemoglobin A$_{1c}$ = 7.3% (56 mmol/mol)
Hematocrit = 35% (0.35)
Creatinine = 1.5 mg/dL (132.6 μmol/L)
Aspartate aminotransferase = 55 U/L (0.92 μkat/L)
Alanine aminotransferase = 72 U/L (1.20 μkat/L)

Which of the following is the best next step in this patient's management?
  A. Measure serum vitamin B$_{12}$
  B. Measure serum vitamin B$_6$
  C. Perform MRI of the spine
  D. Refer for electromyelography and nerve conduction studies

47 An 88-year-old man with type 2 diabetes mellitus, hypertension, dyslipidemia, chronic kidney disease, and coronary artery disease presents for follow-up. He cannot take metformin because of his chronic kidney disease. Although he has intentionally lost 6.6 lb (3 kg) in the past 6 months, his hemoglobin A_{1c} level has increased from 6.7% to 8.3% (50 to 67 mmol/mol). He occasionally has blurred vision and polyuria after a large meal. He has no shortness of breath but does report some ankle swelling at the end of the day.

Current medications include amlodipine, atenolol, aspirin, atorvastatin, isosorbide, furosemide, vitamins B_{12} and D_3, and allopurinol.

On physical examination, his weight is 189 lb (85.9 kg) and height is 65 in (165 cm) (BMI = 31.4 kg/m²). His blood pressure is 143/74 mm Hg, and pulse rate is 68 beats/min. Findings on cardiorespiratory examination are normal. His abdomen is rotund, pedal pulses are 1+, and there is no ankle edema.

Laboratory test results:
    Random glucose = 155 mg/dL (8.6 mmol/L)
    Creatinine = 2.2 mg/dL (194.5 μmol/L)
    Estimated glomerular filtration rate = 30 mL/min
        per 1.73 m²
    Urine protein = 2000 mg/dL
    LDL cholesterol = 53 mg/dL (1.37 mmol/L)
    Aspartate aminotransferase, normal
    Alanine aminotransferase, normal
    Hematocrit = 37% (0.37)

This patient is at high risk for congestive heart failure. You want to add an antihyperglycemic medication to his regimen. Which of the following is most likely to reduce his risk for hospitalization due to heart failure?
    A. Pioglitazone
    B. Saxagliptin
    C. Empagliflozin
    D. Insulin

48 A 63-year-old man with longstanding type 2 diabetes mellitus, nonproliferative diabetes-related retinopathy, hypertension, dyslipidemia, and chronic kidney disease presents for a follow-up visit. His last appointment was just over a year ago.

His medications include metformin, empagliflozin, basal insulin glargine, lisinopril, hydrochlorothiazide, baby aspirin, and simvastatin.

On physical examination, his blood pressure is 132/78 mm Hg, pulse rate is 84 beats/min, and BMI is 24 kg/m². He does not have ankle edema, and you note that he has reduced pedal pulses. He states that when he climbs more than 1 flight of stairs his legs feel "tired." There is no hair on his toes, and the toenails are thickened. His ankle brachial index is 1.4 (normal range, 0.91-1.30).

Laboratory test results:
    Estimated glomerular filtration rate = 53 mL/min
        per 1.73 m²
    LDL cholesterol = 63 mg/dL (1.63 mmol/L)
    HDL cholesterol = 32 mg/dL (0.83 mmol/L)
    Hemoglobin A_{1c} = 7.1% (54 mmol/mol)

Which of the following should be the next step to evaluate for the presence of peripheral arterial disease in this patient?
    A. Transcutaneous oxygen pressure in the foot
    B. Vascular segmental pressures and pulse volume recordings
    C. Systolic toe pressure
    D. Treadmill functional testing

49 A 72-year-old man with a 20-year history of type 2 diabetes mellitus comes to see you because he noticed some redness and skin breakdown on his right foot when he took off his shoes last night. His hemoglobin A_{1c} levels have always been greater than 8.5% (>69 mmol/mol), and he has peripheral neuropathy with insensate feet.

On physical examination, he is afebrile. There is a 1.2-cm ulcer under the right fifth metatarsal head with a depth of 2.4 mm that does not probe to bone. There is mild erythema and warmth of the skin proximal to the ulcer without distal extension, mild surrounding edema, and some serosanguinous discharge.

You arrange for him to be seen by a podiatrist and advise him to start taking antibiotic therapy today.

Which of the following antibiotic regimens should you prescribe?
   A. Clindamycin
   B. Doxycycline
   C. Trimethoprim-sulfamethoxazole
   D. Vancomycin plus ceftazidime

50 A 34-year-old man with type 1 diabetes mellitus is in the clinic waiting room. He seems confused when his name is called and is slurring his words. His fingerstick blood glucose value is 39 mg/dL (2.2 mmol/L). After being treated, he reports that despite using a continuous glucose sensor, he has been having episodes of hypoglycemia with blood glucose readings ranging from 40 to 50 mg/dL (2.2 to 2.8 mmol/L) in the past few months, without any warning symptoms. He has always aimed for tight glycemic control. His hemoglobin A_{1c} level is 5.9% (41 mmol/mol), and he takes multiple daily insulin injections.

Which of the following is the most important advice to give this patient?
   A. Begin a regimen of frequent small meals
   B. Temporarily relax tight glucose targets
   C. Switch to an insulin pump
   D. See the diabetes educator to review symptoms and treatment of hypoglycemia

51 A 29-year-old man with asthma is admitted to the intensive care unit with respiratory failure and bilateral pneumonia requiring endotracheal intubation. There is no history of diabetes mellitus. On admission, his random blood glucose concentration is 183 mg/dL (10.2 mmol/L). After treatment initiation with methylprednisolone, his blood glucose climbs to 302 mg/dL (16.8 mmol/L) and remains elevated over the next 4 hours.

Which of the following is the best approach to manage this patient's hyperglycemia?
   A. Intravenous U100 regular insulin infusion titrated to achieve blood glucose between 140 and 180 mg/dL (7.8-10.0 mmol/L)
   B. Subcutaneous U100 regular insulin every 8 hours, adjusted to maintain blood glucose between 140 and 180 mg/dL (7.8-10.0 mmol/L)
   C. Intravenous U100 regular insulin infusion titrated to achieve blood glucose between 80 and 110 mg/dL (4.4-6.1 mmol/L)
   D. Subcutaneous insulin glargine daily plus insulin aspart every 6 hours, adjusted to a target blood glucose between 140 and 180 mg/dL (7.8-10.0 mmol/L)

52 A 59-year-old man with type 1 diabetes mellitus diagnosed at age 13 years and ischemic cardiomyopathy is hospitalized with an exacerbation of heart failure. He has been on continuous intravenous insulin therapy in the intensive care unit and is now to be transferred to the medical-surgical ward. His estimated total daily dose of insulin is 72 units daily (extrapolated from the drip rate of 3 units per hour in the 6 hours before discontinuation when the rate had stabilized).

Before the intravenous insulin drip is discontinued, which of the following should you order?
   A. Insulin glargine, 29 units twice daily, plus insulin lispro per correction scale before meals if blood glucose is >180 mg/dL (>10.0 mmol/L)
   B. Insulin glargine, 58 units at night, and regular insulin per supplemental scale every 6 hours if blood glucose is >180 mg/dL (>10.0 mmol/L)
   C. Insulin glargine, 29 units at night, plus insulin lispro, 10 units before meals, and a correction dose if blood glucose is >180 mg/dL (>10.0 mmol/L)
   D. Insulin glargine, 58 units in the morning, and insulin lispro, 5 units before meals, and a correction dose if blood glucose is >180 mg/dL (>10.0 mmol/L)

53 A 52-year-old woman with type 2 diabetes mellitus treated at home with metformin and a glucagonlike peptide 1 receptor agonist is currently on postoperative day 1 after a surgical procedure. Before surgery, her blood glucose values ranged from 150 to 180 mg/dL (8.3-10.0 mmol/L) and now they are ranging from 170 to 250 mg/dL (9.4-13.9 mmol/L).

On physical examination, her vital signs are unremarkable. She is nauseated and has been unable to eat meals. She remains on nothing-by-mouth status in the surgical ward.

Which of the following is the best insulin management regimen for this patient?
- A. Once-daily basal insulin, plus correction insulin dose regimen every 4 to 6 hours
- B. Once-daily basal insulin, plus correction insulin dose regimen every 8 to 10 hours
- C. Sliding-scale insulin regimen administered every 4 to 6 hours
- D. A continuous intravenous insulin infusion

54 You are consulted to provide insulin management recommendations for a 53-year-old man who has had type 2 diabetes for 11 years, managed most recently on a regimen of basal insulin plus a glucagonlike peptide 1 receptor agonist. He was involved in a motor vehicle crash and sustained multiple injuries. He has been in the intensive care unit for 6 days and is now to be transferred to a surgical unit. In the intensive care unit, he was managed with an insulin drip and his rate over the last 24 hours has been stable at 1 unit/h (total daily dose 24 units). He is on nothing-by-mouth status. It is anticipated that while he will make a full recovery, it will be at least a few weeks until he can take nutrition by mouth. Continuous enteral nutrition will be initiated. His weight is 193 lb (88 kg), and his BMI is 28 kg/m^2.

Which of the following insulin regimens should be prescribed for glycemic management during continuous enteral tube feeding?
- A. NPH U100 insulin, 8 units at 2300 plus rapid-acting insulin every 4 hours
- B. Insulin glargine U100, 8 units twice daily plus regular insulin every 6 hours
- C. Regular U100 insulin every 4 hours
- D. Insulin glargine U300, 22 units once daily plus rapid-acting insulin every 4 hours

55 You see a 23-year-old man who has had type 1 diabetes mellitus since age 5 years during a hospitalization for diabetic ketoacidosis. He also has bipolar disorder that is well controlled when he takes his medications. He is homeless. Most days, he eats 2 meals at a food kitchen. He has had 4 other hospital admissions for diabetic ketoacidosis this year. His current insulin regimen consists of insulin detemir, 15 units once daily, and insulin glulisine with meals. He keeps his insulins at a shelter where he spends most nights.

Which of the following changes would you recommend in his insulin delivery regimen to help prevent further episodes of diabetic ketoacidosis?
- A. Hybrid closed-loop continuous subcutaneous insulin infusion pump with sensor system
- B. U200 basal insulin degludec once daily plus mealtime insulin
- C. Insulin patch pump system
- D. U500 regular insulin twice daily

56 A 42-year-old woman with a 33-year history of type 1 diabetes mellitus presents for routine follow-up. She has nonproliferative retinopathy. She takes lisinopril, 5 mg daily, for proteinuria. She has been feeling fatigued.

Her insulin regimen includes insulin detemir twice daily and premeal insulin glulisine. She has recently experienced frequent episodes of hypoglycemia that are sometimes, but not always, related to skipped meals. Sometimes she awakens with low blood glucose levels. Over the past few months she has adjusted her basal insulin dose down in 10% increments several times but is still having frequent episodes of hypoglycemia. She has not had much change from her usual lifestyle regimen during this period. She also finds that she gets a bit lightheaded when she stands up rapidly.

On physical examination, her blood pressure is 124/74 mm Hg and pulse rate is 84 beats/min when supine, and her blood pressure is 91/68 mm Hg and pulse rate is 106 beats/min when standing. Her weight is 139 lb (63.2 kg) (BMI = 22 kg/m^2). Findings on heart and lung examinations are unremarkable. Neurologic examination reveals intact sensation to 10-g monofilament on the plantar foot surfaces and delayed ankle reflex recovery.

Pertinent nonfasting laboratory test results:

Serum sodium = 137 mg/dL (137 mmol/L)

Potassium = 4.7 mEq/L (4.7 mmol/L)

Creatinine = 0.9 mg/dL (79.6 μmol/L)

Urinary albumin-to-creatinine ratio = 35 μg/mg

TSH = 8.2 mIU/L

Hemoglobin A_{1c} = 7.8% (62 mmol/mol)

Which of the following is the most likely cause of her orthostatic hypotension?

    A. Adrenal insufficiency

    B. Cardiovascular autonomic neuropathy

    C. Hypothyroidism

    D. Sensorimotor neuropathy

    E. Salt-wasting nephropathy

57 A 43-year-old woman presents for evaluation of an episode of severe hypoglycemia with confusion. She underwent Roux-en-Y gastric bypass surgery several months ago for treatment of morbid obesity complicated by hypertension and type 2 diabetes. Since having surgery and establishing her postoperative meal regimen, she notes that she feels a bit shaky after she eats.

Which of the following is the most likely etiology of her hypoglycemia?

    A. Nesidioblastosis

    B. Increased insulin secretion

    C. Dumping syndrome

    D. Increased insulin sensitivity

58 A 57-year-old woman with morbid obesity and type 2 diabetes mellitus is considering gastric bypass surgery. She has had diabetes for 3 years and is currently treated with metformin and a glucagonlike peptide 1 receptor agonist. Her hemoglobin A_{1c} level is 9.2% (77 mmol/mol) and she has been resistant to starting an injectable medication. She has heard that gastric bypass surgery can result in diabetes remission. She is wondering whether her diabetes is likely to go into remission after the operation.

What will you tell this patient is the best predictor of achieving a hemoglobin A_{1c} level less than 6.0% (<42 mmol/mol) after surgery?

    A. Baseline BMI greater than 32 kg/m^2

    B. Duration of diabetes less than 8 years

    C. Baseline quality of life

    D. Weight loss 2 years after surgery

59 A 55-year-old woman with a history of hypertension and gout presents with a painful swollen lower extremity, and deep venous thrombosis is diagnosed. She is fatigued, has lost 33 lb (15 kg), and has polydipsia and polyuria. Her blood glucose concentration is 253 mg/dL (14.0 mmol/L), and new-onset diabetes mellitus is diagnosed.

On physical examination, she is a thin elderly woman with a swollen, tender right calf and a rash scattered across her feet and ankles (*see image*).

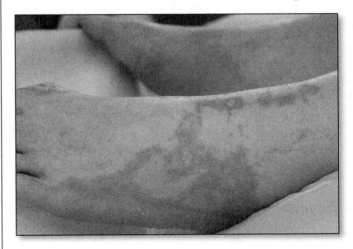

Which of the following is the most likely etiology of her diabetes?

    A. Acromegaly

    B. Rabson-Mendenhall syndrome

    C. Glucagonoma syndrome

    D. Cushing disease

Female Reproduction Board Review

Margaret E. Wierman, MD ● University of Colorado

1 An 18-year-old woman presents with failure to undergo puberty. Her family history is notable for delayed puberty in her mother and maternal aunt who required fertility medications for pregnancy. She has always been thin. She cannot smell coffee.

On physical examination, her height is 65 in (165.1 cm), weight is 142 lb (64.5 kg) (BMI = 23.6 kg/m²), and she has Tanner stage 3 pubic hair. Breast development is Tanner stage 2. Findings on pelvic examination show a small uterus and decreased estrogen effect on the vaginal mucosa.

Laboratory test results:
LH = 2.0 mIU/mL (2.0 IU/L)
FSH = 3.0 mIU/mL (3.0 IU/L)
Prolactin = 15 ng/mL (0.65 nmol/L)
Estradiol = <20 pg/mL (<73.4 pmol/L)

MRI of the pituitary is normal.

A mutation in which of the following genes is the most likely cause of her absent pubertal development?
   A. *KISS1R (GPR54)*
   B. *KAL1*
   C. *NR0B1 (DAX1)*
   D. *FGFR1*
   E. *LEPR*

2 A 17-year-old woman presents with primary amenorrhea. She never had much axillary or pubic hair, but she had normal breast development at age 10 years. She is otherwise healthy, and there is no family history of reproductive disorders. She is on the track team in high school and runs 25 miles weekly.

On physical examination, her BMI is 25 kg/m², height is 69 in (175 cm), and blood pressure is 120/80 mm Hg. She has sparse axillary and pubic hair but normal Tanner stage 5 breast development. Her pelvic examination reveals a blind vaginal vault.

Laboratory test results:
FSH = 7.0 mIU/mL (7.0 IU/L)
LH = 18.0 mIU/mL (18.0 IU/L)

Which of the following is the most likely diagnosis for her pubertal disorder?
   A. Fragile X syndrome
   B. Gonadal dysgenesis
   C. Androgen insensitivity
   D. 5α-Reductase deficiency

3 A 22-year-old Italian woman presents with hyperandrogenic anovulation (hirsutism and irregular menses). She had early development of pubic hair at age 7 years. Menarche was at age 11 years. Her cycles have always been irregular.

On physical examination, her BMI is 25 kg/m². She has hair on her chin, upper lip, and neck; 8 hairs on her areolae; and hair to her umbilicus. She has no clitoromegaly.

Laboratory test results on day 5 of an induced menstrual cycle after medroxyprogesterone withdrawal (5 mg daily for 7 days):
LH = 5.0 mIU/mL (5.0 IU/L)
FSH = 4.0 mIU/mL (4.0 IU/L)
Estradiol = 40 pg/mL (146.8 pmol/L)
Testosterone = 50 ng/dL (1.74 nmol/L)
DHEA-S = 280 µg/dL (7.6 µmol/L)
ACTH = 45 pg/mL (9.9 pmol/L)
Cortisol = 12 µg/dL (331.1 nmol/L)
17-Hydroxyprogesterone = 290 ng/dL (8.8 nmol/L) (reference range, <285 ng/dL [<8.64 nmol/L] in luteal phase and <80 ng/dL [<2.42 nmol/L] in follicular phase)
Prolactin = 18 ng/mL (0.78 nmol/L)

Which of the following diagnoses best explains this patient's clinical presentation?
   A. Polycystic ovary syndrome
   B. Virilizing adrenal tumor
   C. Adrenal Cushing syndrome
   D. Nonclassic congenital adrenal hyperplasia
   E. Sertoli-Leydig–cell tumor of the ovary

4 A 24-year-old woman with Turner syndrome (gonadal dysgenesis) is planning a pregnancy. She will be using a donor egg from her sister and in vitro fertilization. Her height is 59 in (149.9 cm), BMI is 29 kg/m², and blood pressure is 130/80 mm Hg. She is healthy and takes no medications other than oral contraceptives.

Which of the following is the most important pre-pregnancy screening test for this patient?
   A. Brain MRI
   B. Renal ultrasonography
   C. Cardiac MRI
   D. Exercise stress test

5 A 22-year-old woman with polycystic ovary syndrome presents to discuss her contraceptive options. Her menarche was at age 11 years, and her menses have always been irregular. She had onset of hirsutism and acne at age 12 years and both have progressed since adolescence. She is currently using barrier contraceptives and taking spironolactone, 100 mg daily, and metformin, 1000 mg twice daily before meals. Her weight increased during college, and her BMI is now 32 kg/m². Her blood pressure is 130/70 mm Hg. She is concerned about potential risks vs benefits of different contraceptive options in addition to her current therapy.

Which of the following contraceptive methods would be best for this patient?
   A. Oral contraceptive containing norethindrone
   B. Levonorgestrel-releasing intrauterine device
   C. Oral contraceptive containing drospirenone
   D. Depo-medroxyprogesterone
   E. Vaginal ring

6 A 28-year-old woman presents to your office with concerns of hirsutism and male-pattern balding. She had normal menarche at age 12 years and regular menses with 2 uncomplicated pregnancies. Her periods stopped 1 year ago, and she has noticed increased facial hair in a beard-like distribution over the past 18 months, some male-pattern balding, and increased hair on her breasts.

On physical examination, her BMI is 27 kg/m² and blood pressure is 150/90 mm Hg. She is very muscular. She has terminal hairs on her chin in a full-beard distribution, 15 hairs on her areolae, and hair above and below the umbilicus. Her clitoris measures 2.8 × 1.7 cm.

Laboratory test results:
   LDL cholesterol = 151 mg/dL (3.91 mmol/L)
   Testosterone = 350 ng/dL (12.1 nmol/L)
   DHEA-S = 120 µg/dL (3.3 µmol/L) (reference range, 15-200 µg/dL [0.41-5.42 µmol/L])
   Prolactin = 15 ng/mL (0.65 nmol/L)
   FSH = 4.9 mIU/mL (4.9 IU/L)
   LH = 3.8 mIU/mL (3.8 IU/L)
   Hemoglobin A_{1c} = 5.9% (41 mmol/mol)

Which of the following is the most likely diagnosis?
   A. Granulosa-cell ovarian tumor
   B. Exposure to exogenous androgens
   C. Adrenal virilizing tumor
   D. Sertoli-Leydig–cell tumor of the ovary

7 A 20-year-old woman presents to discuss treatment options for hirsutism. She had menarche at age 10 years and has always had irregular menses. Acne and abnormal hair growth began at puberty. Her BMI is 27 kg/m². Excess hair is observed on her upper lip, chin, and neck. No hair is present on her upper chest, upper back, or upper abdomen. She has no temporal recession of her hairline but does have alopecia on the crown of her head.

Laboratory test results:
   Testosterone = 75 ng/dL (2.6 nmol/L)
   DHEA-S = 330 µg/dL (8.9 µmol/L)

Which of the following is the best treatment option for improving hirsutism in this patient?
   A. Spironolactone and ethinyl estradiol, 30 mcg, with norethindrone, 0.5 mg
   B. Flutamide and ethinyl estradiol, 20 mcg, with levonorgestrel, 1 mg
   C. Ethinyl estradiol, 20 mcg, with levonorgestrel, 1 mg
   D. Topical antiandrogen and ethinyl estradiol, 30 mcg, with norethindrone, 1 mg

8 A 32-year-old woman with a history of irregular periods, acne, hirsutism, and progressive weight gain was diagnosed with polycystic ovary syndrome at age 16 years. She was prescribed a levonorgestrel intrauterine device for contraception and spironolactone for hirsutism. She has had progressive weight gain with a current BMI of 33 kg/m². Her blood pressure is 130/80 mm Hg. A urine pregnancy test is negative. She began metformin 6 months ago, and her periods have been more regular for the last 3 months.

Which of the following treatments would most effectively induce ovulation and result in a live birth?
   A. Clomiphene citrate
   B. Letrozole
   C. Spironolactone
   D. Metformin
   E. Progesterone suppositories

9 A 32-year-old woman with polycystic ovary syndrome presents to your office to discuss the health risks associated with her diagnosis. She had early menarche at age 11 years, hirsutism and acne since age 13 years, and weight gain from 120 lb (54.5 kg) to 190 lb (86.4 kg) in her 20s. She has a family history of hypertension and type 2 diabetes mellitus. She has been trying to lose weight on a low-carbohydrate diet, and she started an exercise program to improve her chance for fertility.

For which of the following is she at increased risk?
   A. Obstructive sleep apnea
   B. Stroke
   C. Myocardial infarction
   D. Autoimmune thyroid disease

10 A 26-year-old woman presents to discuss contraceptive options 4 weeks postpartum. Her menarche was at age 12 years, and her periods were regular until her recent pregnancy. Her BMI is 30 kg/m². She has familial hirsutism and intermittent acne. She is planning to breastfeed until her infant is 9 months old.

Which of the following is the best contraceptive option for this patient?
   A. Oral contraceptive containing progestin only
   B. Levonorgestrel-containing intrauterine device
   C. Oral contraceptive containing ethinyl estradiol, 20 mcg, and levonorgestrel, 1 mg
   D. Transdermal patch containing ethinyl estradiol and levonorgestrel

11 A 19-year-old woman calls the overnight on-call physician line with a request for emergency contraception. She has a history of normal puberty and regular menses. Her BMI is 32 kg/m². Her last menstrual period was 17 days ago.

Which of the following is the best option for effective emergency contraception in this patient?
   A. Levonorgestrel, 3.0 mg
   B. Ulipristal acetate (UPA), 10 mg
   C. Ethinyl estradiol, 50 mcg, and levonorgestrel, 0.5 mg
   D. Medroxyprogesterone, 10 mg

12 A 27-year-old woman presents with amenorrhea. Her menarche was at age 14 years. She has never been bothered by acne or excessive hair growth. Her periods were irregular for 18 months after menarche, then regular every 28 days. She was on oral contraceptives from age 16 years until age 25 when she stopped in an attempt to conceive. She had a miscarriage 6 months ago when she was 10 weeks pregnant, which required a dilatation and curettage. Since that time she has had no menstrual bleeding. She runs 2 miles 3 times a week. Her BMI is 20 kg/m².

Which of the following patterns of hormone levels would you expect in this patient?

Answer	FSH	LH	Estradiol	Response to Progestin Withdrawal
A.	Low	Low	Low	No response
B.	High	High	Low	No response
C.	Normal	Normal	Normal	No response
D.	Normal	Normal	Normal	Normal response
E.	Normal	High	Normal	Normal response

13 A 28-year-old woman presents with amenorrhea. She had delayed menarche at age 15 years and had no periods during college. She took an oral contraceptive pill from age 22 to 27 years. She has Hashimoto thyroiditis and takes a stable dosage of levothyroxine. After stopping the oral contraceptive, she had 1 period and then amenorrhea. She exercises 3 times per week for 1.5 hours each session. Her BMI is 20 kg/m². Her gynecologist had ordered timed labs after administering a progestin withdrawal (medroxyprogesterone, 5 mg daily for 7 days).

Blood samples were drawn on day 3 after onset of menstrual bleeding:
FSH = 10 mIU/mL (10 IU/L) (high-normal)
Estradiol = 28 pg/mL (102.8 pmol/L)
Antimullerian hormone = 1.2 ng/mL (8.6 pmol/L)
   (reference range, 1.0-4.0 ng/mL
   [7.1-28.6 pmol/L])
TSH = 2.1 mIU/L

Which of the following is the most likely diagnosis?
A. Polycystic ovary syndrome
B. Autoimmune adrenal insufficiency
C. Hypothalamic amenorrhea (functional amenorrhea)
D. Premature ovarian insufficiency

14 A 28-year-old woman presents to discuss options to treat severe premenstrual dysphoria. Menarche was at age 12 years, and she has regular menses every 28 days. She has always had cramping with menses. Since her mid 20s, and she feels that her mood is much worse the week before her menses, which is consistent with premenstrual syndrome. Recently, she has been unable to work 1 to 2 days per month because of her anxiety and cognitive dysfunction during this time. She recently moved and has a stressful job. She tries to exercise 3 times weekly. Her family history is notable for hypertension, diabetes mellitus, and depression.

On physical examination, her BMI is 28 kg/m², and the rest of the findings are normal.

Which of the following is the best option for treating her premenstrual syndrome?
A. Refer her to a therapist
B. Prescribe a serotonin reuptake inhibitor
C. Prescribe an intermittent serotonin reuptake inhibitor 2 weeks each month before menses
D. Prescribe an antidepressant such as amitriptyline
E. Prescribe a continuous oral contraceptive

15 A 28-year-old female veteran is referred for hormonal treatment of gender dysphoria. The patient recalls always being a tomboy, with a preference for masculine attire and playing with boys. The patient has persistent fantasies of being a man, has cross-dressed full time for 6 months, and believes she was born the wrong sex and wants testosterone therapy. After returning from Afghanistan, she was treated for posttraumatic stress disorder. A mental health provider has evaluated the patient and confirmed the diagnosis of gender dysphoria and verified that there are no active psychiatric issues. She is being treated with depotestosterone, 200 mg intramuscularly every 2 weeks.

While achieving this patient's goals for transition to a male phenotype, which of the following is a risk of the current therapy regimen?
A. Myocardial infarction
B. Diabetes mellitus
C. Breast cancer
D. Colon cancer
E. Weight gain

16 A 44-year-old woman (G3, P2, Ab1) returns to your office to discuss hormonal contraception. She had normal onset of menarche and has always had regular menses. She had 3 uncomplicated pregnancies. She does not smoke cigarettes. She notes heavier periods, and she was recently found to be anemic with a hematocrit level of 32% (0.32). You prescribe iron supplementation. She wonders about the best contraceptive option.

Which of the following methods of contraception would be best for this patient?
- A. Cyclic medroxyprogesterone, 10 days/month
- B. Oral contraceptive with ethinyl estradiol, 50 mcg, with levonorgestrel
- C. Nonhormonal intrauterine device
- D. Diaphragm
- E. Levonorgestrel-releasing intrauterine device

17 A 32-year-old woman presents with a 6-month history of amenorrhea. She has been in excellent health except for a history of type 1 diabetes diagnosed at age 28 years. Her glycemic control has been good, with a hemoglobin A_{1c} value of 7.0% (53 mmol/mol).

Recently, she has noticed dyspareunia, vaginal dryness, and night sweats. Both her mother and maternal aunt had early menopause at age 39 years and age 40 years, respectively. The patient has a 19-year-old brother with a learning disability and cognitive impairment. Her examination findings are normal other than an atrophic vaginal lining.

Laboratory test results:
FSH = 90 mIU/mL (90 IU/L) (reference range, 2.0-12.0 mIU/mL [2.0-12.0 IU/L])
Estradiol = <20 pg/mL (<73.4 pmol/L) (reference range, 22-56 pg/mL [80.8-206.6 pmol/L])
TSH = 3.0 mIU/L
Prolactin = 7 ng/mL (0.30 nmol/L)

Which of the following is the most appropriate next test?
- A. Karyotype analysis
- B. *FMR1* genetic testing
- C. 21-Hydroxylase antibody measurement
- D. TPO antibody measurement
- E. Antimullerian hormone measurement

18 A 51-year-old healthy woman presents with hot flashes, painful intercourse, and insomnia. Her physical examination findings are normal. She wishes to discuss the benefits and risks of menopausal hormone therapy.

Which of the following would be the most common increased risk for this woman if she were prescribed postmenopausal combined estrogen-progestin hormone therapy for 5 years?
- A. Colon cancer
- B. Gallbladder disease
- C. Stroke
- D. Breast cancer
- E. Dementia

19 A 51-year-old woman presents to discuss the pros and cons of hormone therapy in menopause. She had menarche at age 10 years and has always had regular menses. Her last menses was 6 months ago. She never had any children. She is active and works out 3 times a week with aerobic exercise and running. Her family history is notable for osteoporosis and cardiovascular disease. She is having hot flashes 1 to 5 times a day and painful intercourse. Her BMI is 26 kg/m², blood pressure is 110/70 mm Hg, and pulse rate is 68 beats/min.

Laboratory test results:
Total cholesterol = 180 mg/dL (4.66 mmol/L)
LDL cholesterol = 110 mg/dL (2.85 mmol/L)
Hemoglobin A_{1c} = 5.4% (36 mmol/mol)

As you further interview this patient about her personal medical history and family history, which of the following is the most important consideration in discussing the risks of postmenopausal hormone therapy?
- A. Family history of Parkinson disease
- B. Family history of postmenopausal breast cancer
- C. The timing of her first menses, pregnancies, and last menses
- D. History of autoimmune thyroid disease
- E. History of kidney stones

20 A 50-year-old woman presents with worsening hirsutism since menopause 2 years earlier. Her menarche was at age 12 years, and she had regular menses. She had 2 uncomplicated pregnancies. She has gained weight over the years and her BMI is now 32 kg/m². She has noticed increasing hair growth since menopause.

On physical examination, she has increased terminal hair in a beard distribution, hair on her upper chest and upper back, and male-pattern balding.

Laboratory test results:

LH = 32.0 mIU/mL (32.0 IU/L)

FSH = 34.0 mIU/mL (34.0 IU/L)

Testosterone = 180 ng/dL (6.2 nmol/L)

DHEA-S = 280 µg/mL (7.6 µmol/L)

Which of the following is the most likely diagnosis?
   A. Adrenal virilizing tumor
   B. Hyperthecosis ovarii
   C. Granulosa tumor of the ovary
   D. Obesity-induced hyperandrogenism
   E. Sertoli-Leydig–cell tumor of the ovary

21 A 41-year-old healthy woman presents with severe hot flashes and insomnia. She had normal menarche and had regular menses until age 40 years, when she noted some irregularity. Leiomyomata were diagnosed, which required total abdominal hysterectomy and bilateral salpingo-oophorectomy. Since her surgery, she has had intractable hot flashes, trouble sleeping, cognitive issues, and urinary frequency. Her grandmother had breast cancer at age 78 years, her father has hypertension and hyperlipidemia, and her mother has osteoporosis. Her physical examination findings are normal. She runs 3 times a week, has a BMI of 28 kg/m^2, and maintains a healthful diet and lifestyle. You are considering the pros and cons of initiating estrogen-only therapy.

According to findings from the Women's Health Initiative, for which of the following is this patient at increased risk with estrogen-only therapy?
   A. Ovarian cancer
   B. Breast cancer
   C. Deep venous thrombosis
   D. Myocardial infarction
   E. Colon cancer

Male Reproduction Board Review

Frances J. Hayes, MD ● Massachusetts General Hospital

1 A 33-year-old man presents for evaluation of secondary infertility. His wife is 32 years old and they have 2 children. They have been having regular unprotected intercourse for the past year without success. He has a history of a hypophysectomy for a nonsecreting pituitary macroadenoma 5 years earlier, following which he developed secondary hypogonadism. He is currently being treated with a testosterone gel. While on this treatment, he has normal libido and erections.

On physical examination, his BMI is 23 kg/m². He has normal secondary sexual characteristics and a testicular volume of 20 mL bilaterally.

Evaluation after discontinuing testosterone therapy:
Testosterone = 52 ng/dL (1.8 nmol/L)
LH = 1.0 mIU/mL (1.0 IU/L)
FSH = 1.8 mIU/mL (1.8 IU/L)

Semen analyses show normal semen volume with sperm counts of less than 1 million/mL.

Which of the following is the best initial treatment option to induce fertility in this patient?
  A. Intracytoplasmic sperm injection
  B. hCG injections
  C. Pulsatile GnRH therapy
  D. hCG and FSH injections

2 A 35-year-old man is referred to you for evaluation 6 months after his urologist initiated testosterone therapy following bilateral orchidectomy for testicular cancer. He is being treated with intramuscular injections of testosterone enanthate, 300 mg every 3 weeks. He has recovered well from his surgery but reports feeling tired and moody for a few days before each injection.

On physical examination, his vital signs are normal. He has bilateral testicular implants.

A testosterone measurement midway between injections is 750 ng/dL (26.0 nmol/L).

Which of the following is the best next step in this patient's management?
  A. Recommend an antidepressant and continue the same testosterone regimen
  B. Switch to testosterone cypionate at the current dosage
  C. Change the current regimen to 200 mg every 2 weeks
  D. Change the current regimen to 400 mg every 4 weeks

3 A 35-year-old man presents with loss of libido and difficulty getting and sustaining erections. He developed bloody diarrhea 6 months ago and severe ulcerative colitis was diagnosed. His condition did not respond to sulfasalazine and his regimen was switched to prednisone, 60 mg daily. His symptoms improved, allowing a gradual prednisone dosage reduction to 10 mg daily.

On physical examination, his BMI is 30 kg/m². He has cushingoid facies and several ecchymoses on his arms. His testes are 15 mL bilaterally.

Morning testosterone measurements on 2 occasions are 150 ng/dL (5.2 nmol/L) and 180 ng/dL (6.2 nmol/L).

Which of the following hormone profiles is most likely to characterize this patient's hypogonadism?

Answer	LH	FSH	Sex Hormone–Binding Globulin
A.	2.3 mIU/mL (2.3 IU/L)	5.0 mIU/mL (5.0 IU/L)	1.25 μg/mL (12 nmol/L)
B.	2.3 mIU/mL (2.3 IU/L)	5.0 mIU/mL (5.0 IU/L)	7.87 μg/mL (70 nmol/L)
C.	18.1 mIU/mL (18.1 IU/L)	12.3 mIU/mL (12.3 IU/L)	1.25 μg/mL (12 nmol/L)
D.	18.1 mIU/mL (18.1 IU/L)	12.3 mIU/mL (12.3 IU/L)	7.87 μg/mL (70 nmol/L)

4 A 19-year-old man presents for evaluation of painless breast enlargement, which has been present since puberty. He reports having decreased libido but normal erections. He has relatively sparse body hair and shaves 1 to 2 times weekly. He reports no history of testicular pain, swelling, or trauma. He drinks 4 to 6 beers each weekend.

On physical examination, his height is 72 in (183 cm), arm span is 71 in (180 cm), and BMI is 23 kg/m². His blood pressure is 110/70 mm Hg. He has sparse facial hair, normal axillary hair, and Tanner stage 5 pubic hair. There is 4-cm bilateral gynecomastia with no galactorrhea. He has a normal phallus with no hypospadias. His testes are small and firm, measuring 6 mL bilaterally.

Laboratory test results:
Total testosterone = 220 ng/dL (7.6 nmol/L) (reference range, 240-950 ng/dL [8.3-33.0 nmol/L])
FSH = 46.0 mIU/mL (46.0 IU/L) (reference range, 1.0-13.0 mIU/mL [1.0-13.0 IU/L])
LH = 25.0 mIU/mL (25.0 IU/L) (reference range, 1.0-9.0 mIU/mL [1.0-9.0 IU/L])

Which of the following is the most likely cause of this patient's presentation?
A. Inactivating mutation in the gene encoding the FSH receptor
B. Klinefelter syndrome
C. Congenital adrenal hyperplasia due to 17α-hydroxylase deficiency
D. Mumps orchitis

5 A 25-year-old man is referred by his oncologist to discuss options for fertility preservation after a recent diagnosis of Hodgkin lymphoma, which will require treatment with alkylating agents. The patient is currently single but would like to have children in the future. On physical examination, his testes are 25 mL in volume. A semen analysis shows a sperm concentration of 11 million/mL.

Which of the following is the most reliable option for fertility preservation in this patient?
A. Combination of testosterone and progestin to suppress spermatogenesis during chemotherapy
B. Treatment with a GnRH agonist to suppress spermatogenesis during chemotherapy
C. Cryopreservation of spermatogonial stem cells before chemotherapy for future transplantation
D. Sperm cryopreservation before chemotherapy

6 An 18-year-old man is referred for evaluation of bilateral breast enlargement, which has been present for 3 years and has now stabilized. He initially experienced increased sensitivity when jogging, but no longer has any breast tenderness. However, he is very embarrassed by the cosmetic appearance and has given up swimming. He has no nipple discharge. He takes no medication or herbal products and does not use illicit drugs.

On physical examination, the patient is well developed and has facial acne. Palpation of the breasts reveals rubbery, mobile subareolar tissues (3 cm on the left and 3.5 cm on the right). There is no nipple discharge, discoloration, or retraction. Findings on genital examination are age appropriate, with a normal phallus, testes of 15 mL bilaterally, and Tanner stage 5 pubic hair.

Hormonal workup documents normal testosterone, estradiol, LH, FSH, and TSH, and β-hCG is negative.

Which of the following is the best next step in this patient's care?
A. Mammography
B. Reassurance and observation
C. Referral for surgical consultation
D. Aromatase inhibitor therapy

7 A 70-year-old African American man is referred by his primary care physician to discuss testosterone replacement therapy. During workup for decreased libido and erectile dysfunction, hypogonadism was diagnosed and he is eager to start therapy. He has no lower urinary tract symptoms. He has a history of obstructive sleep apnea for which he uses continuous positive airway pressure on a consistent basis and reports no daytime somnolence. He had a myocardial infarction 10 years earlier and is taking an extended-release formulation of isosorbide mononitrate on which he has no angina.

On physical examination, his BMI is 32 kg/m^2 and blood pressure is 125/80 mm Hg. He is well virilized and has normal testes. His prostate feels slightly enlarged but no nodules are palpable.

Laboratory test results:
Testosterone (8 AM) = 170 ng/dL (5.9 nmol/L); 195 ng/dL (6.8 nmol/L) when repeated
LH = 6.9 mIU/mL (6.9 IU/L)
FSH = 9.0 mIU/mL (9.0 IU/L)
Prolactin = 11 ng/mL (0.5 nmol/L)
Transferrin saturation = 30%
Hematocrit = 47% (0.47)
Prostate-specific antigen = 3.3 ng/mL (3.3 µg/L); 3.1 ng/mL (3.1 µg/L) when repeated

Which of the following is the best next step in this patient's management?
A. Start a phosphodiesterase inhibitor
B. Start testosterone replacement therapy
C. Arrange a sleep study
D. Refer him to a urologist

8 A 47-year-old man with HIV infection presents with a 2-year history of increasing fatigue, loss of libido, and erectile dysfunction. He underwent normal puberty and has 2 children. He has experienced no head or testicular trauma. He has no peripheral vision disturbances. His CD$_4$ cell count is currently stable. He states that he does not use androgens.

On physical examination, the patient is normally virilized. His BMI is 26.5 kg/m^2. He has bilateral gynecomastia. His phallus is normal. Both testes are 15 mL.

Laboratory test results:
Total testosterone (8 AM) = 810 ng/dL (28.1 nmol/L); repeated measurement = 750 ng/dL (26.0 nmol/L) (by liquid chromatography tandem mass spectrometry)
LH = 8.7 mIU/mL (8.7 IU/L)
FSH = 7.0 mIU/mL (7.0 IU/L)
TSH = 2.2 mIU/L
Free T$_4$ = 1.1 ng/dL (14.2 pmol/L)
Cortisol (10 AM) = 19.8 µg/dL (546.2 nmol/L)

Which of the following is the best next diagnostic step in this patient's evaluation?
A. Measure free testosterone
B. Determine urinary testosterone-to-epitestosterone ratio
C. Screen for mutations in the androgen receptor gene
D. Refer to evaluate for depression

9 A 25-year-old man is referred to you for evaluation of infertility. He and his wife have been having unprotected intercourse for the past 3 years without a confirmed pregnancy. His wife's workup is normal. The patient underwent normal puberty and reports normal libido and erections.

On physical examination, he is a well-built man with normal muscle mass. His BMI is 25.5 kg/m^2. There is no gynecomastia. His testes are 15 mL bilaterally, and his vas deferens is palpable bilaterally.

Laboratory test results:
Total testosterone = 550 ng/dL (19.1 nmol/L)
FSH = 25.5 mIU/mL (25.5 IU/L)
LH = 3.8 mIU/mL (3.8 IU/L)
Inhibin B = undetectable
Karyotype = 46,XY (100 cells counted)

Two semen analyses (each after 3 days of abstinence) show azoospermia. Semen volume is 2 mL and fructose is positive.

Which of the following genetic abnormalities is this patient most likely to have?
A. Y-Chromosome microdeletion
B. Klinefelter syndrome
C. Mutation in the *KISS1R* gene
D. Mutation in the *CFTR* gene

10 A 20-year-old man is transferred to you by his pediatrician for ongoing management of idiopathic hypogonadotropic hypogonadism. The diagnosis was made at age 18 years during workup for delayed puberty, when he was found to have a serum testosterone level of 55 ng/dL (1.9 nmol/L) and low gonadotropin levels (LH = 0.8 mIU/mL [0.8 IU/L], FSH = 1.1 mIU/mL [1.1 IU/L]). Results of the rest of his pituitary function testing were normal, as was sellar imaging. He has been treated with testosterone from age 18 years, and his levels are normal on treatment. He has a normal sense of smell and normal sexual function but reports fatigue and occasional dizziness.

On physical examination, his height is 75 in (190.5 cm). His blood pressure is 95/60 mm Hg lying down and 80/55 mm Hg standing. He is well virilized and has no gynecomastia. He has pigmentation of buccal mucosa and palmar creases. Testes are 4 mL bilaterally.

Laboratory test results:
Baseline cortisol = 1.0 µg/dL (27.6 nmol/L)
Plasma ACTH = 310 pg/mL (68.2 pmol/L)
    (reference range, 10-80 pg/mL [2.2-17.6 pmol/L])
1 hour after stimulation with 250 mcg of
    intravenous cosyntropin, cortisol = 5.0 µg/dL
    (137.9 nmol/L)

Which of the following is the most likely diagnosis?
  A. Partial hypopituitarism
  B. Autoimmune polyglandular endocrine deficiency syndrome type 1
  C. Adrenal hypoplasia congenita
  D. Kallmann syndrome

11 A 36-year-old man is referred for evaluation of a low serum testosterone level identified during workup of decreasing libido and low energy levels. He has a 10-year-old son. He is taking no medications and is generally healthy.

On physical examination, his BMI is 24 kg/m² and blood pressure is 120/80 mm Hg. He has normal secondary sexual characteristics and no gynecomastia. He has no acne or striae. His testicular volume is 15 mL bilaterally. Muscle strength is normal and he is able to do squats without using his arms to assist.

Laboratory test results:
Total testosterone = 150 ng/dL (5.2 nmol/L)
    (reference range, 300-900 ng/dL
    [10.4-31.2 nmol/L])
Calculated free testosterone, low
LH = 3.0 mIU/mL (3.0 IU/L)
FSH = 3.0 mIU/mL (3.0 IU/L)

Pituitary MRI is normal.

Which of the following is the most appropriate next test?
  A. 24-Hour urinary free cortisol measurement
  B. Karyotype analysis
  C. Urine epitestosterone measurement
  D. Serum prolactin measurement

12 A 75-year-old man on testosterone therapy returns to clinic for follow-up. He was first seen 12 months ago with concerns of reduced libido and fatigue. At that visit, his morning total testosterone level was 200 ng/dL (6.9 nmol/L) and his prostate-specific antigen level was 1.3 ng/mL (1.3 µg/L). His prostate was symmetrically enlarged without nodules. After thorough evaluation, he was started on a 1% testosterone gel, 5 g daily. The patient reports improved sexual function and energy since starting treatment. He has no lower urinary tract symptoms. On physical examination at today's appointment, his prostate examination is unchanged.

Laboratory test results:
Testosterone = 451 ng/dL (15.6 nmol/L)
Prostate-specific antigen = 3.3 ng/mL (3.3 µg/L)
Repeated prostate-specific antigen = 3.0 ng/mL
    (3.0 µg/L)

Which of the following is the best next step in this patient's management?
  A. Refer him to a urologist
  B. Provide reassurance and schedule a follow-up appointment in 12 months
  C. Decrease the dosage of the testosterone gel to 2.5 g daily
  D. Start a 5α-reductase inhibitor

13 An 18-year-old man is referred for evaluation of delayed sexual development. He grew normally in childhood but never experienced a pubertal growth spurt. He has a normal sense of smell. He does not take any medications and does not abuse drugs. He has no family history of anosmia, delayed puberty, or hypogonadism.

On physical examination, his height is 67 in (170 cm), arm span is 70 in (177.8 cm), and BMI is 21 kg/m². He has slight axillary hair and Tanner stage 2 pubic hair but no facial or chest hair. He has no gynecomastia. The right testis measures 2 mL and the left testis measures 3 mL. He has reduced muscle mass. On neurologic examination, his visual fields are full to confrontation and he does not have mirror movements.

Laboratory test results (morning):
Total testosterone = 47 ng/dL (1.6 nmol/L)
Free T_4 = 1.3 ng/dL (16.7 pmol/L)
TSH = 1.41 mIU/L
LH = <0.2 mIU/mL (<0.2 IU/L)
FSH = 0.3 mIU/mL (0.3 IU/L)
Prolactin = 17 ng/mL (0.7 nmol/L)
Cortisol (8 AM) = 18.0 µg/dL (496.6 nmol/L)
IGF-1, low-normal

Which of the following is the most appropriate diagnostic test to perform next?
  A. Genetic testing for a mutation in *KAL1*
  B. GnRH stimulation test
  C. MRI of the sella
  D. Measurement of free testosterone

14 A 36-year-old pharmacist is referred for evaluation of a low serum testosterone level. He reports decreased libido and energy, as well as pain in the small joints of his hands. He is otherwise well and takes no medications. He has a 10-year-old son. He reports never having taken opioids, androgenic anabolic steroids, or corticosteroids.

On physical examination, his BMI is 24 kg/m² and blood pressure is 115/70 mm Hg. He is well virilized with normal secondary sexual characteristics and no gynecomastia. He has normal skin without striae or bruises and has no difficulty rising from a squatting position. Testicular volume is 15 mL bilaterally.

Laboratory test results:
Total testosterone = 150 ng/dL (5.2 nmol/L)
  (reference range, 300-900 ng/dL
  [10.4-31.2 nmol/L])
Calculated free testosterone, low
Serum prolactin = 15 ng/mL (0.7 nmol) (reference range, 5-20 ng/mL [0.2-0.9 nmol/L])
FSH = 3.0 mIU/mL (3.0 IU/L)
LH = 3.0 mIU/mL (3.0 IU/L)
Plasma glucose (fasting) = 101 mg/dL
  (5.6 mmol/L)

X-ray of the hands reveals chondrocalcinosis of the small joints bilaterally. Sellar MRI reveals no pituitary mass.

Which of the following tests is most likely to lead to this patient's specific diagnosis?
  A. Measurement of transferrin saturation
  B. Urine toxicology screen for opioids
  C. Dexamethasone suppression test
  D. Measurement of serum prolactin after serial dilution

15 A 25-year-old man is referred to you for evaluation of hypogonadism 2 months after sustaining a head injury with loss of consciousness after being knocked off his motorcycle. Brain imaging done at the time revealed no hypothalamic, pituitary stalk, or pituitary abnormalities. He has made good progress since his accident, but still has some problems with short-term memory and strength. His libido, which had been quite low after being discharged from hospital, is now beginning to improve and he can get and sustain an erection adequate for intercourse. He is married and would like to start a family in the next 1 to 2 years.

On physical examination, his BMI is 24 kg/m². He has normal secondary sexual characteristics and normal testicular size. On neurologic examination, he has no focal deficits.

Laboratory test results:
Total testosterone = 150 ng/dL (5.2 nmol/L)
  (reference range, 300-900 ng/dL
  [10.4-31.2 nmol/L])
FSH = 3.0 mIU/mL (3.0 IU/L)
LH = 3.0 mIU/mL (3.0 IU/L)

Which of the following is the most appropriate next step in this patient's management?
   A. Start treatment with hCG
   B. Start testosterone replacement
   C. Reevaluate his hypothalamic-pituitary-gonadal axis in 6 to 12 months
   D. Start a phosphodiesterase inhibitor

16 A 65-year-old man is referred to you for evaluation of hypogonadism because he has been complaining of low mood, decreased energy levels, and decreased libido. He had been discharged from the hospital 3 weeks earlier following treatment of pneumonia. His primary care physician saw him last week and measured a serum testosterone concentration, which was low.

On physical examination, his BMI is 26.5 kg/m². He is well virilized, has no gynecomastia, has a normal phallus, and has 25-mL testes bilaterally.

Laboratory test results (sample drawn in the early morning):
   Total testosterone = 240 ng/dL (8.3 nmol/L) (reference range, 300-900 ng/dL [10.4-31.2 nmol/L])
   Serum FSH = 3.0 mIU/mL (3.0 IU/L)
   Serum LH = 4.0 mIU/mL (4.0 IU/L)

Repeated laboratory results (sample drawn in the early morning of today's clinic visit) are similar.

Which of the following is the best next diagnostic study to order?
   A. Serum total testosterone measurement in 3 months
   B. Serum iron studies
   C. Serum prolactin measurement
   D. Free testosterone measurement

17 A 36-year-old man presents for evaluation of a 3-month history of tender gynecomastia. He reports normal energy levels and sexual function. He reports no heat intolerance, diaphoresis, or palpitations. His medical history is remarkable for hepatitis C and premature male-pattern balding for which he takes finasteride, 1 mg daily.

On physical examination, his BMI is 22 kg/m² and pulse rate is 72 beats/min. His thyroid gland is normal. He has tender bilateral gynecomastia

measuring about 3 cm bilaterally. His phallus is normal, and testes are 15 mL bilaterally with no masses palpable.

Laboratory test results:
   Total testosterone = 900 ng/dL (31.2 nmol/L) (reference range, 300-900 ng/dL [10.4-31.2 nmol/L])
   Free testosterone (calculated) = 31 ng/dL (1.08 nmol/L) (reference range, 9.0-30.0 ng/dL [0.31-1.04 nmol/L])
   Estradiol = 90 pg/mL (330.4 pmol/L) (reference range, 10-40 pg/mL [36.7-146.8 pmol/L])
   FSH = 0.5 mIU/mL (0.5 IU/L)
   LH = 0.5 mIU/mL (0.5 IU/L)

Which of the following most likely explains his hormone profile?
   A. Elevated sex hormone–binding globulin due to hepatitis C
   B. Estrogen-secreting testicular tumor
   C. Decreased 5α-reduction due to finasteride
   D. Testosterone abuse

18 A 65-year-old man was prescribed testosterone therapy by his primary care physician to treat hypogonadism. He had a number of questions about the risks and benefits of his treatment that his primary care physician was not able to answer to his satisfaction, so he requested a referral to a specialist. He is generally healthy apart from a history of well-controlled hypertension. He reports nocturia once nightly but no other lower urinary tract symptoms and has a mildly enlarged, smooth prostate without nodules on examination. His pretreatment hematocrit level was 43% and his prostate-specific antigen level was 1.9 ng/mL (1.9 µg/L).

Which of the following adverse effects do you counsel the patient is most likely to occur while he is being treated with testosterone?
   A. Aggressive behavior
   B. Acute urinary retention
   C. Prostate-specific antigen elevation above 4 ng/mL (>4 µg/L)
   D. Erythrocytosis

19 A 40-year-old transgender woman is admitted to the hospital with abdominal pain and is found to have pancreatitis. She has a strong family history of hyperlipidemia and was diagnosed with hypertriglyceridemia in her late teens, for which she was prescribed rosuvastatin and fenofibrate but she has not been taking her medications consistently. At age 18 years, she started hormone therapy with conjugated equine estrogens and spironolactone and started living as a woman. In her late 20s, she had breast augmentation and facial surgery. Six months before admission, type 2 diabetes mellitus was diagnosed, and it has since been managed by diet alone.

Laboratory results:
  Triglycerides = 6050 mg/dL (68.37 mmol/L)
  Lipase = 778 U/L (13.0 µkat/L)
  Glucose = 255 mg/dL (14.2 mmol/L)

She responds well to fluids, insulin, and intensification of her lipid-lowering therapy. Her hormone therapy is held. On review in clinic 6 weeks later, her triglycerides are back to baseline, her blood glucose values are in the range of 100 to 120 mg/dL (5.6-6.7 mmol/L), and she is keen to resume hormone therapy.

Which of the following is the most appropriate management option for this patient?
  A. Resume the previous regimen of conjugated equine estrogen and spironolactone
  B. Start a GnRH agonist with a 0.05-mg estradiol patch
  C. Tell the patient that she is not a candidate for any further hormonal intervention
  D. Switch her estrogen regimen to ethinyl estradiol

20 A 30-year-old man seeks a second opinion for management of infertility. He and his wife have had regular unprotected intercourse for 18 months without a documented pregnancy. His wife's workup is normal. He brings the results of his laboratory testing:

Total testosterone = 250 ng/dL (8.7 nmol/L)
LH = 3.5 mIU/mL (3.5 IU/L)
FSH = 4.0 mIU/mL (4.0 IU/L)
Prolactin = 12 ng/mL (0.5 nmol/L)
Transferrin saturation = 35%

He does not have a copy of his semen analyses, but he was told that they showed no sperm. Adult-onset hypogonadotropic hypogonadism is diagnosed, and hCG injections are initiated. His testosterone level increases to 600 ng/dL (20.8 nmol/L) but he remains azoospermic.

On physical examination, he is an obese, otherwise healthy man who is well virilized. His testes are 20 mL bilaterally, but you have difficulty palpating his vas deferens.

Which of the following is the most appropriate next step?
  A. Add FSH injections
  B. Arrange for transrectal ultrasonography
  C. Increase the hCG dosage
  D. Switch to clomiphene citrate

Thyroid Board Review

Elizabeth N. Pearce, MD, MSc ● Boston University

1 A 34-year-old woman presents for a routine physical examination. There is a family history of Hashimoto thyroiditis in her mother. The patient reports anxiety and recent hair loss, but has no other symptoms. She is not taking any prescription medications. She reports taking biotin, 5000 mcg daily, for hair loss, and is also taking a selenium supplement, 200 mcg daily. Her serum TSH level is documented to be less than 0.01 mIU/L.

Results of repeated blood tests 3 days later:
    TSH = <0.01 mIU/L
    Free T_4 = 3.2 ng/dL (41.2 pmol/L)
    Total T_3 = 374 ng/dL (5.8 nmol/L)
    TSH receptor antibody = >40 U/L (reference range, <1.3 U/L)

Which of the following is the best next step for establishing this patient's diagnosis?
    A. Radioactive iodine uptake and scan
    B. Repeated blood tests after stopping biotin
    C. Thyroid ultrasonography with Doppler assessment of thyroid vascularity
    D. Serum TPO antibody titer

2 A 37-year-old man is noted to have a 3.0-cm left thyroid nodule. Physical examination confirms the thyroid nodule and no cervical adenopathy is noted. His serum TSH concentration is 1.3 mIU/L, and thyroid ultrasonography shows a 3.2-cm solitary hypoechoic nodule without suspicious features.

Which of the following thyroid FNAB findings (see accompanying images) should result in a referral for thyroidectomy?
    A. Figure A
    B. Figure B
    C. Figure C
    D. Figure D

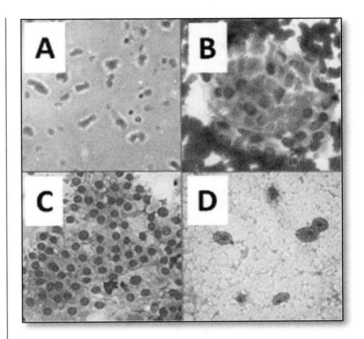

3 A 56-year-old woman with a history of hypothyroidism is referred for evaluation of a high thyroid hormone dosage requirement. She takes levothyroxine on an empty stomach each morning, with no food or other medications for at least 1 hour. Her weight has been stable. Her medical history is notable for Roux-en-Y gastric bypass surgery for obesity at age 30 years.

On physical examination, she has a thyroidectomy scar, delayed deep tendon reflex relaxation phase, and trace pedal edema bilaterally. Her weight is 176 lb (80 kg), and BMI is 32 kg/m².

Her current medications include levothyroxine, 400 mcg daily, and a fish oil supplement twice daily.

Laboratory test results:
    Free T_4 = 0.6 ng/dL (7.7 pmol/L) (reference range, 0.8-1.8 ng/dL [10.30-23.17 pmol/L])
    TSH = 18.2 mIU/L
    Screen for celiac disease, negative

Which of the following is the best next step in this patient's management?
   A. Increase the levothyroxine dosage to 500 mcg daily
   B. Change to once-weekly levothyroxine, 3 mg
   C. Change to liothyronine (T₃)
   D. Switch brands of levothyroxine
   E. Give parenteral levothyroxine

4 A 34-year-old woman presents with symptoms of tachycardia, tremor, heat intolerance, and irregular menses.

On physical examination, her blood pressure is 128/77 mm Hg and pulse rate is 96 beats/min. She has a palpable, nontender, 3-cm right-sided thyroid nodule.

Laboratory test results:
   TSH = <0.01 mIU/L
   Free T$_4$ = 2.9 ng/dL (37.3 pmol/L)
   Total T$_3$ = 320 ng/dL (4.9 nmol/L)
   TPO antibodies = 37 IU/mL (37 kIU/L)
   Thyroid stimulating immunoglobulin = <120%

Her radioactive iodine uptake is 26% at 24 hours (*see image*). In discussing therapeutic options, she makes it clear that her primary concern is to avoid the need for lifelong medication.

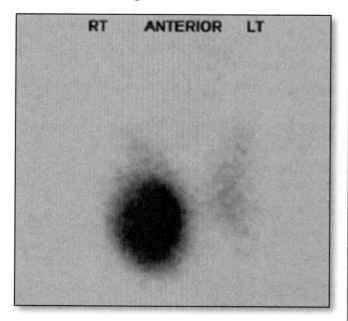

Which of the following therapeutic options would be most appropriate for this patient?
   A. Radioactive iodine treatment
   B. Methimazole
   C. Thyroid lobectomy
   D. Ethanol injection
   E. Radiofrequency ablation

5 A 58-year-old woman with stage IV medullary thyroid cancer is referred for consideration of further therapy. Medullary thyroid cancer was diagnosed 8 years earlier and she has had a persistent postoperative elevation of serum calcitonin. Distant metastases to the lungs and ribs were detected 1 year ago, with disease progression over the past 6 months. Physical examination reveals a well-healed thyroidectomy scar but findings are otherwise unremarkable.

Laboratory test results:
   Serum calcitonin = 15,000 pg/mL (4380 pmol/L) (reference range, <10 pg/mL [<2.9 pmol/L])
   Carcinoembryonic antigen = 65 ng/mL (65 μg/L) (reference range, 0.2-4.7 ng/mL [0.2-4.7 μg/L])

Which of the following is the most appropriate next step in this patient's management?
   A. Radiolabeled calcitonin antibody therapy
   B. Chemotherapy with adriamycin and cisplatin
   C. Radiotherapy to the lung and rib lesions
   D. Tyrosine kinase inhibitor therapy
   E. Somatostatin analogue therapy

6 A 74-year-old woman with fatigue and weight gain is referred for evaluation of subclinical hypothyroidism. The patient has gained 10 lb (4.5 kg) over the past 2 years since retirement, and frequently requires a midday nap. Her medical history is notable for hyperlipidemia, which has been managed by diet alone.

On physical examination, she has minimal goiter without nodules. The rest of her examination findings are normal.

Laboratory test results:
   Serum TSH = 8.9 mIU/L
   Free T$_4$ = 1.3 ng/dL (16.7 pmol/L)
   LDL cholesterol = 160 mg/dL (4.14 mmol/L)
   HDL cholesterol = 38 mg/dL (0.98 mmol/L)
   TPO antibodies, elevated

On repeated testing 3 months later, her TSH value is essentially unchanged.

Which potential effect of initiating levothyroxine treatment for this patient is most strongly supported by current evidence?
   A. Weight loss
   B. Improved cognitive function
   C. Less fatigue
   D. Iatrogenic subclinical hyperthyroidism
   E. Increased HDL cholesterol

7 A 35-year-old man presents with a new palpable 2-cm thyroid nodule. Thyroid ultrasonography demonstrates the following finding in the right thyroid lobe (*see image, arrow*).

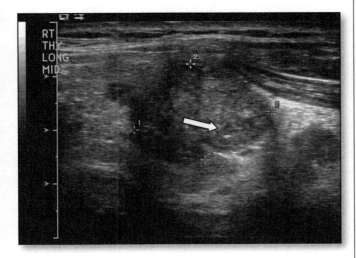

On the basis of the ultrasound pattern observed, what is the likelihood of thyroid cancer?
   A. 70%-90%
   B. 20%-40%
   C. 10%-20%
   D. <3%

8 A 23-year-old man is seen for follow-up of hypothyroidism. He has been treated with levothyroxine, 150 mcg daily, since age 15 years. His dosage has been stable for several years, and his most recent TSH value 10 months ago was 1.34 mIU/L. He reports strict adherence to his levothyroxine regimen. He notes that since his last visit he has entered body-building competitions and has started using a regimen of anabolic steroids and aromatase inhibitors that he obtains over the Internet.

Which of the following patterns is most likely in this patient?

Answer	TSH	Total T$_4$	Total T$_3$	Free T$_4$
A.	10.0 mIU/L	15.0 µg/dL (193.1 nmol/L)	280 ng/dL (4.3 nmol/L)	0.7 ng/dL (9.0 pmol/L)
B.	1.2 mIU/L	15.0 µg/dL (193.1 nmol/L)	280 ng/dL (4.3 nmol/L)	1.4 ng/dL (18.0 pmol/L)
C.	1.2 mIU/L	10.0 µg/dL (128.7 nmol/L)	150 ng/dL (2.3 nmol/L)	1.4 ng/dL (18.0 pmol/L)
D.	1.2 mIU/L	5.0 µg/dL (64.4 nmol/L)	70 ng/dL (1.1 nmol/L)	1.4 ng/dL (18.0 pmol/L)
E.	0.01 mIU/L	5.0 µg/dL (64.4 nmol/L)	70 ng/dL (1.1 nmol/L)	2.8 ng/dL (36.0 pmol/L)

Reference ranges: TSH, 0.5-5.0 mIU/L; total T$_4$, 5.5-12.5 µg/dL (94.02-213.68 nmol/L); total T$_3$, 70-200 ng/dL (1.08-3.08 nmol/L); free T$_4$, 0.8-1.8 ng/dL (10.30-23.17 pmol/L)

9 A 42-year-old woman comes to see you after recently moving to your area. She underwent transsphenoidal resection of a nonfunctional pituitary adenoma 5 years ago. There is a history of type 1 diabetes in her mother. Her medications include hydrocortisone, 10 mg in the morning and 5 mg in the afternoon, and an oral contraceptive. She describes mild fatigue and difficulty losing weight.

Laboratory test results:
   TSH = 5.6 mIU/L
   Free T$_4$ = 0.6 ng/dL (7.7 pmol/L)

Levothyroxine is initiated at a dosage of 50 mcg daily. Six week later, her fatigue is unchanged.

Laboratory test results:
   TSH = 0.16 mIU/L
   Free T$_4$ = 0.9 ng/dL (11.6 pmol/L)

Which of the following is the best next step?
   A. Discontinue levothyroxine
   B. Discontinue levothyroxine and add methimazole, 5 mg daily
   C. Continue the current levothyroxine dosage and add levotriiodothyronine, 5 mcg daily
   D. Continue the current levothyroxine dosage and increase the hydrocortisone dosage to 15 mg in the morning and 5 mg in the afternoon
   E. Increase the levothyroxine dosage to 88 mcg daily

10 A 47-year-old man presents with palpitations. His weight has recently decreased from 240 to 210 lb (109 to 95.5 kg). He has otherwise been healthy and has had no recent illnesses.

On physical examination, his thyroid is nontender and there is no goiter. He has a fine tremor of his outstretched hands, and his pulse rate is 94 beats/min. He has no stigmata of Graves disease.

Laboratory test results:
    TSH = <0.01 mIU/L
    Free T_4 = 4.1 ng/dL (52.8 pmol/L)
    Total T_3 = 280 ng/dL (4.3 nmol/L)
    Thyroglobulin antibody = <4 IU/mL
    Radioactive iodine uptake = 1% at 24 hours

A spot urinary iodine concentration on the day of the radioactive iodine uptake test is 94 µg/L (while a reference range is not available, the most recent median US urinary iodine concentration in adults is 144 µg/L).

Which of the following tests is most likely to reveal the diagnosis?
    A. Radioactive iodine uptake/scan after a low-iodine diet
    B. Serum thyroglobulin measurement
    C. Assessment of serum erythrocyte sedimentation rate
    D. Thyroid ultrasonography with color Doppler
    E. Thyroid-stimulating immunoglobulin measurement

11 A 47-year-old woman is found to have a left thyroid nodule. Thyroid ultrasonography shows a 2.5-cm hypoechoic nodule without calcification or hypervascularity, with no suspicious lymph nodes. The patient undergoes FNAB of the dominant nodule with cytologic findings of follicular neoplasm (Bethesda class IV). Repeated FNAB with molecular analysis reveals a *RET/PTC* rearrangement.

Which of the following is the most appropriate next step in this patient's management?
    A. Repeated thyroid ultrasonography in 6 months
    B. Repeated FNAB in 6 months
    C. Repeated molecular analysis in 6 months
    D. Referral for diagnostic lobectomy
    E. Referral for total thyroidectomy

12 A 28-year-old man undergoes thyroidectomy with central neck dissection for a 2.5-cm papillary thyroid cancer. The tumor shows microscopic local invasion but no aggressive histology and 1 of 12 central lymph nodes contains tumor. The patient undergoes radioiodine remnant ablation using 100 mCi of ^{131}I, and a posttreatment scan shows no uptake outside of the thyroid bed. Surveillance testing at 6 months reveals a stimulated thyroglobulin concentration of 15 ng/mL (15 µg/L) with negative thyroglobulin antibodies, no abnormal uptake on radioiodine whole-body scan, and no adenopathy on neck ultrasonography. No additional therapy is given. Six months later, a suppressed thyroglobulin level is 0.5 ng/mL (0.5 µg/L), stimulated thyroglobulin is 5 ng/mL (5 µg/L), thyroglobulin antibodies are negative, and neck ultrasonography is unchanged.

Which of the following should be the next step in this patient's management?
    A. Thyroglobulin testing using a different assay
    B. PET-CT scan
    C. CT of the chest
    D. MRI of the neck
    E. Repeated surveillance testing in 1 year

13 A 34-year-old woman is found to have a TSH concentration of 0.17 mIU/L on laboratory tests performed as part of routine physical examination. She has no hyperthyroid symptoms. She is otherwise healthy and is not currently taking any medications or supplements. There is a small goiter on examination with no bruit and no palpable nodules. She has no signs of Graves eye disease. Her resting pulse rate is 84 beats/min.

Laboratory test results 4 months later:
    TSH = 0.23 mIU/L
    Free T_4 = 1.5 ng/dL (19.3 pmol/L)
    Total T_3 = 167 ng/dL (2.6 nmol/L)
    Thyroid-stimulating immunoglobulin = 134% (mildly elevated)

She has 2 children and is not planning additional pregnancies.

Which of the following is the best option?
  A. Repeat thyroid function tests in 6 months
  B. Start atenolol, 25 mg daily
  C. Start methimazole, 5 mg daily
  D. Schedule radioactive iodine treatment
  E. Schedule total thyroidectomy

14 A 48-year-old man with a history of a 3.0-cm papillary thyroid cancer treated 1 year ago with thyroidectomy and radioiodine ablation is referred for follow-up. Physical examination reveals a 1.5-cm, level 3 lymph node on the left side. Neck ultrasonography shows bilateral cervical adenopathy. His serum thyroglobulin concentration is 3.2 ng/mL (3.2 µg/L) at baseline, and it rises to 19.2 ng/mL (19.2 µg/L) after recombinant human TSH. A whole-body scan is negative. PET-CT shows uptake in the neck corresponding to the palpable lymph node, but FNAB shows only reactive changes.

Which of the following is the best next step in this patient's management?
  A. Left lateral radical neck dissection
  B. PET-CT after recombinant human TSH
  C. MRI of the neck
  D. FNAB again and measurement of thyroglobulin in aspirate
  E. Surveillance testing again in 1 year

15 A 57-year-old man with Graves disease develops agranulocytosis while taking methimazole. Methimazole is stopped and cell counts recover, but he develops nausea and vomiting and presents to the emergency department.

On physical examination, his temperature is 103°F (39.4°C), pulse rate is 140 beats/min and irregular, and crackles are heard to the mid lung fields. Free T_4 and T_3 levels are 3 times the upper normal limit. He is admitted to the intensive care unit and receives antipyretics, intravenous propranolol, hydrocortisone, and oral potassium iodide therapy. His condition continues to deteriorate and urgent thyroidectomy is planned.

Which additional measure could be considered for this patient before thyroidectomy?
  A. Hemodialysis
  B. Replacement of propranolol with atenolol
  C. Plasmapheresis
  D. Intravenous immunoglobulin therapy

16 A 73-year-old man with tall-cell variant of papillary thyroid cancer invading the strap muscles and extending to the trachea undergoes total thyroidectomy. The surgeon scrapes tumor off the trachea, but is unable to remove tumor surrounding the recurrent laryngeal nerve. The patient receives therapeutic radioiodine therapy using 200 mCi ^{131}I. A whole-body scan obtained 10 days after radioiodine shows only faint uptake in the thyroid bed.

Which of the following is the most appropriate next step in this patient's management?
  A. External beam radiation therapy to the thyroid bed
  B. Tyrosine kinase inhibitor therapy
  C. Repeated radioiodine therapy in 3 to 6 months, using dosimetry
  D. Chemotherapy with doxorubicin and cisplatin
  E. No treatment unless disease progresses

17 A 26-year-old woman with Graves hyperthyroidism has been treated with methimazole, 10 mg daily, for 15 months. On palpation, her thyroid gland is at the upper limit of normal size. There is no bruit. She does not smoke cigarettes. She is interested in stopping methimazole.

Current laboratory test results:
  TSH = 0.6 mIU/L
  Total T_3 = 169 ng/dL (2.6 nmol/L)
  Free T_4 = 1.5 ng/dL (18.0 pmol/L)
  TPO antibodies = 369 IU/mL (369 kIU/L)
    (reference range, <2.0 IU/mL [<2.0 kIU/L])
  Thyroid-stimulating immunoglobulin = 334%
    (reference range, ≤120%)

Which of the following characteristics of this patient predicts a likelihood that her Graves hyperthyroidism will recur if methimazole is stopped?

    A. Age

    B. TPO antibody titer

    C. Thyroid-stimulating immunoglobulin level

    D. Thyroid size

    E. Smoking status

18 A 75-year-old woman is admitted to the medical intensive care unit with progressive obtundation and is found to be in myxedema coma. She is treated with intravenous levothyroxine therapy, stress-dose dexamethasone, and empiric antibiotics while awaiting blood culture results. After 48 hours, the patient has gradually improved sensorium but develops progressive hypotension with narrowing of the pulse pressure and diminished heart sounds. Electrocardiography shows low voltage in all leads.

Laboratory test results:

    Free T_4 = 1.0 ng/dL (12.9 pmol/L)

    TSH = 12.8 mIU/L

    Serum cortisol = 2.8 µg/dL (77.3 nmol/L)

    Creatine kinase = 280 U/L (4.7 µkat/L) with 12% MB fraction but normal troponin levels

Which of the following is the most likely cause of this patient's change in clinical status?

    A. Adrenal insufficiency

    B. Cardiac ischemia

    C. Inadequate thyroid hormone replacement

    D. Cardiomyopathy

    E. Cardiac tamponade

19 A 72-year-old man reports left-sided neck pain and palpitations for 2 weeks. Physical examination reveals firm enlargement (about 1.5 times normal size) and tenderness over the left thyroid lobe. Laboratory testing shows an elevated free T_4 level and suppressed TSH level. Radioactive iodine uptake is 2% at 24 hours. Subacute thyroiditis is diagnosed and he is prescribed ibuprofen therapy.

Three weeks later the patient notes persistent pain, now accompanied by dysphagia, and a further increase in size of the left thyroid lobe (now 3 times normal size). Thyroid function test results are essentially unchanged. Ultrasonography reveals an enlarged and heterogeneous left thyroid lobe with increased vascularity.

Which of the following should be the next step in this patient's management?

    A. Perform FNAB

    B. Start methimazole

    C. Change ibuprofen to prednisone

    D. Perform contrast CT of the neck

    E. Refer for thyroidectomy

20 You recently palpated a new thyroid nodule in a 38-year-old man with a history of hypothyroidism. Ultrasound-guided FNAB of his palpable nodule is interpreted as suspicious for papillary carcinoma. He undergoes total thyroidectomy without complications. Surgical pathology shows a 2.3-cm intrathyroidal, fully encapsulated papillary carcinoma with clear margins, no lymphovascular invasion, and no positive lymph nodes. Three months ago, his TSH level was 0.5 mIU/L on levothyroxine, 137 mcg daily. His dosage was increased to 150 mcg daily at the time of his surgery.

Current laboratory test results 1 week postoperatively:

    TSH = 0.2 mIU/L

    Thyroglobulin (measured using a radioimmunoassay) = 13 ng/mL (13 µg/L)

    Thyroglobulin antibody = <4.0 IU/mL

Which of the following is the best next step?

    A. Repeated thyroglobulin measurement using a immunometric assay

    B. Repeated thyroglobulin and thyroglobulin antibody measurements in 6 weeks using the same radioimmunoassay

    C. Measurement of thyroglobulin in serially diluted sera

    D. PET/CT scan

    E. Radioactive iodine ablation

21 A 76-year-old woman is admitted to the intensive care unit with hypotension due to sepsis. Despite aggressive therapy, the patient's condition continues to deteriorate. One month earlier, the patient had a normal thyroid laboratory panel.

Which of the following patterns is expected in this patient?

Answer	TSH	Total T$_4$	Total T$_3$	Free T$_4$
A.	10.0 mIU/L	7.0 µg/dL (90.1 nmol/L)	70 ng/dL (1.1 nmol/L)	0.7 ng/dL (9.0 pmol/L)
B.	7.5 mIU/L	5.5 µg/dL (70.8 nmol/L)	55 ng/dL (0.8 nmol/L)	0.8 ng/dL (10.3 pmol/L)
C.	0.2 mIU/L	2.5 µg/dL (31.2 nmol/L)	25 ng/dL (0.4 nmol/L)	0.5 ng/dL (6.4 pmol/L)
D.	5.0 mIU/L	12.0 µg/dL (154.4 nmol/L)	70 ng/dL (1.1 nmol/L)	2.2 ng/dL (28.3 pmol/L)
E.	0.01 mIU/L	12.0 µg/dL (154.4 nmol/L)	360 ng/dL (5.5 nmol/L)	2.2 ng/dL (28.3 pmol/L)

Reference ranges: TSH, 0.5-5.0 mIU/L; total T$_4$, 5.5-12.5 µg/dL (70.8-160.9 nmol/L); total T$_3$, 70-200 ng/dL (1.1-3.1 nmol/L); free T$_4$, 0.8-1.8 ng/dL (10.3-23.2 pmol/L).

22 A 26-year-old woman presents for evaluation. She is currently 15 weeks' pregnant with her first child. At an initial antenatal visit at 11 weeks' gestation, her serum TSH level was 0.03 mIU/L.

Laboratory test results at a follow-up obstetric visit 2 days ago:
  Serum TSH = 0.11 mIU/L
  Free T$_4$ index = 3.6 (reference range, 1-4)
  Total T$_3$ = 280 ng/dL (4.3 nmol/L)
  Thyroid-stimulating immunoglobulin = 140%

She reports mild fatigue but is otherwise feeling well. She had some morning sickness earlier in her pregnancy, but this has resolved in the last 3 weeks. On physical examination, her pulse rate is 92 beats/min. On palpation, her thyroid gland is nontender and 20 g in size without nodules. She has no proptosis.

Which of the following is the best option?
  A. Start methimazole, 5 mg daily
  B. Start propylthiouracil, 50 mg 3 times daily
  C. Start atenolol
  D. Repeat thyroid function tests in 4 to 6 weeks
  E. Plan thyroidectomy in the second trimester

23 A 56-year-old man is referred for evaluation of a neck mass. The patient notes dysphagia with solid foods and positional dyspnea when lying on his right side. Medical history is noncontributory. On physical examination, he has a large goiter extending below the clavicle on the left. His serum TSH level is 0.2 mIU/L, and radioiodine uptake is 12% at 24 hours. CT of the neck is shown (*see image*).

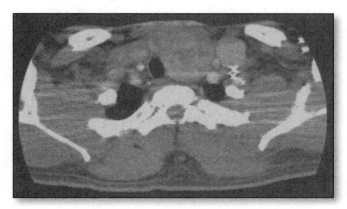

Which of the following is the best next step in this patient's management?
  A. Levothyroxine suppressive therapy
  B. Radioiodine therapy using recombinant human TSH
  C. Thermal ablation therapy
  D. Thyroidectomy from collar incision
  E. No intervention until symptoms progress

24 A 46-year-old man with a history of papillary thyroid cancer diagnosed 5 years ago is found to have multiple new macroscopic lung and bone metastases. A CT-guided lung biopsy confirms metastatic papillary thyroid cancer. The patient undergoes treatment with radioiodine and is noted to have minimal uptake in the lung lesions. The lesions are strongly avid for FDG-PET.

Which of the following most closely approximates the predicted 10-year survival for this patient?
  A. 90%
  B. 70%
  C. 40%
  D. 30%
  E. 10%

25 A 55-year-old man presents with new fatigue. He has a history of atrial fibrillation for which he had been taking amiodarone for 14 months. The amiodarone treatment was discontinued 2 months ago. Serum TSH was normal (1.47 mIU/L) at the time that the amiodarone was stopped.

He has a minimally enlarged thyroid on physical examination, without palpable nodules. His pulse rate is 92 beats/min. He has a fine tremor of his outstretched hands.

Laboratory test results:
TSH = <0.01 mIU/L
Total T_3 = 263 ng/dL (4.1 nmol/L)
Free T_4 = 4.7 ng/dL (60.5 pmol/L)

Which of the following is the best test for establishing this patient's underlying thyroid pathophysiology?
A. Radioactive iodine uptake
B. Serum IL-6 measurement
C. Serum TPO antibody measurement
D. Thyroid ultrasonography with color Doppler

26 An 81-year-old Hispanic woman undergoing evaluation for syncope is referred for abnormalities identified on thyroid function testing. She has hypertension and takes hydrochlorothiazide.

On physical examination, her pulse rate is 90 beats/min and she has a normal thyroid. She has a fine tremor, but normal deep tendon reflexes.

Thyroid function test results:
Total T_4 = 17.0 μg/dL (218.8 nmol/L) (reference range, 5.5-12.5 μg/dL [94.02-213.68 nmol/L])
Free T_4 = 1.8 ng/dL (23.2 pmol/L) (reference range, 0.8-1.8 ng/dL [10.30-23.17 pmol/L])
Total T_3 = 156 ng/dL (2.4 nmol/L) (reference range, 70-200 ng/dL [1.08-3.08 nmol/L])
Free T_3 = 3.1 pg/mL (4.8 pmol/L) (reference range, 2.3-4.2 pg/mL [3.53-6.45 pmol/L])
TSH = 2.0 mIU/L

Which of the following is the most likely diagnosis?
A. Selenium deficiency
B. Familial thyroxine-binding globulin excess
C. Familial dysalbuminemic hyperthyroxinemia
D. Thyroid hormone resistance
E. TSH-secreting pituitary adenoma

27 A 63-year-old man with metastatic renal cell carcinoma is prescribed sunitinib therapy. The patient has no history of thyroid dysfunction, and baseline thyroid function is normal.

Which of the following thyroid abnormalities is most likely to occur in this patient after starting sunitinib?
A. Primary hypothyroidism
B. Secondary hypothyroidism
C. Primary hyperthyroidism
D. Secondary hyperthyroidism
E. "Euthyroid sick" syndrome

28 A 33-year-old man with a history of Graves disease treated 6 months earlier with radioiodine is noted to have progressive monocular vision loss.

On physical examination, he has bilateral periorbital edema and conjunctival erythema, with Hertel measurements of 22 mm proptosis on the right side and 24 mm on the left side. Extraocular eye muscle testing shows restricted upward and lateral gaze on the left side. An afferent pupillary defect is present on the left side, and visual acuity measurement is 20/40 on the right and 20/400 on the left.

Laboratory test results:
Serum TSH = 0.9 mIU/L
Free T_4 = 1.2 ng/dL (15.4 pmol/L) (reference range, 0.8-1.8 ng/dL [10.3-23.2 pmol/L])
Thyroid-stimulating immunoglobulin = positive at 290%

The patient is given pulse therapy with solumedrol with no improvement.

Which of the following would be the best next step in this patient's management?
- A. Orbital radiotherapy
- B. Rituximab
- C. Strabismus surgery
- D. Teprotumumab
- E. Orbital decompression surgery

29 A 35-year-old woman with Hashimoto thyroiditis and vitamin D deficiency is referred for advice regarding levothyroxine dosing. Two years ago, her condition was well controlled on 100 mcg daily of levothyroxine, but in order to maintain a normal TSH value, her physician has repeatedly increased her dosage, and she currently takes 300 mcg daily. The patient uses a pill sorter to take her prescription each morning on an empty stomach. She waits until lunch before taking a multivitamin with iron and a calcium supplement. Her weight is stable and she has no diarrhea or abdominal pain. Physical examination reveals a small, firm goiter but is otherwise unremarkable.

Laboratory test results:
  Serum TSH = 11.6 mIU/L
  Free T_4 = 1.0 ng/dL (12.9 pmol/L) (reference range, 0.8-1.8 ng/dL [10.3-23.2 pmol/L])
  Complete blood cell count, normal
  Liver enzymes, normal
  Serum albumin, normal

Which of the following should be the next step in the evaluation of this patient's increasing levothyroxine dosage requirement?
- A. Move the timing of when she takes the calcium tablets and multivitamins to just before the evening meal
- B. Screen for occult celiac disease
- C. Measure TSH with a different assay
- D. Change to T_4/T_3 combination therapy

30 An 18-year-old man has a palpable 2-cm neck mass (*see CT images 1 and 2, arrows*). Results from thyroid function tests are normal. Ultrasonography (*image 3*) confirms a cystic mass juxtaposed to the hyoid bone.

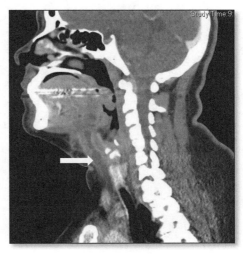

Image 1, sagittal view

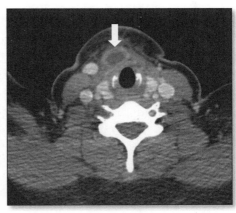

Image 2, coronal view

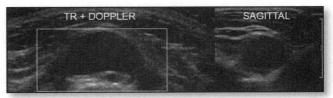

Image 3

Which of the following statements is correct?
- A. The mass will resolve spontaneously
- B. The risk of thyroid cancer is 50%
- C. The risk of future infection is 50%
- D. Radioiodine therapy will shrink the mass
- E. The mass will shrink with levothyroxine

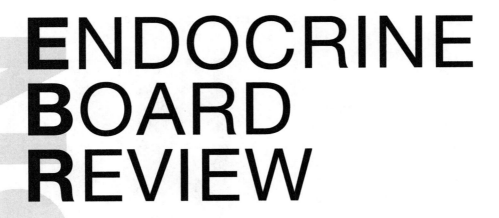

ENDOCRINE
BOARD
REVIEW

Diabetes Mellitus, Section 1 Board Review

Serge A. Jabbour, MD ● Thomas Jefferson University

1 ANSWER: D) Lifestyle intervention

Lifestyle intervention (Answer D) is preferred over metformin (Answer C) on the basis of findings from available studies, mainly the landmark Diabetes Prevention Program. In the Diabetes Prevention Program, 3234 obese patients (average BMI, 34 kg/m^2) aged 25 to 85 years (average age, 51 years) at high risk for diabetes (based on BMI ≥24 kg/m^2 and fasting and 2-hour plasma glucose concentrations of 96 to 125 mg/dL [5.3-6.9 mmol/L] and 140 to 199 mg/dL [7.8-11.1 mmol/L], respectively) were randomly assigned to one of the following groups:

- Intensive lifestyle changes with the aim of reducing weight by 7% through a behavioral modification program aimed at a low-fat diet and exercise for 150 minutes per week.
- Treatment with metformin (850 mg twice daily) plus information on diet and exercise.
- Placebo plus information on diet and exercise.

After an average follow-up of 3 years, fewer patients in the intensive lifestyle group developed diabetes, as diagnosed by fasting plasma glucose and 2-hour postload glucose concentrations (14% vs 22% and 29% in the metformin and placebo groups, respectively). The intensive lifestyle and metformin interventions reduced the cumulative incidence of diabetes by 58% and 31%, respectively. Lifestyle intervention was effective in men and women in all age groups and in all ethnic groups.

In a follow-up observational study (the Diabetes Prevention Program Outcomes Study), the benefit of the lifestyle intervention was shown to persist more than 10 years. In this study, 85% of patients originally enrolled in the Diabetes Prevention Program joined the long-term follow-up and were offered group-implemented lifestyle intervention. Patients originally assigned to metformin continued receiving it (unblinded). During a cumulative 10 years of follow-up, the incidence of diabetes in the lifestyle and metformin groups was significantly reduced by 34% and 18%, respectively, compared with placebo.

The Actos Now for Prevention of Diabetes study assessed the ability of pioglitazone (30 to 45 mg daily) to reduce the risk of developing diabetes in 600 patients with impaired glucose tolerance and 1 or more components of the metabolic syndrome. After a median follow-up period of 2.4 years, fewer patients randomly assigned to pioglitazone developed diabetes (5.0% vs 16.7% with placebo; hazard ratio, 0.28; 95% confidence interval, 0.16-0.49). Weight gain was significantly greater with pioglitazone (3.9 vs 0.77 kg), and edema was more frequent (12.9% vs 6.4%). Pioglitazone (Answer E) should not be used for diabetes prevention in this patient because of potential adverse effects (fluid retention, weight gain, heart failure), especially since he already has 2+ edema on examination.

There are no studies on dapagliflozin (Answer B) or exenatide (Answer A) with respect to diabetes prevention.

EDUCATIONAL OBJECTIVE:
Identify prediabetes (impaired fasting glucose and impaired glucose tolerance) and recommend the best way to prevent progression to diabetes.

REFERENCE(S):

Knowler WC, Barrett-Connor E, Fowler SE, et al; Diabetes Prevention Program Research Group. Reduction in the incidence of type 2 diabetes with lifestyle intervention or metformin. *N Engl J Med*. 2002;346(6):393-403.

Diabetes Prevention Program Research Group, Knowler WC, Fowler SE, et al. 10-year follow-up of diabetes incidence and weight loss in the

Diabetes Prevention Program Outcomes Study [published correction appears in *Lancet*. 2009; 374(9707):2054]. *Lancet*. 2009;374(9702): 1677-1686.

DeFronzo RA, Tripathy D, Schwenke DC, et al; ACT NOW Study. Pioglitazone for diabetes prevention in impaired glucose tolerance [*N Engl J Med*. 2011;365(2):189 and *N Engl J Med*. 2011; 365(9):869]. *N Engl J Med*. 2011;364(12): 1104-1115.

2 **ANSWER: C) Assessment for urine ketones**
In patients with type 1 diabetes, the urine should be tested for ketones if the blood glucose concentration is above 300 mg/dL (>16.7 mmol/L) for unexplained reasons, especially if the person feels unwell at the time. Testing for ketonuria should also be performed during periods of illness or stress or if there are symptoms compatible with ketoacidosis such as nausea, vomiting, and abdominal pain. If ketonuria is present in the setting of hyperglycemia, diabetic ketoacidosis should be suspected and the patient should be ideally sent to the emergency department for more testing (serum ketones, electrolytes, bicarbonate, pH, etc) and treated accordingly with intravenous fluids and insulin drip if diabetic ketoacidosis is indeed present.

While basal rate testing (Answer A), diabetes education (Answer B), and a continuous glucose sensor (Answer D) are all needed to help this patient achieve a lower hemoglobin A_{1c}, none of these options is the best immediate step to take now. These steps can be done over weeks to months. Therapy for stress management (Answer E) is appropriate if she is willing to explore it, but again, this is not immediately necessary.

EDUCATIONAL OBJECTIVE:
Determine when checking urine ketones is appropriate in a patient with type 1 diabetes mellitus.

REFERENCE(S):
Weber C, Kocher S, Neeser K, Joshi SR. Prevention of diabetic ketoacidosis and self-monitoring of ketone bodies: an overview. *Curr Med Res Opin*. 2009;25(5):1197-1207.

Goldstein DE, Little RR, Lorenz RA, et al. Tests of glycemia in diabetes. *Diabetes Care*. 2004;27(7): 1761-1773.

3 **ANSWER: A) 1.5 L of 0.9% NaCl over the first hour, and intravenous insulin bolus of 10 units then 10 units per hour**
This patient meets the criteria for the hyperosmolar hyperglycemic state (also known as hyperosmotic hyperglycemic nonketotic state). The diagnostic criteria are a plasma glucose concentration greater than 600 mg/dL (>33.3 mmol/L), effective serum osmolality greater than 320 mOsm/kg (>320 mmol/kg), arterial pH greater than 7.30, serum bicarbonate greater than 18 mEq/L (>18 mmol/L), and severe dehydration with absence of or minimal ketoacidosis.

The most common precipitating factors for hyperosmolar hyperglycemic state are infection (often pneumonia or urinary tract infection) and discontinuation of or inadequate insulin therapy. Compromised water intake due to underlying medical conditions, particularly in older patients, can promote the development of severe dehydration and the hyperosmolar hyperglycemic state. Other conditions and factors associated with the hyperosmolar hyperglycemic state include acute major illnesses such as myocardial infarction, cerebrovascular accident, sepsis, or pancreatitis, etc.

The hyperosmolar hyperglycemic state is treated with fluids and insulin. Because of severe dehydration, isotonic 0.9% NaCl is initiated at a rate of 15 to 20 mL/kg over the first hour (thus, Answers C, D, and E are incorrect). A decision is then made as to whether to continue the 0.9% NaCl or switch to 0.45% NaCl depending on volume status and corrected serum sodium. In fact, in this patient, the corrected serum sodium was 148 mEq/L (148 mmol/L) (serum sodium may be corrected by adding 1.6 mg/dL to the measured serum sodium for each 100 mg/dL of glucose above 100 mg/dL [>5.6 mmol/L]). Administration of hypertonic saline at 3% (Answer E) might worsen the hypernatremia and hyperosmolarity.

Intravenous insulin treatment can be initiated with an intravenous bolus of regular insulin (0.1 units/kg body weight) followed within 5 minutes by a continuous infusion of regular insulin of 0.1 units/kg per hour (bolus of 10 units and 10 units as a drip in this patient who weighs 220 lb [100 kg]) (thus, Answer B is incorrect). Alternatively, the bolus dose can be omitted if a higher dose of continuous intravenous regular insulin (0.14 units/kg per hour) is initiated.

The best approach for this patient is to administer 1.5 L of 0.9% NaCl over the first hour, and then an intravenous insulin bolus of 10 units followed by 10 units per hour (Answer A).

EDUCATIONAL OBJECTIVE:
Manage the hyperosmolar hyperglycemic state.

REFERENCE(S):
Kitabchi AE, Umpierrez GE, Miles JM, Fisher JN. Hyperglycemic crises in adult patients with diabetes. *Diabetes Care*. 2009;32(7):1335-1343.

Nyenwe EA, Kitabchi AE. Evidence-based management of hyperglycemic emergencies in diabetes mellitus. *Diabetes Res Clin Pract*. 2011;94(3): 340-351.

4 ANSWER: D) Polysomnography

In both men and women, the strongest risk factor for obstructive sleep apnea is obesity. The prevalence of obstructive sleep apnea progressively increases as BMI and associated markers (eg, neck circumference, waist-to-hip ratio) increase. In a prospective study of nearly 700 adults with 4-year longitudinal follow-up, a 10% increase in weight was associated with a 6-fold increase in the risk of incident obstructive sleep apnea. In a population-based study of more than 1000 adults who underwent polysomnography, moderate-to-severe obstructive sleep apnea (apnea-hypopnea index ≥15 events/h) was present in 11% of patients who were normal weight, 21% of those who were overweight (BMI, 25-30 kg/m^2), and 63% of those who were obese (BMI >30 kg/m^2).

Most patients with obstructive sleep apnea first come to the attention of a clinician because of daytime sleepiness, or the bed partner reports loud snoring, gasping, snorting, or interruptions in breathing while sleeping. Diagnostic testing for obstructive sleep apnea should be performed in any patient with unexplained excessive daytime sleepiness, which is the clinically relevant symptom of obstructive sleep apnea that is most responsive to treatment. In the absence of excessive daytime sleepiness, diagnostic testing is pursued if the patient snores and either works in a mission-critical profession (eg, airline pilots, bus drivers, and truck drivers) or has 2 or more additional clinical features of obstructive sleep apnea.

Full-night, attended, in-laboratory polysomnography (Answer D) is considered the gold-standard diagnostic test for obstructive sleep apnea. It involves monitoring the patient during a full night's sleep. Patients in whom obstructive sleep apnea is diagnosed and who choose positive airway pressure therapy are subsequently brought back for another study, during which their positive airway pressure device is titrated. Split-night, attended, in-laboratory polysomnography is similar, except the diagnostic portion of the study is performed during the first part of the night only. Those patients in whom obstructive sleep apnea is diagnosed during the first part of the night and who choose positive airway pressure therapy can have their positive airway pressure device titrated during the second part of the night.

There is no role for an ACTH stimulation test (Answer A). This patient has weight gain (not weight loss), has no other symptoms suggestive of adrenal insufficiency, and has normal blood pressure and electrolytes.

Total testosterone can be lower than normal because of obesity. Obesity decreases the serum concentration of sex hormone–binding globulin, thereby decreasing the serum total testosterone concentration, usually without lowering the free testosterone concentration. The binding abnormality is proportional to the degree of obesity and is corrected by weight loss. Therefore, before diagnosing hypogonadism, serum free testosterone should be measured by equilibrium dialysis. If it is normal, pituitary MRI (Answer B) and prolactin measurement (Answer C) are not necessary. The patient also has normal libido, which is consistent with a normal gonadal axis; the erectile dysfunction is most likely due to his diabetes and other comorbidities.

Free T$_4$ measurement (Answer E) is incorrect because the normal TSH level excludes primary hypothyroidism unless he has central hypothyroidism. However, there is no indication that he does (no history of pituitary surgery, no radiation, and no obvious pituitary hormone abnormalities).

5 ANSWER: E) Pioglitazone

Nonalcoholic fatty liver disease (NAFLD) is observed worldwide and is the most common liver disorder in Western industrialized countries, where the major risk factors for NAFLD (central obesity, type 2 diabetes mellitus, dyslipidemia, and metabolic syndrome) are common.

One of the management options for NAFLD includes optimization of blood glucose control in those with diabetes. In addition, certain antidiabetes agents have been shown to improve liver histology such as steatosis, lobular inflammation, hepatocellular ballooning, and fibrosis.

The effect of thiazolidinediones on histologic parameters in nonalcoholic steatohepatitis (NASH) was examined in a meta-analysis of 4 randomized trials that compared thiazolidinediones with placebo in 334 patients with NASH. The analysis found that compared with placebo, thiazolidinediones were more likely to improve hepatic histologic parameters such as ballooning degeneration, lobular inflammation, and steatosis. Improvement in fibrosis was not seen when all thiazolidinediones were examined, but when the analysis was limited to 3 studies that used pioglitazone (Answer E), there was a significant improvement in fibrosis among patients treated with pioglitazone compared with placebo.

The effectiveness of metformin (Answer A) for the treatment of NASH was evaluated in a meta-analysis that included 3 randomized trials of metformin with histologic data available both before and after treatment. There was no difference between the patients who received metformin and the control patients with regard to histologic response (steatosis, ballooning, inflammation, or fibrosis) or changes in alanine aminotransferase levels.

There are no available data on changes in liver histology in patients with NASH and type 2 diabetes regarding dulaglutide (Answer C), dapagliflozin (Answer B), or sitagliptin (Answer D).

Another option to treat NASH is liraglutide. In a randomized trial, 52 patients with NASH (one-third had type 2 diabetes) were assigned to either receive liraglutide or placebo for 48 weeks. An end-of-treatment biopsy was performed in 23 patients in the liraglutide arm and in 22 patients in the placebo arm. NASH resolved in 9 patients (39%) who received liraglutide and in 2 patients (9%) who received placebo. With regard to fibrosis progression, patients who received liraglutide were less likely to have progression of fibrosis.

EDUCATIONAL OBJECTIVE:
Explain the effect of various antidiabetes agents on nonalcoholic steatohepatitis.

REFERENCE(S):
  Portillo-Sanchez P, Cusi K. Treatment of nonalcoholic fatty liver disease (NAFLD) in patients with type 2 diabetes mellitus. *Clin Diabetes Endocrinol.* 2016;2(9):1-9.
  Rakoski MO, Singal AG, Rogers MA, Conjeevaram H. Meta-analysis: insulin sensitizers for the treatment of non-alcoholic steatohepatitis. *Aliment Pharmacol Ther.* 2010;32(10):1211-1221.
  Armstrong MJ, Gaunt P, Aithal GP, et al. Liraglutide safety and efficacy in patients with non-alcoholic steatohepatitis (LEAN): a multicentre, double-blind, randomised, placebo-controlled phase 2 study. *Lancet.* 2016;387(10019):679-690.

6 **ANSWER: A) 2-Hour oral glucose tolerance test**

A 2-hour oral glucose tolerance test (Answer A) (with measurement of fasting and 2-hour glucose) is recommended for all women with polycystic ovary syndrome at initial diagnosis. If this is not feasible, fasting glucose should be measured together with glycated hemoglobin (hemoglobin A_{1c}). This approach is consistent with a number of professional organizations' guidelines (eg, the American College of Obstetricians and Gynecologists, American Association of Clinical Endocrinologists, the Endocrine Society, the Androgen Excess Society) and with a consensus panel representing the European Society of Human Reproduction and Embryology and the American Society of Reproductive Medicine.

The rationale for an oral glucose tolerance test is that a standard fasting glucose measurement (Answer D) lacks the sensitivity to detect impaired glucose tolerance or early type 2 diabetes that will be present on an oral glucose tolerance test in a substantial number of women with polycystic ovary syndrome.

Limited studies have shown poor sensitivity of hemoglobin A_{1c} (Answer C) measurement for detecting impaired glucose tolerance.

In a retrospective observational study at an academic tertiary-care medical center, 208 premenopausal women with polycystic ovary syndrome underwent clinical evaluation (Ferriman-Gallwey score, BMI, waist circumference, blood pressure), hormone analyses (testosterone, sex hormone–binding globulin, fasting lipids, insulin, glucose, hemoglobin A_{1c}), transvaginal ultrasonography, and 2-hour oral glucose tolerance tests measuring capillary blood glucose at 0 minutes and 120 minutes, insulin, and C-peptide. The main outcome measures were the results of the oral glucose tolerance test and hemoglobin A_{1c} values. Type 2 diabetes was diagnosed in 20 patients based on results of oral glucose tolerance testing. The sensitivity and specificity of a hemoglobin A_{1c} value of 6.5% or greater ($\geq$48 mmol/mol) for the diagnosis of diabetes were 35% and 99%, respectively, compared with the diagnosis established by oral glucose tolerance testing.

Patients with polycystic ovary syndrome and normal glucose tolerance should be rescreened at least once every 2 years or more frequently if additional risk factors are identified. Patients with impaired glucose tolerance should be screened annually for development of type 2 diabetes.

No tests of insulin resistance are necessary to diagnose polycystic ovary syndrome, nor are they needed to select treatments. There is currently no validated test for measuring insulin resistance in a clinical setting, including insulin levels (Answer B) or glucose-to-insulin ratios (Answer E).

EDUCATIONAL OBJECTIVE:
Guide the screening for prediabetes and type 2 diabetes in women with polycystic ovary syndrome.

REFERENCE(S):

Velling Magnussen L, Mumm H, Andersen M, Glintborg D. Hemoglobin A1c as a tool for the diagnosis of type 2 diabetes in 208 premenopausal women with polycystic ovary syndrome. *Fertil Steril*. 2011;96(5):1275-1280.

Salley KE, Wickham EP, Cheang KI, Essah PA, Karjane NW, Nestler JE. Glucose intolerance in polycystic ovary syndrome--a position statement of the Androgen Excess Society. *J Clin Endocrinol Metab*. 2007;92(12):4546-4556.

American Association of Clinical Endocrinologists Polycystic Ovary Syndrome Writing Committee. American Association of Clinical Endocrinologists Position Statement on Metabolic and Cardiovascular Consequences of Polycystic Ovary Syndrome. *Endocr Pract*. 2005;11(2):126-134.

Legro RS, Arslanian SA, Ehrmann DA, et al; Endocrine Society. Diagnosis and treatment of polycystic ovary syndrome: an Endocrine Society Clinical Practice Guideline. *J Clin Endocrinol Metab*. 2013;98(12):4565-4592.

7 **ANSWER: E) TPO antibodies**

Up to 20% of patients with type 1 diabetes mellitus have positive antithyroid antibodies (TPO and/or thyroglobulin antibodies) (Answer E). Patients with circulating antibodies may be euthyroid, or they may develop autoimmune hypothyroidism, with a prevalence of about 2% to 5% in patients with type 1 diabetes. Rarely, children and adolescents with type 1 diabetes may be hyperthyroid, with a reported prevalence of about 1%, with circulating thyroid-stimulating immunoglobulins (Answer B).

About 5% of patients with type 1 diabetes mellitus develop celiac disease (gluten-sensitive enteropathy diagnosed by a positive small-bowel biopsy sample), and 7% to 10% have tissue transglutaminase antibodies (Answer A).

Less than 1% to 2% of children and adolescents with type 1 diabetes have autoimmune adrenalitis with circulating antibodies to steroid 21-hydroxylase (Answer C).

Autoimmune polyglandular syndrome type 1, also referred to as the autoimmune polyendocrinopathy-candidiasis-ectodermal dystrophy (APECED) syndrome, is a rare autosomal recessive disorder. Hypoparathyroidism or chronic mucocutaneous candidiasis is usually the first manifestation, characteristically appearing during childhood or early adolescence, and always by the early 20s. Adrenal insufficiency usually develops later, at age 10 to 15 years. Hypoparathyroidism may or may not occur in association with parathyroid gland antibodies (Answer D) that are directed against the calcium-sensing receptor.

EDUCATIONAL OBJECTIVE:
List the prevalence of various autoimmune conditions (mostly Hashimoto) in patients with type 1 diabetes mellitus.

REFERENCE(S):

Warncke K, Fröhlich-Reiterer EE, Thon A, et al; DPV Initiative of the German Working Group for Pediatric Diabetology; German BMBF Competence Network for Diabetes Mellitus. Polyendocrinopathy in children, adolescents, and young adults with type 1 diabetes: a multicenter analysis of 28,671 patients from the German/Austrian DPV-Wiss database. *Diabetes Care.* 2010;33(9):2010-2012.

Dost A, Rohrer TR, Fröhlich-Reiterer E, et al; DPV Initiative and the German Competence Network Diabetes Mellitus. Hyperthyroidism in 276 children and adolescents with type 1 diabetes from Germany and Austria. *Horm Res Paediatr.* 2015;84(3):190-198.

Likhari T, Magzoub S, Griffiths MJ, Buch HN, Gama R. Screening for Addison's disease in patients with type 1 diabetes mellitus and recurrent hypoglycaemia. *Postgrad Med J.* 2007;83(980):420-421.

⑧ ANSWER: D) Psychological evaluation

Eating disorders are relatively common in patients with diabetes, especially in female adolescents and young adults with type 1 diabetes. Eating disorders have a deleterious effect on glycemic control and on long-term outcome in these patients. One study evaluated 91 females with type 1 diabetes (mean age, 15 years) at baseline and at follow-up 4 to 5 years later. The following findings were noted:

- Twenty-six (29%) had a self-reported eating disorder at baseline, which persisted in 16 (18%) at follow-up.
- Among the patients with normal eating patterns at baseline, 15% had disordered eating at follow-up.
- Dieting or omission of insulin for weight loss and bulimia nervosa were the most common eating disorders. Bulimia nervosa is characterized by recurrent episodes of binge eating and inappropriate compensatory behaviors (such as self-induced vomiting), as well as frequent comorbid psychopathology. Insulin omission leading to weight loss is a unique purging behavior available to patients with type 1 diabetes, observed mainly in females.

Eating disorders are suspected in a patient with type 1 diabetes when there is poor glycemic control associated with recurrent episodes of diabetic ketoacidosis (due to omission of insulin) and recurrent hypoglycemia (deliberately inducing hypoglycemia through intentional insulin overdosing to justify eating sweets and high-carbohydrate meals, often followed by self-induced vomiting), frequently missed medical appointments, refusal to be weighed, and preoccupation with appearance. It is important to evaluate patients with diabetes, especially young women, for an eating disorder (or misreporting of insulin administration) and arrange appropriate psychological counseling and support when indicated (Answer D). Pharmacotherapy (Answer E) can be used at a later stage; first-line treatment is a selective serotonin reuptake inhibitor.

Switching to insulin pump therapy (Answer A) would not help, as her eating disorder must be addressed first. Her ACTH level, electrolytes, and blood pressure are normal, making Addison disease an extremely unlikely diagnosis. Thus, an ACTH stimulation test (Answer B) is unnecessary. Tissue transglutaminase antibody assessment is highly sensitive and specific for celiac disease, while the standard gliadin antibody tests (Answer C) have lower diagnostic accuracy and are no longer recommended because they yield many false-positive results leading to unnecessary endoscopy with biopsy.

EDUCATIONAL OBJECTIVE:
Screen for eating disorders in patients with type 1 diabetes mellitus.

REFERENCE(S):
Pinhas-Hamiel O, Hamiel U, Levy-Shraga Y. Eating disorders in adolescents with type 1 diabetes: challenges in diagnosis and treatment. *World J Diabetes*. 2015;6(3):517-526.

Leffler D, Schuppan D, Pallav K, et al. Kinetics of the histological, serological and symptomatic responses to gluten challenge in adults with coeliac disease. *Gut*. 2013;62(7):996-1004.

Mannucci E, Rotella F, Ricca V, Moretti S, Placidi GF, Rotella CM. Eating disorders in patients with type 1 diabetes: a meta-analysis. *J Endocrinol Invest*. 2005;28(5):417-419.

9 ANSWER: A) Now
Although the mainstay of diabetes prevention should always focus on lifestyle management, including diet and physical activity counseling, the screening guidelines vary. Current guidelines (American Diabetes Association, World Health Organization) suggest a BMI criterion of 23 kg/m² for type 2 diabetes screening in Asian Americans (decreased from 25 kg/m² in the general population) because data demonstrate that Asian Americans are at greater risk for diabetes at a lower BMI than non-Asian populations. Using a BMI criterion between 23 and 24 kg/m², sensitivity of detection is 80% for essentially all Asian American populations. Although a BMI cutoff lower than 23 kg/m² has been proposed, the specificity for diabetes detection is considerably less at 13.1%. Therefore, this patient should be screened for type 2 diabetes now (Answer A). Delaying screening (Answers B, C, and D) will not serve his best interests. Of note,

current American Diabetes Association guidelines recommend beginning screening at age 45 years, independent of BMI.

EDUCATIONAL OBJECTIVE:
Select the appropriate criteria for type 2 diabetes mellitus/prediabetes screening in patients of diverse racial/ethnic backgrounds.

REFERENCE(S):
American Diabetes Association. Standards of medical care in diabetes--2017. *Diabetes Care*. 2017;40(Suppl 1):S1-S135.

WHO Expert Consultation. Appropriate body-mass index for Asian populations and its implications for policy and intervention strategies [published correction appears in *Lancet*. 2004;363(9412): 902]. *Lancet*. 2004;363(9403):157-163.

10 ANSWER: E) Iron deficiency
Although the international standardization of the hemoglobin A_{1c} assay has decreased potential technical errors in interpreting results, there are a number of biologic and patient-specific factors that may cause misleading results.

Hemoglobin A_{1c} values are influenced by red blood cell survival. Thus, falsely high values in relation to mean blood glucose values can be obtained when red blood cell turnover is low, resulting in a disproportionate number of older red cells. This problem can occur in patients with iron, vitamin B_{12}, or folate deficiency anemia (thus, Answer E is correct).

In contrast, rapid red blood cell turnover leads to a greater proportion of younger red cells and falsely low hemoglobin A_{1c} values. Examples include patients with hemolysis (Answer C); patients treated for iron, vitamin B_{12}, or folate deficiency; and patients treated with erythropoietin.

It should be noted that hemoglobin A_{1c} values tend to be lower in pregnancy (Answer D) because the average blood glucose concentration is about 20% lower in pregnant women than in nonpregnant women, and in the first half of pregnancy there is a rise in red cell mass and a slight increase in red blood cell turnover.

Laboratory error (Answer B) is unlikely to happen twice—both of the patient's hemoglobin A_{1c} values were high at 7.8% (62 mmol/mol) and 8.5% (69 mmol/mol).

High nighttime blood glucose values (Answer A) would not likely occur suddenly and without a rise in fasting blood glucose.

EDUCATIONAL OBJECTIVE:
Identify iron deficiency anemia as a cause of falsely high hemoglobin A_{1c} values.

REFERENCE(S):
National Glycohemoglobin Standardization Program (NGSP) Web site. Factors that interfere with HbA1c test results. Available at: http://www.ngsp.org/factors.asp. Accessed for verification May 2017.

Ahmad J, Rafat D. HbA1c and iron deficiency: a review. *Diabetes Metab Syndr*. 2013;7(2):118-122.

Silva JF, Pimentel AL, Camargo JL. Effect of iron deficiency anaemia on HbA1c levels is dependent on the degree of anaemia. *Clin Biochem*. 2016; 49(1-2):117-120.

11 ANSWER: E) Proteinuria

The turnover of serum proteins, mainly albumin, is more rapid than that of hemoglobin; thus, serum fructosamine (glycated proteins, mostly albumin) values reflect mean blood glucose values over a much shorter period (1 to 2 weeks). There is generally a good correlation between serum fructosamine and hemoglobin A_{1c} values. Fructosamine responds more rapidly with changes in blood glucose control than does hemoglobin A_{1c}. Falsely low fructosamine values in relation to mean blood glucose values occur with rapid albumin turnover, for example, in patients with protein-losing enteropathy or nephrotic syndrome (Answer E). Sickle cell disease (Answer B), hemolysis (Answer C), and hypothyroidism (Answer D) do not falsely lower fructosamine. Laboratory errors (Answer A) do rarely occur, but in this case, the heavy proteinuria explains the normal fructosamine value.

EDUCATIONAL OBJECTIVE:
Identify nephrotic syndrome as a cause of falsely low fructosamine values.

REFERENCE(S):
Vetter SW. Glycated serum albumin and AGE receptors. *Adv Clin Chem*. 2015;72:205-275.

Koga M. Glycated albumin; clinical usefulness. *Clin Chim Acta*. 2014;433:96-104.

Parrinello CM, Selvin E. Beyond HbA1c and glucose: the role of nontraditional glycemic markers in diabetes diagnosis, prognosis, and management. *Curr Diab Rep*. 2014;14(11):548.

12 ANSWER: A) Both temperature and altitude

Several physical factors influence the accuracy of blood glucose strips; the most common are altitude and temperature (thus, Answer A is correct and Answers B, C, and D are incorrect).

Persons with diabetes who intend to participate in activities at high altitude or, in particular, at low temperature, should be informed that blood glucose meters may give totally unreliable false low or high readings. Glucose dehydrogenase–based meters perform better than the glucose oxidase–based meter at high altitude. However, at low temperature, all tested meters perform with similar magnitudes of discrepancy.

Temperature can affect readings indirectly as well, by influencing circulation to the skin (cold temperature), which may particularly affect results of alternate site testing.

EDUCATIONAL OBJECTIVE:
Identify environmental factors that can affect the accuracy of blood glucose meter readings.

REFERENCE(S):
Öberg D, Östenson CG. Performance of glucose dehydrogenase-and glucose oxidase-based blood glucose meters at high altitude and low temperature. *Diabetes Care*. 2005;28(5):1261.

Ginsberg BH. Factors affecting blood glucose monitoring: sources of errors in measurement. *J Diabetes Sci Technol*. 2009;3(4):903-913.

Olansky L, Kennedy L. Finger-stick glucose monitoring: issues of accuracy and specificity. *Diabetes Care*. 2010;33(4):948-949.

13
ANSWER: C) Acetaminophen

When you examine the graphs from the patient's continuous glucose monitoring, week 1 glucose levels show many spikes and week 2 control is fairly stable. This should lead you to suspect a difference in schedule or activities (lifestyle management issues) during the less well-controlled week (not an answer option) *or* interference between the continuous glucose monitor and acetaminophen (Answer C) when taken for headaches. Acetaminophen falsely elevates continuous glucose monitoring values for up to 8 hours when using the Dexcom sensor, but this is not observed with other continuous glucose sensors. Biotin (Answer A) does not interfere with continuous glucose monitoring values. If his basal insulin rates and/or boluses were low (Answers B and D), his glucose spikes would occur all the time as opposed to his fairly stable tracing in week 2.

EDUCATIONAL OBJECTIVE:
Correctly interpret data from a continuous glucose-monitoring device.

REFERENCE(S):
DeSalvo D, Buckingham B. Continuous glucose monitoring: current use and future directions. *Curr Diab Rep*. 2013;13(5):657-662.

Liebl A, Henrichs HR, Heinemann L, Freckmann G, Biermann E, Thomas A, et al; Continuous Glucose Monitoring Working Group of the Working Group Diabetes Technology of the German Diabetes Association. Continuous glucose monitoring: evidence and consensus statement for clinical use. *J Diabetes Sci Technol*. 2013;7(2):500-519.

Gilliam LK, Hirsch IB. Practical aspects of real-time continuous glucose monitoring. *Diabetes Technol Ther*. 2009;11(Suppl 1):75-82.

Maahs DM, DeSalvo D, Pyle L, et al. Effect of acetaminophen on CGM glucose in an outpatient setting. *Diabetes Care*. 2015;38(10):e158-e159.

14
ANSWER: E) Diabetic ketoacidosis

Sodium-glucose cotransporter 2 (SGLT-2) inhibitors are associated with euglycemic diabetic ketoacidosis and ketosis (Answer E), perhaps as a consequence of their noninsulin-dependent glucose clearance, hyperglucagonemia, and volume depletion. Patients with type 1 or type 2 diabetes who experience nausea, vomiting, or malaise or develop a metabolic acidosis in the setting of SGLT-2 inhibitor therapy should be promptly evaluated for the presence of urine and/or serum ketones. SGLT-2 inhibitors should only be used with great caution, extensive counseling, and close monitoring in the setting of type 1 diabetes for which their use is off-label. SGLT-2 inhibitors are being studied in patients with type 1 diabetes regarding efficacy and safety. Three SGLT-2 inhibitors are approved in the United States: canagliflozin, dapagliflozin, and empagliflozin. Dapagliflozin and empagliflozin are not associated with higher rates of fractures (Answer A), hyperkalemia (Answer B), hyponatremia (Answer D), or bladder tumors (Answer C) in studies done in patients with type 2 diabetes. Canagliflozin has been associated with hyperkalemia (in patients with moderate renal impairment and on drugs that can interfere with potassium excretion) and an increased risk of bone fractures (mainly upper extremities).

EDUCATIONAL OBJECTIVE:
Counsel patients about sodium-glucose cotransporter 2 inhibitors and diabetic ketoacidosis in the setting of type 1 diabetes mellitus (off-label use).

REFERENCE(S):
Peters AL, Buschur EO, Buse JB, Cohan P, Diner JC, Hirsch IB. Euglycemic diabetic ketoacidosis: a potential complication of treatment with sodium-glucose cotransporter 2 inhibition. *Diabetes Care*. 2015;38(9):1687-1693.

Erondu N, Desai M, Ways K, Meininger G. Diabetic ketoacidosis and related events in the canagliflozin type 2 diabetes clinical program. *Diabetes Care*. 2015;38(9):1680-1686.

U.S. Food and Drug Administration. FDA Drug Safety Communication: FDA revises labels of SGLT2 inhibitors for diabetes to include warnings about too much acid in the blood and serious urinary tract infections. December 4, 2015. Available at: http://www.fda.gov/Drugs/DrugSafety/ucm475463.htm. Accessed for verification May 2017.

15
ANSWER: C) Review the electronic medical record to see when the prescriptions for insulin and syringes were last filled

Diabetic ketoacidosis is a common, life-threatening complication of diabetes, accounting for as many as 4% to 9% of all hospital admissions for patients with diabetes. There are many precipitating causes for development of diabetic ketoacidosis, the most common being undertreatment or omission of insulin doses, the presence of comorbid conditions, illicit drug use, and previously undiagnosed diabetes. This patient reports adherence to her insulin regimen, but she is upset about her weight gain over the past 2 years and is stressed about her upcoming college exams, so the possibility of nonadherence should be seriously considered. Checking the electronic medical record for prescription refills (Answer C) is one way of assessing a patient's adherence.

Although this patient's serum creatinine is elevated, there is clear evidence of volume depletion, and this is a more likely reason for her azotemia than acute kidney injury (thus, Answer A is incorrect). Atypical antipsychotic agents have been linked to weight gain and rarely to diabetic ketoacidosis, but these instances have been in the setting of type 2 diabetes (thus, Answer B is incorrect). This patient's total daily insulin dose (0.5 units/kg per day) should be adequate to prevent the development of diabetic ketoacidosis if she were taking all her doses (thus, Answer D is incorrect). In fact, if you increase her dose and she begins taking it as prescribed, it could cause dangerous hypoglycemia.

EDUCATIONAL OBJECTIVE:
Differentiate among the common precipitating causes of diabetic ketoacidosis.

REFERENCE(S):
Steenkamp DW, Alexanian SM, McDonnell ME. Adult hyperglycemic crisis: a review and perspective. *Curr Diab Rep*. 2013;13(1):130-137.

Guenette MD, Hahn M, Cohn TA, Teo C, Remington GJ. Atypical antipsychotics and diabetic ketoacidosis: a review. *Psychopharmacology (Berl)*. 2013;226(1):1-12.

Kitabchi AE, Umpierrez GE, Miles JM, Fisher JN. Hyperglycemic crises in adult patients with diabetes. *Diabetes Care*. 2009;32(7):1335-1343.

Kitabchi AE, Umpierrez GE, Fisher JN, Murphy MB, Stentz FB. Thirty years of personal experience in hyperglycemic crises: diabetic ketoacidosis and hyperglycemic hyperosmolar state. *J Clin Endocrinol Metab*. 2008;93(5):1541-1552.

16
ANSWER: B) Zinc transporter 8 (ZnT8) antibody testing

In first-degree relatives of individuals with type 1 diabetes, screening before overt clinical symptoms develop, as occurred in this patient, can detect the disease in a clinically silent phase. Multiple positive antibodies are highly predictive of future disease development, while positivity for only 1 autoantibody may not indicate high risk. Several serum antibodies can be detected before the manifestation of autoimmune hyperglycemia, including islet-cell antibodies, insulin autoantibodies, glutamic acid decarboxylase antibodies, and antibodies to tyrosine phosphatase-like proteins. Analysis of zinc transporter 8 (ZnT8) antibodies increases the diagnostic sensitivity of islet autoantibodies for type 1 diabetes; 26% of patients with antibody-negative type 1 diabetes (negative for insulin, glutamic acid decarboxylase, tyrosine phosphatase-like proteins, and islet-cell antibodies) have ZnT8 autoantibodies (thus, Answer B is correct).

Oral glucose tolerance testing (Answer A) may uncover hyperglycemia, but it is not helpful in characterizing the type of diabetes. This patient is much more likely to have type 1 diabetes than MODY, both statistically and because of the family history, and testing for *GCK* gene mutations (Answer C) would not confirm the diagnosis of type 1 diabetes. The major susceptibility alleles for type 1 diabetes are HLA-DR3 and HLA-DR4 (Answer D), and finding them is supportive, but not specific (approximately 5% of children with this genotype develop type 1A diabetes vs approximately 0.3% of children overall), and does not confirm the diagnosis as strongly as ZnT8 antibodies.

EDUCATIONAL OBJECTIVE:
Select the best test to confirm the diagnosis of type 1 diabetes mellitus.

REFERENCE(S):

Mrena S, Virtanen SM, Laippala P, et al. Models for predicting type 1 diabetes in siblings of affected children. *Diabetes Care.* 2006;29(3):662-667.

Greenbaum CJ, Cuthbertson D, Krischer JP; Disease Prevention Trial of Type 1 Diabetes Study Group. Type 1 diabetes manifested solely by 2-h oral glucose tolerance test criteria. *Diabetes.* 2001;50(2):470-476.

Andersson C, Vaziri-Sani F, Delli A, et al; BDD Study Group. Triple specificity of ZnT8 autoantibodies in relation to HLA and other islet autoantibodies in childhood and adolescent type 1 diabetes. *Pediatr Diabetes.* 2013;14(2):97-105.

Vaziri-Sani F, Delli AJ, Elding-Larsson H, et al. A novel triple mix radiobinding assay for the three ZnT8 (ZnT8-RWQ) autoantibody variants in children with newly diagnosed diabetes. *J Immunol Methods.* 2011;371(1-2):25-37.

Vermeulen I, Weets I, Asanghanwa M, et al; Belgian Diabetes Registry. Contribution of antibodies against IA-2β and zinc transporter 8 to classification of diabetes under 40 years of age. *Diabetes Care.* 2011;34(8):1760-1765.

Gorus FK, Balti EV, Vermeulen I, et al. Screening for insulinoma antigen 2 and zinc transporter 8 autoantibodies: a cost-effective and age-dependent strategy to identify rapid progressors to clinical onset among relatives of type 1 diabetic patients. *Clin Exp Immunol.* 2012;171(1):82-90.

17 ANSWER: A) Start insulin

This patient presents with a form of type 1 diabetes that may be seen in adults, latent autoimmune diabetes in adults (LADA). Patients with LADA progress to the need for insulin very slowly, over years, or more rapidly, as in this patient. LADA may be present in up to 30% of patients with a clinical diagnosis of type 2 diabetes.

Compared with type 2 diabetes, LADA is generally associated with a lower BMI, lower triglycerides, higher HDL cholesterol, and lower prevalence of hypertension. The Immunology of Diabetes Society has proposed the following criteria for LADA: age at onset of at least 30 years, positive for at least one type 1 diabetes autoantibody, and not requiring insulin within the first 6 months after diagnosis. Many experts feel the latter criterion is too subjective. This patient's continued symptomatic hyperglycemia and lack of response to metformin are clues to the correct diagnosis. Failure to recognize it can delay appropriate treatment. The diagnosis is confirmed by the seropositivity of the antibodies (glutamic acid decarboxylase antibodies being the most sensitive immune parameter), especially if the titer is high. This patient requires insulin (Answer A) to control his hyperglycemia; no other intervention has been well studied or shown to be effective in treating LADA. Thus, adding a sulfonylurea (Answer D), a sodium-glucose cotransporter 2 (Answer B), or a glucagonlike peptide 1 receptor agonist (Answer C) is incorrect.

EDUCATIONAL OBJECTIVE:
Diagnose latent autoimmune diabetes in adults (LADA) in a patient misdiagnosed as having type 2 diabetes and review treatment implications.

REFERENCE(S):

Liao Y, Xiang Y, Zhou Z. Diagnostic criteria of latent autoimmune diabetes in adults (LADA): a review and reflection. *Front Med.* 2012;6(3):243-247.

Naik RG, Brooks-Worrell BM, Palmer JP. Latent autoimmune diabetes in adults. *J Clin Endocrinol Metab.* 2009;94(12):4635-4644.

18 ANSWER: B) Change carbohydrate ratio to 1:16

When initiating pramlintide, the current mealtime insulin dose should be reduced by 50% to avoid hypoglycemia. Pramlintide is a synthetic analogue of human amylin cosecreted with insulin by pancreatic β cells; it reduces postprandial glucose increases via the following mechanisms: (1) prolongation of gastric emptying time, (2) reduction of postprandial glucagon secretion, and (3) reduction of caloric intake through centrally mediated appetite suppression. The main adverse effect is nausea (28%-48%), alleviated by slow titration of the drug. Because of its mechanism of action and gastrointestinal adverse effects, mealtime insulin is reduced by 50% upon initiation (thus, Answer B is correct and Answer C is incorrect). Basal insulin and sensitivity factors should not be changed (thus, Answers A, D, and E are incorrect).

EDUCATIONAL OBJECTIVE:
Correctly prescribe pramlintide and reduce the mealtime insulin dose upon initiation.

REFERENCE(S):

Symlin [prescribing information]. San Diego, CA: Amylin Pharmaceuticals, Inc; 2007. Available at: http://www.accessdata.fda.gov/drugsatfda_docs/label/2007/021332s006lbl.pdf. Accessed for verification May 2017.

Messer C, Green D. A review of pramlintide in the management of diabetes. *Clin Med Ther.* 2009:1:305-311.

19 **ANSWER: A) He should consider a brief period of weightlifting before jogging to reduce the chance of hypoglycemia**

With an adequate concentration of insulin on board, aerobic activity is most often associated with a slight increase, no change, or a mild decrease in blood glucose during or shortly after the activity. Anaerobic exercise, however, often induces a rise in blood glucose levels because of the excess release of catecholamines (14- to 18-fold rise). Aerobic exercise is associated with a more modest rise (2- to 4-fold) in catecholamines. Hypoglycemia is certainly still possible with aerobic exercise such as jogging, especially if the jogging is strenuous, and there is no magic number for the ideal pre-jog glucose value that will guarantee against it (thus, Answer C is incorrect). Recent evidence has shown that including small amounts of anaerobic activity (eg, weightlifting) during aerobic exercise may reduce the drop in blood glucose levels associated with moderate-intensity aerobic exercise (thus, Answer A is correct). Eating big snacks defeats the purpose of jogging and could lead to weight gain. Increasing his basal rate after jogging is not necessary as the hyperglycemia is a rebound effect from his hypoglycemic events (thus, Answer B is incorrect). Physical activity is recommended for all patients with diabetes and should not be prohibited or avoided because of hypoglycemia (thus, Answer D is incorrect).

EDUCATIONAL OBJECTIVE:
Advise patients with type 1 diabetes mellitus about the effects of exercise on the risk of hypoglycemia.

REFERENCE(S):

Lumb AN, Gallen IW. Diabetes management for intense exercise. *Curr Opin Endocrinol Diabetes Obes.* 2009;16(2):150-155.

Yardley JE, Sigal RJ, Perkins BA, Riddell MC, Kenny GP. Resistance exercise in type 1 diabetes. *Can J Diabetes.* 2013;37(6):420-426.

Cryer PE. Mechanisms of hypoglycemia-associated autonomic failure in diabetes. *N Engl J Med.* 2013;369(4):362-372.

Davis SN, Tate D, Hedrington MS. Mechanisms of hypoglycemia and exercise-associated autonomic dysfunction. *Trans Am Clin Climatol Assoc.* 2014;125:281-291.

20 **ANSWER: C) 6.0%**

The risk of type 1 diabetes mellitus in children appears to be on the rise and can be affected by a number of factors including geography, age, sex, family history, and environment. The risk of developing type 1 diabetes increases from 0.4% in individuals with no family history of the disease to 4% to 8% in offspring of an affected parent (thus, Answer C is correct). Having an affected father confers a higher risk than having an affected mother. The risk rises to as high as 30% when both parents have type 1 diabetes.

EDUCATIONAL OBJECTIVE:
Counsel patients about the magnitude of risk of type 1 diabetes mellitus in the offspring of an affected parent.

REFERENCE(S):

van Esch SC, Cornel MC, Snoek FJ. "I am pregnant and my husband has diabetes. Is there a risk for my child?" A qualitative study of questions asked by email about the role of genetic susceptibility to diabetes. *BMC Public Health.* 2010;10:688.

Mehers KL, Gillespie KM. The genetic basis for type 1 diabetes. *Br Med Bull.* 2008;88(1):115-129.

Aly TA, Ide A, Jahromi MM, et al. Extreme genetic risk for type 1A diabetes. *Proc Natl Acad Sci U S A.* 2006;103(38):14074-14079.

21 ANSWER: C) Convert the insulin regimen to U500 insulin

Insulin is the preferred therapeutic option for patients with persistent hyperglycemia that fails to respond to other agents. However, in patients requiring more than 200 units of insulin a day, the volume of insulin becomes problematic, both in terms of patient comfort and pharmacokinetics because large-volume insulin injections are uncomfortable and poorly absorbed. For patients taking very large insulin doses, U500 insulin (Answer C) should be considered. Although the formulation of U500 is similar to that of regular insulin, the duration of action is longer, permitting adequate delivery with 2 or 3 injections per day. Use of U500 has been shown to lead to the same or better glucose control, fewer injections, and lower-volume injections than U100 insulin. A critical aspect of successful use of U500 insulin is patient education: careful explanation of the amount of insulin given per unit volume, recalibration of dosing per syringe, and instructions for administration errors are very important. Fortunately, U500 pens are now available and patients with severe insulin resistance who are good candidates for U500 insulin are not prone to hypoglycemia.

Given the severity of this patient's hyperglycemia, switching to insulin degludec, even at a higher dose (Answer D), or adding metformin (Answer A) is unlikely to achieve a target hemoglobin A_{1c} level less than 7.0% (<53 mmol/mol). Switching to an insulin pump (Answer B) is not desirable because large volumes of insulin, either by injection or pump, are poorly absorbed and are unlikely to achieve the target hemoglobin A_{1c} level.

EDUCATIONAL OBJECTIVE:
Treat extreme insulin resistance with U500 insulin.

REFERENCE(S):
Hood RC, Arakaki RF, Wysham C, Li YG, Settles JA, Jackson JA. Two treatment approaches for human regular U-500 insulin in patients with type 2 diabetes not achieving adequate glycemic control on high-dose U-100 insulin therapy with or without oral agents: a randomized, titration-to-target clinical trial. *Endocr Pract*. 2015;21(7): 782-793.

Quinn SL, Lansang MC, Mina D. Safety and effectiveness of U-500 insulin therapy in patients with insulin-resistant type 2 diabetes mellitus. *Pharmacotherapy*. 2011;31(7):695-702.

Lane WS, Cochran EK, Jackson JA, et al. High-dose insulin therapy: is it time for U-500 insulin? *Endocr Pract*. 2009;15(1):71-79.

Garg R, Johnston V, McNally PG, Davies MJ, Lawrence IG. U-500 insulin: why, when and how to use in clinical practice. *Diabetes Metab Res Rev*. 2007;23(4):265-268.

22 ANSWER: B) Decrease insulin glargine to 40 units at bedtime; discontinue repaglinide

Individuals with severely insulin-deficient type 2 diabetes mellitus can experience hypoglycemia unawareness or hypoglycemia-associated autonomic failure. Hypoglycemia unawareness is characterized by a reduction in the sympathoadrenal and autonomic responses and is more common in those with longer duration of type 2 diabetes and in older adults. This syndrome can lead to a prolonged exposure to hypoglycemia, resulting in loss of consciousness, seizures, or brain damage. However, it is possible to improve the control of glycemia and reduce the frequency of hypoglycemia with short-term relaxation of glycemic targets. This hypoglycemia avoidance includes reducing insulin therapy for several weeks to allow one's blood glucose levels to run a little higher, thereby increasing sensitivity to symptoms. Accordingly, this patient's insulin dosage should be decreased by 10% to 20% and insulin secretagogues should be discontinued (Answer B). Although approaches that discontinue the insulin secretagogue are preferred, replacing glargine with the same dose of insulin detemir (Answer C) or NPH (Answer D) would not resolve the issue. An approach that continues the use of an insulin secretagogue (Answer A) should be avoided.

EDUCATIONAL OBJECTIVE:
Manage hypoglycemia in type 2 diabetes mellitus.

REFERENCE(S):

American Diabetes Association. Standards of medical care in diabetes--2016. *Diabetes Care.* 2016;39(Suppl 1):S39-S46.

Cryer PE. Diverse causes of hypoglycemia-associated autonomic failure in diabetes. *N Engl J Med.* 2004;350(22):2272-2279.

23 ANSWER: E) Hepatic glucose output and β-cell dysfunction

Glucagonlike peptide 1 is an incretin produced from the proglucagon gene in L cells of the small intestine and is secreted in response to nutrients. Glucagonlike peptide 1 is deficient in patients with type 2 diabetes. Dipeptidyl-peptidase 4 inhibitors are a class of oral diabetes drugs that inhibit the enzyme dipeptidyl-peptidase 4. This is a ubiquitous enzyme expressed on the surface of most cell types that deactivates glucagonlike peptide 1; therefore, its inhibition could potentially affect glucose regulation through multiple effects.

Incretin-based therapies include dipeptidyl-peptidase 4 inhibitors and glucagonlike peptide 1 receptor agonists. Dipeptidyl-peptidase 4 inhibitors, through increasing endogenous glucagonlike peptide 1, can stimulate glucose-dependent insulin secretion from the β cells and can lower glucagon secretion, thereby lowering hepatic glucose output (Answer E). Glucagonlike peptide 1 receptor agonists exert the same effects and, in addition, slow gastric emptying and decrease food intake.

Dipeptidyl-peptidase 4 inhibitors have no effect on insulin action (Answer A), gastric emptying (Answers B and D), or satiety (Answer C).

EDUCATIONAL OBJECTIVE:
Summarize the pathogenesis of type 2 diabetes mellitus and the mechanism of action of incretin therapies.

REFERENCE(S):

Demuth HU, McIntosh CH, Pederson RA. Type 2 diabetes--therapy with dipeptidyl peptidase IV inhibitors. *Biochim Biophys Acta.* 2005;1751(1): 33-44.

Koliaki C, Doupis J. Incretin-based therapy: a powerful and promising weapon in the treatment of type 2 diabetes mellitus. *Diabetes Ther.* 2011;2(2):101-121.

24 ANSWER: D) Discontinuation of insulin and initiation of glimepiride

Monogenic forms of diabetes comprise a heterogeneous group of disorders. They are caused by single gene mutations and are characterized by impaired insulin secretion. It is estimated that up to 5% of all diabetes cases are monogenic and affected patients are often undiagnosed or are misclassified as having type 1 or type 2 diabetes.

Accurate diagnosis is important because of the special implications for treatment, prognosis, and familial risk. Monogenic diabetes includes MODY (maturity-onset diabetes of the young), mitochondrial diabetes, and neonatal diabetes. Many gene mutations have been identified that cause diabetes by disturbing the coupling of blood glucose concentration and insulin secretion.

The patient in this vignette has MODY, characterized by (1) young age at diagnosis, often under 25 years, (2) a marked family history of diabetes in every generation due to autosomal dominant inheritance, (3) absence of obesity and signs of insulin resistance, (4) commonly mild hyperglycemia without the need for insulin therapy and negative results for β-cell antibodies. The diagnosis can be confirmed by genetic testing where available. MODY 3 (*HNF1A* mutation [hepatocyte nuclear factor-1-alpha gene on chromosome 12]), the most prevalent MODY form, presents with early glycosuria and hyperglycemia, which is often postprandial. Optimal treatment for MODY 3 is sulfonylureas (thus, Answer D is correct and Answer A is incorrect). One study documented a significantly greater drop in hemoglobin A_{1c} level with a sulfonylurea compared with metformin (thus, Answer C is incorrect). Almost 70% of patients previously treated with insulin are successfully switched to sulfonylureas once an *HNF1A* mutation is identified. Patients with MODY 3 are at risk for microvascular and macrovascular complications of type 1 and type 2 diabetes mellitus. In addition, patients with diabetes caused by an *HNF1A* mutation appear to have an increased risk of cardiovascular mortality compared with unaffected family members. There are no data on using sodium-glucose cotransporter 2 inhibitors in patients with MODY (thus, Answer B is incorrect).

EDUCATIONAL OBJECTIVE:
Diagnose monogenic diabetes mellitus that was initially misdiagnosed as type 1 diabetes and assess the treatment implications.

REFERENCE(S):

Henzen C. Monogenic diabetes mellitus due to defects in insulin secretion. *Swiss Med Wkly.* 2012;142:w13690.

Thanabalasingham G. Diagnosis and management of maturity onset diabetes of the young (MODY). *BMJ.* 2011;343:d6044.

Wherrett DK, Bundy B, Becker DJ, et al; Type 1 Diabetes TrialNet GAD Study Group. Antigen-based therapy with glutamic acid decarboxylase (GAD) vaccine in patients with recent-onset type 1 diabetes: a randomised double-blind trial. *Lancet.* 2011;378(9788):319-327.

Shepherd M, Shields B, Ellard S, Rubio-Cabezas O, Hattersley AT. A genetic diagnosis of HNF1A diabetes alters treatment and improves glycaemic control in the majority of insulin-treated patients. *Diabet Med.* 2009;26(4):437-441.

25 **ANSWER: D) C-peptide, glutamic acid decarboxylase antibodies, and insulinoma-associated protein 2 antibodies**

Ketosis-prone diabetes, previously referred to as Flatbush diabetes or type 1b diabetes, has been increasingly recognized since the mid-1990s. In the United States, 20% to 50% of newly diagnosed patients are black or Hispanic. Although these patients present with diabetic ketoacidosis, predicting the duration of insulin therapy has been a therapeutic challenge. To facilitate the understanding of the diagnosis and insulin management subsequent to the acute diabetic ketoacidosis episode, 4 classification systems have been developed focusing on β-cell autoimmunity measured by glutamic acid decarboxylase and insulinoma-associated protein 2 antibodies and β-cell function measured by the C-peptide level (thus, Answer D is correct). The system of classification that most accurately (99% sensitivity and 96% specificity) predicts the need for insulin treatment 12 months after presentation with diabetic ketoacidosis is known as the Aβ system. Other classification systems measure BMI as a surrogate for β-cell function, but do not include β-cell autoimmunity (thus, Answer A is incorrect).

The American Diabetes Association classification measures only β-cell autoimmunity and does not include hemoglobin A_{1c} (thus, Answer B is incorrect). None of the 4 classification systems measures β-cell function with hemoglobin A_{1c} (thus, Answer C is incorrect).

EDUCATIONAL OBJECTIVE:
Choose the appropriate classification system for predicting duration of insulin therapy in ketosis-prone diabetes.

REFERENCE(S):

Banerji MA, Dham S. A comparison of classification schemes for ketosis-prone diabetes. *Nat Clin Pract Endocrinol Metab.* 2007;3(7):506-507.

Balasubramanyam A, Garza G, Rodriguez L, et al. Accuracy and predictive value of classification schemes for ketosis-prone diabetes. *Diabetes Care.* 2006;29(12):2575-2579.

Mauvais-Jarvis F, Sobngwi E, Porcher R, et al. Ketosis-prone type 2 diabetes in patients of sub-Saharan African origin: clinical pathophysiology and natural history of beta-cell dysfunction and insulin resistance. *Diabetes.* 2004;53(3): 645-653.

26 **ANSWER: A) Repaglinide**

New-onset diabetes after transplant (NODAT) occurs in approximately one-third of all patients who receive a renal transplant. Risk factors include increased age, obesity, African American or Hispanic ethnicity, family history of diabetes, and certain antirejection medications, including glucocorticoids. NODAT can be defined as the presence of diabetes symptoms (including polyuria, polydipsia, and unexplained weight loss) and a random plasma glucose value of 200 mg/dL or greater (≥11.1 mmol/L), a fasting plasma glucose value of 126 mg/dL or greater (≥7.0 mmol/L), or a 2-hour plasma glucose value of 200 mg/dL or greater (≥11.1 mmol/L) *any time after transplant.*

A stepwise approach is recommended for managing NODAT, beginning with lifestyle management and treatment with antihyperglycemic oral agents. Meglitinides (Answer A) are a good option because the risk of hypoglycemia is lower than that associated with sulfonylureas. Pioglitazone (Answer B) is not used in the setting of possible heart failure (shortness of breath, lower extremities edema). Dapagliflozin (Answer C) is not indicated when the estimated glomerular filtration rate is less than 60 mL/min per 1.73 m^2. Insulin therapy (Answer D) is initiated if oral agents have not been effective or have been accompanied by unacceptable adverse effects.

EDUCATIONAL OBJECTIVE:
Identify new-onset diabetes after transplant and recommend appropriate treatment.

REFERENCE(S):

Kasayama S, Tanaka T, Hashimoto K, Koga M, Kawase I. Efficacy of glimepiride for the treatment of diabetes occurring during glucocorticoid therapy. *Diabetes Care*. 2002;25(12):2359-2360.

Türk T, Pietruck F, Dolff S, Kribben A, et al. Repaglinide in the management of new-onset diabetes mellitus after renal transplantation. *Am J Transplant*. 2006;6(4):842-846.

Sharif A. Should metformin be our antiglycemic agent of choice post-transplantation? *Am J Transplant*. 2011;11(7):1376-1381.

27 **ANSWER: D) Insulin**
Cystic fibrosis–related diabetes (CFRD) is the result of a primary defect of insulin secretion due in part to nonautoimmune destruction of β cells (mainly) and also α cells in the pancreas, so both insulin and glucagon secretion are defective. However, histologic studies have reported variability in the degree of islet-cell destruction. This indicates there are other factors contributing to the insulin deficiency in CFRD, perhaps "collateral damage" from fibrosis and fatty infiltration or islet amyloid. The presence of CFRD strongly correlates with poorer clinical status, reflected by reduced pulmonary function and nutritional status, increased frequency of acute pulmonary exacerbations, and significant sputum pathogens. Annual screening for CFRD in all patients with cystic fibrosis is recommended beginning by 10 years of age, consistent with guidelines from the American Diabetes Association, Cystic Fibrosis Foundation, Pediatric Endocrine Society, and International Society for Pediatric and Adolescent Diabetes (ISPAD). The best test for screening and diagnosis of CFRD is the oral glucose tolerance test.

The recommended treatment of CFRD is insulin (Answer D), as this clearly has beneficial nutritional effects and probably improves pulmonary function and survival. Although hemoglobin A$_{1c}$ is not recommended as a screening test for CFRD, it is helpful in monitoring treatment, and it should be measured every 3 months in patients on insulin therapy. For patients with CFRD, experts suggest trying to maintain hemoglobin A$_{1c}$ as low as possible, ideally in the lower part of the normal range (eg, <5.5% [<37 mmol/mol]). This target is designed to optimize lung function and reduce pulmonary exacerbations.

Use of oral hypoglycemic agents (Answer B) to augment insulin production is largely unsuccessful. No data exist regarding treatment of CFRD with sodium-glucose cotransporter 2 inhibitors, glucagonlike peptide 1 receptor agonists (Answer C), or dipeptidyl-peptidase 4 inhibitors. Metformin (Answer A) is not expected to work either, and it might not be safe because cystic fibrosis is affecting this patient's liver function.

EDUCATIONAL OBJECTIVE:
Recommend the best treatment for cystic fibrosis–related diabetes mellitus.

REFERENCE(S):

Moran A, Pillay K, Becker DJ, Acerini CL; International Society for Pediatric and Adolescent Diabetes. ISPAD Clinical Practice Consensus Guidelines 2014. Management of cystic fibrosis-related diabetes in children and adolescents. *Pediatr Diabetes*. 2014;15(Suppl 20):65-76.

O'Shea D, O'Connell J. Cystic fibrosis related diabetes. *Curr Diab Rep*. 2014;14(8):511.

Kelly A, Moran A. Update on cystic fibrosis-related diabetes [published correction appears in *J Cyst Fibros*. 2014;13(1):119]. *J Cyst Fibros*. 2013;12(4):318-331.

28 **ANSWER: B) Total iron-binding capacity and serum ferritin measurements**
When diabetes is diagnosed, the possibility of secondary diabetes should be considered. Secondary diabetes occurs when a separate condition leads to hyperglycemia; these are considered distinct from routine type 1 or type 2 diabetes, although clinical features are often shared.

Broad categories of secondary diabetes include medication-induced (eg, corticosteroids), other endocrinopathies (eg, acromegaly), pancreatic diseases (eg, pancreatitis), infections (eg, cytomegalovirus), and genetic conditions (eg, Rabson-Mendenhall syndrome). One relatively common condition that should be considered is hemochromatosis, or iron overload. Primary hemochromatosis is the most common genetic disorder in the United States, affecting approximately 1 in every 200 to 300 Americans. It is more common in persons of Western European heritage. It results from increased absorption of iron through the gastrointestinal tract, with excess iron deposition in many tissues (pancreas, liver, pituitary, etc). Traditional teaching has been that hyperglycemia results from iron deposition in the pancreas, leading to islet-cell dysfunction. However, recent data suggest that the pathogenesis involves primarily insulin resistance with secondary β-cell decompensation, as in routine cases of type 2 diabetes. Secondary hemochromatosis includes conditions characterized by increased red blood cell breakdown or a history of many blood transfusions (thalassemia, sideroblastic anemia, hemolytic anemia). The clues in this case include amenorrhea (due to hypogonadotropic hypogonadism from pituitary iron deposition) and hepatic dysfunction and enlargement. The initial approach to diagnosis is assessing markers of iron stores, which can be performed by measuring the total iron-binding capacity and serum ferritin (Answer B). These 2 tests are used to calculate the transferrin saturation, a more useful indication of iron stores than either measure alone.

Glutamic acid decarboxylase antibodies (Answer A) would be elevated if this were type 1 diabetes or latent autoimmune diabetes of adults, but these diagnoses seem unlikely. Pancreatic CT (Answer C) should be considered if a pancreatic neoplasm were being considered, but there are no suggestive symptoms in this vignette. Pituitary MRI (Answer D) is done after documenting secondary hypogonadism (after checking free testosterone, LH, and FSH).

EDUCATIONAL OBJECTIVE:
Diagnose hemochromatosis as a cause of secondary diabetes mellitus.

REFERENCE(S):
Bacon BR, Adams PC, Kowdley KV, Powell LW, Tavill AS; American Association for Study of Liver Diseases. Diagnosis and management of hemochromatosis: 2011 practice guideline by the American Association for the Study of Liver Diseases. *Hepatology*. 2011;54(1):328-343.

Hatunic M, Finucane FM, Brennan AM, Norris S, Pacini G, Nolan JJ. Effect of iron overload on glucose metabolism in patients with hereditary hemochromatosis. *Metabolism*. 2010;59(3):380-384.

29 ANSWER: B) Aripiprazole

The key features in this case are rapid weight gain and development of hypertriglyceridemia since initiation of olanzapine therapy. Atypical antipsychotic agents, such as olanzapine, are now frequently used to treat thought disorders because of a lower risk of extrapyramidal adverse effects than with traditional antipsychotic drugs. However, several compounds in this drug class have metabolic consequences, including weight gain, hyperlipidemia, insulin resistance, and impaired glucose metabolism. The drugs most frequently implicated are clozapine and olanzapine. Although definitive epidemiologic data are not available, up to 30% to 40% of patients treated with clozapine and olanzapine are reported to develop weight gain and associated metabolic disorders.

In this patient, the temporal association of olanzapine initiation and the onset of weight gain with subsequent hypertension and hypertriglyceridemia suggest that use of this medication is the proximate cause of her problems. Given that there are other antipsychotic drugs that have lesser metabolic effects, it is important to communicate with the physician treating the schizophrenia in order to discuss the likely role of olanzapine in this case and explore alternative treatments. Because clozapine (Answer A) is associated with the same problems as olanzapine, switching to this medication is incorrect. Risperidone (Answer D) and quetiapine (Answer C) have intermediate effects; aripiprazole (Answer B), ziprasidone, and amisulpride have little or no association with metabolic abnormalities. Thus, aripiprazole is the best option.

EDUCATIONAL OBJECTIVE:
Manage the metabolic complications of atypical antipsychotic medications.

REFERENCE(S):

De Hert M, Detraux J, van Winkel R, Yu W, Correll CU. Metabolic and cardiovascular adverse effects associated with antipsychotic drugs. *Nat Rev Endocrinol*. 2011;8(2):114-126.

Newcomer JW. Metabolic considerations in the use of antipsychotic medications: a review of recent evidence. *J Clin Psychiatry*. 2007;68(Suppl 1): 20-27.

30 ANSWER: D) Refer to a nutritionist
The American College of Cardiology/ American Heart Association Blood Cholesterol and the National Lipid Association Guidelines recommend statin treatment for individuals with diabetes aged 40 to 75 years with LDL-cholesterol levels between 70 and 189 mg/dL (1.81 and 4.90 mmol/L) and without clinical atherosclerotic cardiovascular disease (thus, Answer B is incorrect because this patient is 32 years old). After 20 years of diabetes, it is extremely unlikely that a relatively minor reduction in hemoglobin A_{1c} from 7.2% to less than 7.0% (Answer A) would have any impact on her cardiovascular disease risk. Her previous degree of glycemic control is much more important. Without clinical albuminuria, adding an ACE inhibitor (Answer C) would not be expected to result in a cardiovascular disease benefit in a normotensive, normoalbuminuric patient with type 1 diabetes. Her BMI is elevated and her lipids are abnormal, suggesting a poor diet. She would greatly benefit from seeing a nutritionist (Answer D).

EDUCATIONAL OBJECTIVE:
Determine when statin use is appropriate as part of cardiovascular risk reduction in patients with type 1 diabetes mellitus.

REFERENCE(S):

American Diabetes Association. Standards of medical care in diabetes--2016. *Diabetes Care*. 2016;39(Suppl 1):S60-S71.

Stone NJ, Robinson J, Lichtenstein AH, et al. 2013 ACC/AHA Guideline on the Treatment of Blood Cholesterol to Reduce Atherosclerotic Cardiovascular Risk in Adults: a report of the American College of Cardiology/American Heart Association Task Force on Practice Guidelines. *Circulation*. 2014;129(25 Suppl 2):S1-S45.

Jacobson TA, Ito MK, Maki KC, et al. National Lipid Association recommendations for patient-centered management of dyslipidemia: part 1 - executive summary. *J Clin Lipidol*. 2014;8(5):473-488.

Nathan DM, Cleary PA, Backlund JY, et al; Diabetes Control and Complications Trial/Epidemiology of Diabetes Interventions and Complications (DCCT/EDIC) Study Research Group. Intensive diabetes treatment and cardiovascular disease in patients with type 1 diabetes. *N Engl J Med*. 2005;353(25):2643-2653.

Adrenal Board Review

Richard J. Auchus, MD, PhD ● University of Michigan

1 **ANSWER: C) Perform CT with fine cuts of the adrenals**

This patient has resistant hypertension and hypokalemia, and the index of suspicion for primary aldosteronism is very high. Case detection with the aldosterone-to-renin ratio is indicated and was indeed ordered. Of all medications, mineralocorticoid receptor antagonists are the most likely to interfere with screening because these drugs have a tendency to raise renin. However, if renin remains suppressed, the screen is valid despite the presence of any medications. The revised Endocrine Society guidelines recommend eliminating confirmatory testing from the evaluation when renin is suppressed, hypokalemia is present, and the aldosterone concentration is greater than 20 ng/dL (>554.8 pmol/L), as is the case in this patient (*see image*). Thus, the next step is adrenal CT (Answer C).

If the renin had not been low, the screen would not be interpretable and would require repeated testing. Volume and the renin-aldosterone axis might take up to 6 weeks to re-equilibrate after stopping spironolactone, but typically only 2 weeks, and in this case it is not required (Answer A). Similarly, discontinuation of other antihypertensive agents (Answer B) is not required for diagnosis if the renin is suppressed, and MRI (Answer D) is inferior to CT due to low resolution. The patient is tolerating spironolactone, so changing to eplerenone (Answer E), which is more expensive, is not necessary. In fact, all of the subsequent steps of the evaluation can be performed without stopping spironolactone, as long as the renin remains suppressed on that dosage. If the patient cannot or does not wish to pursue surgical management, one should continue medical therapy

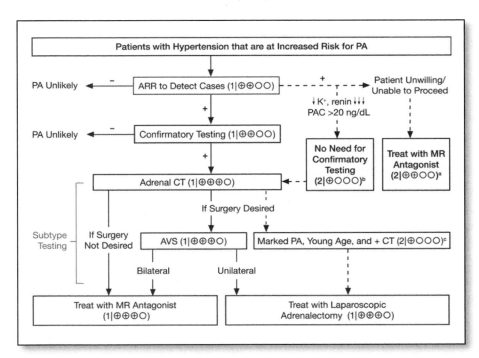

Reprinted from Funder JW, Carey RM, Mantero F, et al. The management of primary aldosteronism: case detection, diagnosis, and treatment: an Endocrine Society Clinical Practice Guideline. *J Clin Endocrinol Metab.* 2016;101(5):1889-1916.

with a mineralocorticoid receptor antagonist. If he develops gynecomastia and/or erectile dysfunction from spironolactone, then substitution of eplerenone is appropriate.

EDUCATIONAL OBJECTIVE:
Interpret screening for primary aldosteronism.

REFERENCE(S):
Funder JW, Carey RM, Mantero F, et al. The management of primary aldosteronism: case detection, diagnosis, and treatment: an Endocrine Society Clinical Practice Guideline. *J Clin Endocrinol Metab.* 2016;101(5):1889-1916.

Haase M, Riester A, Kropil P, et al. Outcome of adrenal vein sampling performed during concurrent mineralocorticoid receptor antagonist therapy. *J Clin Endocrinol Metab.* 2014;99(12):4397-4402.

Vaidya A, Malchoff CD, Auchus RJ, AACE Adrenal Scientific Committee. An individualized approach to the evaluation and management of primary aldosteronism. *Endocr Pract.* 2017;23(6):680-689.

2 **ANSWER: B) Follicular-phase progesterone**
Few women with classic 21-hydroxylase deficiency ever attempt to bear children (<25% of all and <10% of those with null *CYP21A2* alleles). For those who do attempt to have children, however, fecundity rates are close to that of the general population (>90%). Of the parameters that matter for achieving fertility, neither androgens nor the precursor 17-hydroxyprogesterone—which is characteristically elevated in this disease—are targets of therapy in this situation (thus, Answers A, C, D, and E are incorrect). Women with 21-hydroxylase deficiency can ovulate despite elevated adrenal-derived androgens. However, high adrenal-derived progesterone in the follicular phase (Answer B) has the same effect as progestin-only contraceptives, primarily unfavorable cervical mucus and endometrial receptivity. The goal is a follicular-phase progesterone concentration less than 0.6 ng/mL (<2.0 nmol/L).

EDUCATIONAL OBJECTIVE:
Titrate therapy for a woman with classic 21-hydroxylase deficiency who is attempting to bear children.

REFERENCE(S):
Auchus RJ, Arlt W. Approach to the patient: the adult with congenital adrenal hyperplasia. *J Clin Endocrinol Metab.* 2013;98(7):2645-2655.

Arlt W, Willis DS, Wild SH, et al; United Kingdom Congenital Adrenal Hyperplasia Adult Study Executive (CaHASE). Health status of adults with congenital adrenal hyperplasia: a cohort study of 203 patients. *J Clin Endocrinol Metab.* 2010; 95(11):5110-5121.

Casteràs A, De Silva P, Rumsby G, Conway GS. Reassessing fecundity in women with classical congenital adrenal hyperplasia (CAH): normal pregnancy rate but reduced fertility rate. *Clin Endocrinol (Oxf).* 2009;70(6):833-837.

3 **ANSWER: B) Measure plasma metanephrines and perform a 1-mg overnight dexamethasone suppression test**
Because of hypertension and hypokalemia, this patient was evaluated for primary aldosteronism, and the screening aldosterone-to-renin ratio is positive. Ordinarily, one would proceed to confirmatory testing, followed by CT, and then adrenal venous sampling to localize the source(s) of aldosterone. In this case, however, the weight gain, hyperglycemia, plethora, and dermal atrophy are suggestive of hypercortisolism as well. Proximal myopathy and striae are late manifestations in the development of Cushing syndrome and are insensitive findings. Because CT was performed, we know that she has a fairly large adrenal tumor—significantly larger than those that usually cause primary aldosteronism. On careful inspection, one can discern that the contralateral adrenal gland is somewhat atrophic, suggesting hypercortisolism from the adrenal tumor. When the diameter of adrenal cortical tumors is greater than 2.4 cm, the risk of hypercortisolism rises, and if the tumor is removed without testing cortisol dynamics, adrenal crisis might occur postoperatively. In addition, the CT scan in this vignette was done only with contrast, so one cannot use density to determine

whether the tumor is lipid-rich and thus exclude pheochromocytoma.

Spironolactone (Answer A) will treat the mineralocorticoid excess but not glucocorticoid manifestations and this patient needs further evaluation. Left adrenalectomy (Answer D) is incorrect because the possibilities of hypercortisolism and pheochromocytoma must be excluded before performing surgery for a tumor of that size. Adrenal venous sampling (Answer C) and a saline infusion test (Answer E) are routine in the evaluation of primary aldosteronism, but with the concern of hypercortisolism and the presence of a large adrenal tumor, measuring plasma metanephrines and performing a 1-mg overnight dexamethasone suppression test (Answer B) are the correct next steps.

In this case, the plasma metanephrines were normal, and the overnight dexamethasone suppression test resulted in a cortisol concentration of 4.4 µg/dL (121.4 nmol/L). Subsequent testing documented an ACTH concentration of 6 pg/mL (1.3 pmol/L), DHEA-S concentration of 22 µg/dL (0.6 µmol/L) (reference range, 44-352 µg/dL [1.2-9.5 µmol/L]), and normal urinary free cortisol excretion. Thus, the diagnosis of ACTH-independent hypercortisolism was established, which trumps the evaluation of primary aldosteronism and indicates that the adrenal tumor should be removed with perioperative glucocorticoid coverage. Coproduction of aldosterone and cortisol from adrenal cortical adenomas, particularly larger tumors, is well described. It is possible, although unlikely, that the primary aldosteronism is bilateral and unrelated to the adrenal tumor, so the patient should be rescreened for primary aldosteronism after adrenalectomy. If it persists, spironolactone would be an appropriate treatment.

EDUCATIONAL OBJECTIVE:
Suspect cortisol co-production in large aldosterone-producing adenomas.

REFERENCE(S):
Spath M, Korovkin S, Antke C, Anlauf M, Willenberg HS. Aldosterone- and cortisol-co-secreting adrenal tumors: the lost subtype of primary aldosteronism. *Eur J Endocrinol*. 2011;164(4):447-455.

Morelli V, Reimondo G, Giordano R, et al. Long-term follow-up in adrenal incidentalomas: an Italian multicenter study. *J Clin Endocrinol Metab*. 2014;99(3):827-834.

Fallo F, Bertello C, Tizzani D, et al. Concurrent primary aldosteronism and subclinical cortisol hypersecretion: a prospective study. *J Hypertens*. 2011;29(9):1773-1777.

4 ANSWER: D) Low plasma ACTH, low serum DHEA-S, low cortisol after dexamethasone

Most patients who demonstrate clinical evidence of glucocorticoid excess have iatrogenic Cushing syndrome from pharmacologic use of glucocorticoids. The history in these patients shows onset of symptoms shortly after the commencement of treatment. Even twice-daily inhaled glucocorticoids can cause some clinical features of Cushing syndrome such as fat redistribution and growth suppression in children. The half-life of synthetic glucocorticoids is markedly increased upon co-administration of P450 3A4 inhibitors such as ritonavir, as well as macrolide antibiotics, ketoconazole or itraconazole, and less so with diltiazem and verapamil. Given the known drug-drug interaction and temporal sequence, the probability that fluticasone is the cause of this patient's Cushing syndrome is overwhelming, and he will have suppression of the hypothalamic-pituitary adrenal axis (Answer D).

Although he might have an abnormality on sellar MRI, the history of rapid onset is inconsistent with Cushing disease (Answer A), which occurs over years. The possibility of coincidental ectopic ACTH syndrome (Answer B) in this setting is extraordinarily low. Coincidental ACTH-independent hypercortisolism of rapid onset is even less likely. If cortisol is suppressed from exogenous glucocorticoids, ACTH will be suppressed immediately, and DHEA-S will be suppressed within 4 weeks if not sooner (thus, Answers C and E are incorrect).

EDUCATIONAL OBJECTIVE:
Explain how P450 3A4 inhibitors increase the half-life of synthetic glucocorticoids and might cause iatrogenic Cushing syndrome.

REFERENCE(S):

Danaher PJ, Salsbury TL, Delmar JA. Metabolic derangement after injection of triamcinolone into the hip of an HIV-infected patient receiving ritonavir. *Orthopedics*. 2009;32(6):450.

Taylor RL, Grebe SK, Singh RJ. Quantitative, highly sensitive liquid chromatography-tandem mass spectrometry method for detection of synthetic corticosteroids. *Clin Chem*. 2004;50(12):2345-2352.

5 ANSWER: C) Serum 17-hydroxyprogesterone measurement

The presence of macroscopic fat in a large, heterogeneous adrenal mass is pathognomonic for a myelolipoma. These benign tumors are composed of blood vessel, marrow, and mesenchyme cell elements and do not make steroids. The pathogenesis of these tumors is not known, but bilateral tumors are very rare, except in patients with longstanding, poorly controlled 21-hydroxylase deficiency. This man was born in a rural area where newborn screening for 21-hydroxylase deficiency is not performed, and he has a history and electrolyte pattern suggestive of incomplete adrenal insufficiency. Because he is male, genital ambiguity would not have been present at birth. His history is typical of that of men with classic but incomplete ("simple virilizing" or "non–salt-wasting") 21-hydroxylase deficiency who are not identified at birth and can survive many years in the absence of a severe illness. Thus, the diagnosis will be established with a 17-hydroxyprogesterone measurement (Answer C).

Pheochromocytomas are heterogeneous but lack macroscopic fat. Thus, measurement of plasma metanephrines (Answer B) is incorrect. This patient has evidence of adrenal insufficiency, not Cushing syndrome, so testing for hypercortisolism (Answer D) is not useful. Paradoxically, DHEA-S (Answer A) is typically low or normal in patients with classic 21-hydroxylase deficiency and will not be diagnostic. Tuberculosis or other infectious causes of adrenal insufficiency can demonstrate enlarged bilateral adrenal glands, but macroscopic fat is not present, so a purified protein derivative skin test (Answer E) is incorrect.

EDUCATIONAL OBJECTIVE:
Describe the imaging characteristics of bilateral myelolipomas and recognize that 21-hydroxylase deficiency is a risk factor for their development.

REFERENCE(S):

Nermoen I, Rorvik J, Holmedal SH, et al. High frequency of adrenal myelolipomas and testicular adrenal rest tumours in adult Norwegian patients with classical congenital adrenal hyperplasia because of 21-hydroxylase deficiency. *Clin Endocrinol (Oxf)*. 2011;75(6):753-759.

Ravichandran R, Lafferty F, McGinniss MJ, Taylor HC. Congenital adrenal hyperplasia presenting as massive adrenal incidentalomas in the sixth decade of life: report of two patients with 21-hydroxylase deficiency. *J Clin Endocrinol Metab*. 1996;81(5):1776-1779.

6 ANSWER: E) Refer for inferior petrosal sinus sampling

This woman has convincing biochemical and clinical evidence of ACTH-dependent Cushing syndrome. In most young women with this clinical picture, the etiology is Cushing disease due to an ACTH-producing pituitary adenoma, but ectopic ACTH syndrome cannot be excluded. In addition, this patient's ACTH level is quite high for pituitary Cushing disease, and the MRI does not clearly identify a tumor. Thus, before referring to surgery (Answer B), the source of ACTH should be identified with inferior petrosal sinus sampling (Answer E).

Although oral contraceptives can cause false-positive results on dexamethasone suppression testing due to increased corticosteroid-binding globulin, the magnitude of post-dexamethasone cortisol is typically less than 5.0 µg/dL (<138 nmol/L), and the test is unnecessary given the salivary cortisol values, which are readily interpretable (thus, Answer A is incorrect). Likewise, additional demonstration of hypercortisolemia such as urinary free cortisol excretion (Answer C) is not necessary and will not identify the source of ACTH. Mifepristone therapy is indicated for patients with Cushing syndrome that is not curable with surgery or in patients who are not surgical candidates and in whom diabetes or glucose intolerance is present. This patient is a surgical candidate and is not hyperglycemic; furthermore, the starting dosage of mifepristone is 300 mg daily (thus, Answer D is incorrect).

EDUCATIONAL OBJECTIVE:
Evaluate ACTH-dependent hypercortisolism.

REFERENCE(S):
Nieman LK, Biller BM, Findling JW, et al. The diagnosis of Cushing's syndrome: an Endocrine Society Clinical Practice Guideline. *J Clin Endocrinol Metab*. 2008;93(5):1526-1540.
Ilias I, Torpy DJ, Pacak K, Mullen N, Wesley RA, Nieman LK. Cushing's syndrome due to ectopic corticotropin secretion: twenty years' experience at the National Institutes of Health. *J Clin Endocrinol Metab*. 2005;90(8):4955-4962.

7 **ANSWER: B) Intravenous low-osmolar iodinated contrast**

Patients with known or suspected pheochromocytomas are vulnerable to catecholamine crises, and certain medications precipitate an abrupt burst of catecholamine secretion. Pregnant women with pheochromocytoma are particularly vulnerable to such crises, and this population often requires treatment for nausea. Perhaps the most consistently dangerous agents are dopamine (D2-receptor) antagonists such as metoclopramide (Answer A). Intravenous glucocorticoid administration (Answer C) has been documented to precipitate crises, and a few cases of crises have occurred during oral dexamethasone suppression testing for evaluation of an adrenal mass. Glucagon (Answer D) is sometimes used during CT scanning to relax the bowels, but glucagon is contraindicated when pheochromocytoma is suspected. A glucagon stimulation test had been developed for pheochromocytoma testing, but the dangers of this test and the widespread availability of measurement of plasma or urine metanephrines have made this test obsolete. Inhalational anesthetics (Answer E) commonly precipitate a surge in catecholamines during surgery, and preoperative adrenergic blockade is used to mitigate the clinical consequences of this surge. Additional drugs that should be avoided are monoamine oxidase inhibitors, phenothiazines, and cosyntropin, as all of these agents have been associated with crises. In general, β-adrenergic blockers should be avoided until α-adrenergic blockade and volume expansion have commenced to avoid hypotension.

An old teaching claimed that iodinated contrast agents precipitate crises, but a well-designed study showed that catecholamines do not rise with current low-osmolar contrast media (Answer B). It is possible that a patient with metastatic disease and high tumor burden and who has just received chemotherapy or radionuclide therapy might have a catecholamine surge with low-osmolar contrast, which does not apply to this patient.

EDUCATIONAL OBJECTIVE:
List the drugs and diagnostic agents that should be avoided in patients with suspected pheochromocytoma.

REFERENCE(S):
Eisenhofer G, Rivers G, Rosas AL, Quezado Z, Manger WM, Pacak K. Adverse drug reactions in patients with phaeochromocytoma: incidence, prevention and management. *Drug Saf*. 2007; 30(11):1031-1062.
Baid SK, Lai EW, Wesley RA, et al. Brief communication: radiographic contrast infusion and catecholamine release in patients with pheochromocytoma [published correction appears in *Ann Intern Med*. 2009;150(4):292]. *Ann Intern Med*. 2009;150(1):27-32.
Barrett C, van Uum SH, Lenders JW. Risk of catecholaminergic crisis following glucocorticoid administration in patients with an adrenal mass: a literature review. *Clin Endocrinol (Oxf)*. 2015; 83(5):622-628.

8 **ANSWER: D) Serum DHEA-S concentration 120 µg/dL (3.3 µmol/L) (reference range, 38-523 µg/dL [1.0-14.2 µmol/L])**

The hypothalamic-pituitary-adrenal axis displays a prominent circadian rhythm, and these diurnal fluctuations in ACTH and cortisol production both guide and impede testing. A random serum cortisol measurement can be used to exclude adrenal insufficiency when it is above roughly 14 µg/dL (>386.2 nmol/L). ACTH is high in primary adrenal insufficiency and low in secondary adrenal insufficiency, and hence ACTH alone cannot diagnose adrenal insufficiency. Chances are best for obtaining a convincingly high value in the early morning. Lower random values in the afternoon are typical, and while the laboratory might report a "normal range" for cortisol and ACTH in the afternoon, this normal range cannot be used to conclusively exclude adrenal insufficiency. Because cortisol has a short half-life of 30 to 60 min, dynamic testing is most commonly used to exclude adrenal insufficiency in the afternoon. Alternatively, DHEA-S is also a measure of adrenal cortex function because it is produced in parallel with cortisol under ACTH stimulation. In contrast to cortisol, the half-life of DHEA-S is long (approximately 1 day), so little diurnal fluctuation is observed. Consequently, it is more likely that a conclusively normal DHEA-S value than cortisol value will be obtained in the afternoon, and a normal DHEA-S value in the absence of DHEA consumption excludes both primary and secondary adrenal insufficiency (thus, Answer D is correct and Answer E is incorrect). A single dose of methylprednisolone will not suppress adrenal function for more than 1 to 2 days, so random testing 2 weeks later is an appropriate screen. The caveat with DHEA-S testing is that an age-related decline occurs, such that normal values are low when patients are older than about 64 years.

An afternoon serum cortisol value of 8.0 µg/dL (220.7 nmol/L) (Answer A) might be in the "normal range" for that time of day, but the value would have to exceed roughly 14 µg/dL (>386.2 nmol/L) to exclude adrenal insufficiency. Random afternoon salivary cortisol testing (Answer B) has not been validated as a test of adrenal function, and ACTH values alone (Answer C) cannot be used to exclude adrenal insufficiency.

EDUCATIONAL OBJECTIVE:
Use DHEA-S measurement in the evaluation of adrenal function.

REFERENCE(S):

Nasrallah MP, Arafah BM. The value of dehydroepiandrosterone sulfate measurements in the assessment of adrenal function. *J Clin Endocrinol Metab.* 2003;88(11):5293-5298.

Fischli S, Jenni S, Allemann S, et al. Dehydroepiandrosterone sulfate in the assessment of the hypothalamic-pituitary-adrenal axis. *J Clin Endocrinol Metab.* 2008;93(2):539-542.

Al-Aridi R, Abdelmannan D, Arafah BM. Biochemical diagnosis of adrenal insufficiency: the added value of dehydroepiandrosterone sulfate measurements. *Endocr Pract.* 2011;17(2): 261-270.

Stewart PM, Corrie J, Seckl JR, Edwards CR, Padfield PL. A rational approach for assessing the hypothalamo-pituitary-adrenal axis. *Lancet.* 1988;1(8596):1208-1210.

9 **ANSWER: E) Acromegaly**
The mucosal lentigines shown in the photograph are characteristic of Carney complex, which most commonly results from mutations in the tumor suppressor gene *PRKA1A*, encoding the regulatory subunit of protein kinase A. Carney complex is inherited in an autosomal dominant manner, and its manifestations are caused by loss or mutation of the wild-type *PRKA1A* allele in a cell of a susceptible tissue, leading to constant and unregulated elevation of cyclic AMP. In the adrenal cortex, cyclic AMP drives the growth of adrenal cells into clusters of cell clones that show autonomous cortisol production. Thus, the Cushing syndrome associated with this condition is due to micronodular adrenocortical hyperplasia. Often the adrenal glands appear normal or just slightly irregular on CT scans because multiple small adenomas (<1 cm) form in both glands. Patients with Carney complex can develop several additional tumors such as pituitary adenomas, which most commonly produce GH (thus, Answer E is correct). Other tumors include thyroid adenomas, Sertoli-cell tumors of the testes in men, and uterine tumors in women.

Familial clustering of paragangliomas (Answer A) occurs primarily in kindreds with mutations in the succinate dehydrogenase (*SDH*) genes, and these susceptibility genes are not associated with ACTH-independent hypercortisolism. Primary hyperparathyroidism (Answer B) and gastrinoma (Answer C) are primarily components of multiple endocrine neoplasia type 1 and some other genetic disorders, none of which feature ACTH-independent hypercortisolism. Primary aldosteronism (Answer E) has

3 familial forms, but these occur in isolation without ACTH-independent hypercortisolism.

EDUCATIONAL OBJECTIVE:
List the endocrinopathies associated with Carney complex and distinguish them from manifestations of other genetic endocrine tumor syndromes.

REFERENCE(S):
Bertherat J, Horvath A, Groussin L, et al. Mutations in regulatory subunit type 1A of cyclic adenosine 5'-monophosphate-dependent protein kinase (PRKAR1A): phenotype analysis in 353 patients and 80 different genotypes. *J Clin Endocrinol Metab*. 2009;94(6):2085-2091.

Kirschner LS. PRKAR1A and the evolution of pituitary tumors. *Mol Cell Endocrinol*. 2010; 326(1-2):3-7.

10 ANSWER: B) Perform bilateral adrenalectomy

This woman has a metastatic, low-grade foregut neuroendocrine tumor with a pancreatic primary tumor. Originally, this tumor showed only features of gastrinoma, and predictably, she showed slow progression and good hormonal control with depot octreotide. With time, clones from this tumor can acquire the capacity to produce other hormones, and this patient shows rapidly progressive hypercortisolism suggestive of ectopic ACTH syndrome. Pancreatic neuroendocrine tumors that produce ACTH often co-secrete gastrin, so the index of suspicion is high for ectopic ACTH syndrome, which the history, physical examination findings, and laboratory findings corroborate. The most important point in this patient's management is that the tumor burden is not her most pressing immediate problem; rather, it is her hypercortisolism. She is at high risk for psychosis, opportunistic infections, and venous thrombosis. Prompt control of her Cushing syndrome is indicated with medical and/ or surgical management. Bilateral adrenalectomy (Answer B) is the best step now.

Biopsy of the liver mass (Answer A) will only reveal a low-grade neuroendocrine tumor. Given the delayed onset of Cushing syndrome with the preexisting tumor, it is likely that not all of the cells will stain for ACTH, and the biopsy findings would not add to the management plan. Although octreotide dose-response spans a wide range, ACTH production this high is very likely not to respond to a simple doubling of the dose (Answer C). Anthracycline-based chemotherapy (Answer D) for neuroendocrine tumors is reserved for high-grade tumors such as small cell lung cancer and is not indicated for this low-grade malignancy. Liver MRI (Answer E) is better than CT for demonstrating subtle metastases, but in this case it will not change management since the primary objective is to control the hypercortisolism. In the case of ectopic ACTH syndrome with an occult tumor source, ^{111}In-pentotreotide scintigraphy can be useful, but it rarely identifies tumors smaller than 1 cm in diameter and is rarely positive if the CT is nondiagnostic. A newer somatostatin analogue imaging agent, ^{68}Ga-DOTATATE, provides high-resolution PET/CT images and might be more sensitive than ^{111}In-pentotreotide scintigraphy.

EDUCATIONAL OBJECTIVE:
Manage the ectopic ACTH syndrome resulting from a metastatic neuroendocrine tumor.

REFERENCE(S):
Kamp K, Alwani RA, Korpershoek E, Franssen GJ, de Herder WW, Feelders RA. Prevalence and clinical features of the ectopic ACTH syndrome in patients with gastroenteropancreatic and thoracic neuroendocrine tumors. *Eur J Endocrinol*. 2016;174(3):271-280.

Ejaz S, Vassilopoulou-Sellin R, Busaidy NL, et al. Cushing syndrome secondary to ectopic adrenocorticotropic hormone secretion: the University of Texas MD Anderson Cancer Center Experience. *Cancer*. 2011;117(19):4381-4389.

Isidori AM, Kaltsas GA, Pozza C, et al. The ectopic adrenocorticotropin syndrome: clinical features, diagnosis, management, and long-term follow-up. *J Clin Endocrinol Metab*. 2006;91(2):371-317.

Ilias I, Torpy DJ, Pacak K, Mullen N, Wesley RA, Nieman LK. Cushing's syndrome due to ectopic corticotropin secretion: twenty years' experience at the National Institutes of Health. *J Clin Endocrinol Metab*. 2005;90(8):4955-4962.

11

ANSWER: C) Adrenocortical carcinoma

Functional benign adrenal adenomas nearly always produce a single active hormone as their final product. Large cortisol-producing adenomas sometimes co-secrete aldosterone, but usually one hormone excess is dominant, while the second is mild. In contrast, overt, clinically manifested excess of more than one active steroid, such as androgen and mineralocorticoid excess, is characteristic of adrenal cancer. Furthermore, the rapid progression of androgen excess alone, with very high testosterone and virilization (voice deepening), is worrisome for an adrenal or ovarian tumor. Coexistence of mineralocorticoid excess, disproportionate to the cortisol and aldosterone concentrations, suggests elevation of cortisol precursors, primarily corticosterone and 11-deoxycorticosterone. Adrenal carcinomas tend to be relatively deficient in 11β-hydroxylase activity, leading to elevation of 11-deoxycortisol and further upstream intermediates, which can account for the robust androgen and mineralocorticoid excess with normal or modestly elevated cortisol.

Macronodular adrenocortical hyperplasia (Answer A) typically manifests with pure cortisol excess, and the mineralocorticoid excess is due to cortisol and parallels cortisol production. DHEA-S is typically normal in hypercortisolemic patients with macronodular hyperplasia rather than suppressed as is often the case in hypercortisolemic patients with unilateral adrenal cortical adenomas, but this preservation of DHEA-S does not account for the profound androgen excess in this patient. While mild or nonclassic 11β-hydroxylase deficiency (Answer B) has been described, these patients have mild androgen excess and rarely have hypertension; the abrupt onset in this vignette is also inconsistent with a genetic etiology. Licorice ingestion (Answer D) can cause hypertension despite normal amounts of cortisol, but it does not lead to androgen excess. Glycyrrhetinic acid, derived from the glycyrrhizzic acid found in licorice, inhibits 11β-hydroxysteroid dehydrogenase type 2, not 11β-hydroxylase. Anabolic steroid abuse (Answer E) could account for the androgen excess but not the mineralocorticoid excess.

EDUCATIONAL OBJECTIVE:
Suspect adrenal cortical carcinoma on the basis of clinical features.

REFERENCE(S):

Arlt W, Biehl M, Taylor AE, et al. Urine steroid metabolomics as a biomarker tool for detecting malignancy in adrenal tumors. *J Clin Endocrinol Metab*. 2011;96(12):3775-3784.

Messer CK, Kirschenbaum A, New MI, Unger P, Gabrilove JL, Levine AC. Concomitant secretion of glucocorticoid, androgens, and mineralocorticoid by an adrenocortical carcinoma: case report and review of literature. *Endocr Pract*. 2007;13(4): 408-412.

12

ANSWER: B) Successful study: left adrenal gland is the source (left adenoma)

For adrenal venous sampling, the cortisol concentrations in the adrenal vein samples are used to determine whether the adrenal veins were accessed and to correct for the fractional dilution of the adrenal vein blood with mixed venous blood. This ratio of cortisol in the adrenal vein blood to the cortisol in the mixed venous blood is often called the selectivity index. The selectivity index on both sides should be greater than 2 if adrenal venous sampling is performed without cosyntropin and greater than 3 (typically at least 5) if performed with cosyntropin infusion. Otherwise, the sample does not contain sufficient adrenal vein blood to interpret the results. The study should not be interpreted unless both selectivity indices are greater than these minimum values, with the one exception discussed below. The right side, which is more difficult to access, more often fails the selectivity test than the left side. When access to the right side is successful, the steroids in the right-side sample are usually more concentrated than in the left-side sample due to the dilution of the left adrenal vein specimen from the inferior phrenic vein. In this case, the selectivity index on the right side is greater than 100, and although the selectivity index on the left side is only 8, this value is sufficient for a valid study (thus, Answers A, D, and E are incorrect).

Although the absolute value of aldosterone in the right adrenal vein sample is much higher than in the left adrenal vein sample, the cortisol-corrected aldosterone (aldosterone-to-cortisol ratio) is higher on the left by a factor of 4.1, which identifies the left adrenal as the dominant source of aldosterone (thus, Answer B is correct and Answer C is incorrect). If the aldosterone-to-cortisol ratio in one adrenal vein is much lower than in the mixed venous blood, which is called "contralateral suppression," aldosterone production can usually be confidently localized to the other adrenal, even if that implicated adrenal vein was not accessed adequately. In this case, there is also contralateral suppression on the right side, which supports a left-dominant interpretation.

EDUCATIONAL OBJECTIVE:
Interpret results of adrenal venous sampling.

REFERENCE(S):
Rossi GP, Auchus RJ, Brown M, et al. An expert consensus statement on the use of adrenal vein sampling for the subtyping of primary aldosteronism. *Hypertension.* 2014;63(1):151-160.
Funder JW, Carey RM, Mantero F, et al. The management of primary aldosteronism: case detection, diagnosis, and treatment: an Endocrine Society Clinical Practice Guideline. *J Clin Endocrinol Metab.* 2016;101(5):1889-1916.
Vaidya A, Malchoff CD, Auchus RJ; AACE Adrenal Scientific Committee. An individualized approach to the evaluation and management of primary aldosteronism. *Endocr Pract.* 2017;23(6): 680-689.

13 **ANSWER: A) Prescribe α-adrenergic blockade and refer for left adrenalectomy**
The classic presentation of pheochromocytoma involves paroxysmal hypertension with sweating and palpitations. In order to produce such symptoms, however, the tumor must be fairly large, and catecholamine production (as assessed with plasma or urine metanephrines) must be at least 5- or 10-fold elevated. Today, about 10% of pheochromocytomas are discovered incidentally as adrenal nodules found on cross-sectional imaging performed for other reasons. The imaging features of pheochromocytomas include higher-than-lipid density (>10 Hounsfield units) on precontrast CT scans and low (<60% absolute) contrast washout at 15 minutes, as is the case for this patient's tumor. Measurement of plasma metanephrines is a very sensitive test for pheochromocytoma, although fraught with false-positive results. A typical false-positive result is a plasma normetanephrine concentration less than 1.5 times the upper normal limit, whereas any elevation of plasma metanephrines must be taken seriously. His screening metanephrines are convincingly positive and of the magnitude that does not typically result in symptoms. He received α-adrenergic blockade and underwent adrenalectomy (Answer A), and the tumor was documented to be a pheochromocytoma.

For a patient with an incidental adrenal nodule, renin and aldosterone measurement (Answer B) are indicated only if hypertension and/or hypokalemia are present, which is not the case here. Neither adrenal MRI (Answer C) nor additional biochemical testing is needed as the diagnosis is already established. Pheochromocytomas grow and can be malignant, so waiting to perform a repeated CT scan in 12 months (Answer D), as is often done when biochemical testing is negative, is unwise. Biopsy of an adrenal mass (Answer E) is rarely indicated, except in a patient with suspected adrenal metastasis from an occult or recurrent malignancy, and biopsy should never be performed when plasma or urine metanephrines are elevated because of the potential for precipitating a catecholamine crisis.

EDUCATIONAL OBJECTIVE:
Diagnose an incidentally discovered pheochromocytoma.

REFERENCE(S):
Young WF Jr. Endocrine hypertension: then and now. *Endocr Pract.* 2010;16(5):888-902.
Sawka AM, Jaeschke R, Singh RJ, Young WF Jr. A comparison of biochemical tests for pheochromocytoma: measurement of fractionated plasma metanephrines compared with the combination of 24-hour urinary metanephrines and catecholamines. *J Clin Endocrinol Metab.* 2003;88(2): 553-558.
Eisenhofer G, Goldstein DS, Walther MM, et al. Biochemical diagnosis of pheochromocytoma: how to distinguish true- from false-positive test results. *J Clin Endocrinol Metab.* 2003;88(6): 2656-2666.

14
ANSWER: A) Cosyntropin stimulation test measuring 17-hydroxyprogesterone

The evaluation of androgen excess should be very simple. If cortisol production is normal and the history indicates androgen excess in early childhood, then nonclassic 21-hydroxylase deficiency should be considered. Note that "premature adrenarche" is a descriptive term that requires the exclusion of 21-hydroxylase deficiency, which was not previously the case. A morning 17-hydroxyprogesterone concentration less than 200 ng/dL (<6.1 nmol/L) excludes nonclassic 21-hydroxylase deficiency, and a value greater than 1000 ng/dL (>30.3 nmol/L) establishes the diagnosis. Serum 17-hydroxyprogesterone varies with the time of day and across the menstrual cycle. Given this patient's suspicious history and an equivocal random value of 300 ng/dL (9.1 nmol/L), a formal cosyntropin stimulation test for 17-hydroxyprogesterone (Answer A) is warranted.

Adrenal-directed CT (Answer C) is recommended if the testosterone concentration is markedly elevated (>150 ng/dL [>5.2 nmol/L]). Nonclassic 3β-hydroxysteroid dehydrogenase/isomerase deficiency is exceedingly rare and is only considered in unusual cases after nonclassic 21-hydroxylase deficiency has been excluded; furthermore, the best parameter for this diagnosis is the 17-hydroxypregnenolone-to-cortisol ratio, which must be measured together (thus, Answer B is incorrect). Plasma ACTH measurement (Answer D) will not aid in this patient's diagnosis. In a patient with childhood-onset androgen excess sufficient to advance bone age, a diagnosis should be pursued. Thus, no further testing (Answer E) is incorrect.

EDUCATIONAL OBJECTIVE:
Guide the biochemical evaluation of adrenal androgen excess.

REFERENCE(S):
Auchus RJ. The classic and nonclassic conenital adrenal hyperplasias. *Endocr Pract*. 2015;21(4): 383-389.

Witchel SF. Nonclassic congenital adrenal hyperplasia. *Curr Opin Endocrinol Diabetes Obes*. 2012;19(3):151-158.

Carbunaru G, Prasad P, Scoccia B, et al. The hormonal phenotype of nonclassic 3 beta-hydroxysteroid dehydrogenase (HSD3B) deficiency in hyperandrogenic females is associated with insulin-resistant polycystic ovary syndrome and is not a variant of inherited HSD3B2 deficiency. *J Clin Endocrinol Metab*. 2004;89(2):783-794.

15
ANSWER: A) Right adrenalectomy

This patient has early but conclusive ACTH-independent hypercortisolism. Her ACTH is low, and both serum cortisol after dexamethasone administration and 24-hour urinary free cortisol are elevated. In patients with a unilateral hyperfunctional adrenocortical adenoma, DHEA-S is often low, due to absence of ACTH stimulation. In contrast, her DHEA-S is normal, and her CT shows bilateral nodularity, consistent with macronodular adrenocortical hyperplasia. Unlike micronodular hyperplasia, these tumors are synthetically inefficient and must become large in order to cause hypercortisolemia. Unlike in primary aldosteronism, the amount of cortisol produced is always proportionate to the size of the nodules. Several studies have demonstrated that when one adrenal is significantly smaller than the other and cortisol excess is modest, as in this case, debulking or cytoreduction by removing the larger gland produces a remission of hypercortisolemia, which can last for several years. Although the contralateral gland is likely to grow over time, the duration can be many years, so unilateral adrenalectomy (Answer A) to delay iatrogenic adrenal insufficiency is preferred.

Bilateral adrenalectomy (Answer B) will render the patient adrenal insufficient and is less desirable than restoration of normal cortisol dynamics. Pasireotide (Answer C) and cabergoline (Answer D) are used to treat ACTH-dependent Cushing syndrome. Spironolactone (Answer E) might help to control the patient's blood pressure but will not treat the glucocorticoid-related morbidities.

The hyperplastic cells in macronodular adrenocortical hyperplasia often express ectopic G-protein–coupled receptors, and as a consequence, many of these patients demonstrate aberrant cortisol production in response to atypical stimuli such as vasopressin, serotonin, or LH. A significant minority of cases (20%-35%) demonstrates familial disease with autosomal dominant inheritance. Approximately half of these families have mutations in the *ARMC5* gene (armadillo repeat containing 5 gene). Mutations in the *APC* gene (adenomatous polyposis coli gene) and *PDE11A* gene (phosphodiesterase 11A gene) have also been implicated in the pathogenesis of the adrenal hyperplasia in these patients.

EDUCATIONAL OBJECTIVE:
Manage asymmetric macronodular adrenocortical hyperplasia with mild hypercortisolemia.

REFERENCE(S):
Young WF Jr, du Plessis H, Thompson GB, et al. *World J Surg.* 2008;32(5):856-862.

Perogamvros I, Vassiliadi DA, Karapanou O, Botoula E, Tzanela M, Tsagarakis S. Biochemical and clinical benefits of unilateral adrenalectomy in patients with subclinical hypercortisolism and bilateral adrenal incidentalomas. *Eur J Endocrinol.* 2015;173(6):719-725.

Hsiao HP, Kirschner LS, Bourdeau I, et al. Clinical and genetic heterogeneity, overlap with other tumor syndromes, and atypical glucocorticoid hormone secretion in adrenocorticotropin-independent macronodular adrenal hyperplasia compared with other adrenocortical tumors. *J Clin Endocrinol Metab.* 2009;94(8):2930-2937.

Assié G, Libé R, Espiard S, et al. ARMC5 mutations in macronodular adrenal hyperplasia with Cushing's syndrome. *N Engl J Med.* 2013;369(22): 2105-2114.

16 **ANSWER: C) Perform an** **^{18}F-fluorodeoxyglucose (FDG)-PET scan**
The evaluation of an incidental adrenal nodule most often involves small tumors (<2 cm) and a focus on detecting subtle autonomous hormone excess. Thus, the recommended initial screening is for hypercortisolism (1-mg overnight dexamethasone suppression test), pheochromocytoma (urine or plasma metanephrines measurement), and, if the patient is hypertensive or hypokalemic, measurement of serum aldosterone and plasma renin activity. In this vignette, the situation is a little different. The patient has a history of colon cancer and development of an adrenal mass in the last year. His blood pressure is normal, and the imaging characteristics (27 Hounsfield units, 35% washout) are inconsistent with a lipid-rich cortical neoplasm. Thus, one should be suspicious of metastasis to the adrenal.

A right adrenalectomy (Answer A) is premature until a diagnosis is made. For example, if metastatic cancer is found in the adrenal, then additional disease might be present elsewhere, and systemic chemotherapy rather than surgery would be appropriate. MRI (Answer B) might provide additional evidence for or against a lipid-rich adenoma, but the tumor in this clinical context is concerning, and the CT results cannot be ignored. Waiting a year to repeat the CT (Answer D) is inappropriate given the imaging characteristics and the relatively rapid development of the mass. Because he does not have hypertension or hypokalemia, there is no need to screen for primary aldosteronism (Answer E). An ^{18}F-fluorodeoxyglucose (FDG)-PET scan (Answer C) will determine whether the mass has high metabolic activity characteristic of malignancy, and this is the best step now. Also, because it is a whole-body imaging study, it will evaluate for disease elsewhere. Biopsy of the right adrenal mass would also be an appropriate option in this setting, but the FDG-PET scan has the added benefit of screening for disease elsewhere.

EDUCATIONAL OBJECTIVE:
Recommend appropriate use of an ^{18}F-fluorodeoxyglucose-PET scan in the evaluation of an adrenal mass.

REFERENCE(S):
Kandathil A, Wong KK, Wale DJ, et al. Metabolic and anatomic characteristics of benign and malignant adrenal masses on positron emission tomography/computed tomography: a review of literature. *Endocrine.* 2015;49(1):6-26.

Boland GW, Blake MA, Holalkere NS, Hahn PF. PET/CT for the characterization of adrenal masses in patients with cancer: qualitative versus quantitative accuracy in 150 consecutive patients. *AJR Am J Roentgenol.* 2009;192(4):956-962.

17 ANSWER: C) *VHL*

The susceptibility genes for pheochromocytoma and paraganglioma are shown (*see table*).

The *SDH* genes often cause paragangliomas, and the *NF1*, *TMEM127*, *MYX*, and *MAX* genes are rare causes of genetic pheochromocytoma (thus, Answers D and E are incorrect). *RET* mutations (Answer A), which cause multiple endocrine neoplasia type 2A and 2B, are a more common cause of bilateral pheochromocytoma, although tumors associated with these syndromes produce epinephrine and metanephrine. Pheochromocytoma is not a characteristic tumor of multiple endocrine neoplasia type 1 (Answer B). Classic von Hippel–Lindau syndrome involves retinal and cerebellar hemangiomas, pancreatic islet-cell tumors, and renal cell cancer, but pheochromocytoma can also be part of the syndrome. In some patients and in some kindreds, isolated familial pheochromocytoma is the major manifestation. In contrast to the biochemical profile of pheochromocytomas associated with multiple endocrine neoplasia 2A and 2B, the adrenal pheochromocytomas in von Hippel–Lindau syndrome produce norepinephrine and normetanephrine. Thus, given this patient's laboratory test results, the gene most likely responsible for pheochromocytoma in this kindred is *VHL* (Answer C).

EDUCATIONAL OBJECTIVE:
Compare the genetics and hormonal function of different familial pheochromocytoma syndromes.

REFERENCE(S):

Pacak K, Wimalawansa SJ. Pheochromocytoma and paraganglioma. *Endocr Pract*. 2015;21:406-412.

Fishbein L, Merrill S, Fraker DL, Cohen DL, Nathanson KL. Inherited mutations in pheochromocytoma and paraganglioma: why all patients should be offered genetic testing. *Ann Surg Oncol*. 2013;20(5):1444-1450.

Syndrome	Gene(s)	Tumor Locations	Hormone Products	Other Features
Familial paraganglioma type 1	*SDHD*	Head & neck PGL, multiple; mediastinal PGL; rarely AM	NE, DA, or none	Clear cell RCC, GIST, pituitary adenoma, pulmonary chondroma
Familial paraganglioma type 2	*SDHAF2*	Head & neck PGL, multiple; rarely AM	Unknown	Unknown
Familial paraganglioma type 3	*SDHC*	Head & neck PGL; mediastinal PGL	NE or none	Clear cell RCC
Familial paraganglioma type 4	*SDHB*	Abdominal & pelvic PGL; mediastinal PGL; rarely AM	NE, DA, or none	Often malignant PGL; clear cell RCC, GIST, pituitary adenoma, neuroblastoma, pulmonary chondroma
Familial paraganglioma	*SDHA*	Head & neck or other PGL; AM	Unknown	Unknown
Multiple endocrine neoplasia type 2A and 2B	*RET*	AM, bilateral	E>>NE	Medullary thyroid carcinoma, hyperparathyroidism; marfanoid habitus & mucosal ganglioneuromas (2B only)
Neurofibromatosis type 1	*NF1*	AM	E or E & NE	Café-au-lait spots, neurofibromas, carcinoid tumors, peripheral nerve sheath tumors
von Hippel–Lindau syndrome	*VHL*	AM, bilateral; rarely PGL	NE>>DA	Retinal hemangiomas, hemangioblastomas, clear cell RCC, pancreatic islet cell tumors, other
Familial pheochromocytoma	*TMEM127*	AM	NE & E	Unknown
Familial pheochromocytoma	*MAX*	AM, bilateral	NE & E	Moderate risk malignant
Familial pheochromocytoma	*HRAS*	AM	NE or E	Unknown
Familial pheochromocytoma/PGL	*HIF2A*	PGL, multiple; less commonly AM	NE	Polycythemia, duodenal somatostatinoma
Familial pheochromocytoma/PGL	*PHD1 & PHD2*	AM, bilateral; PGL, multiple	NE	Polycythemia
Fumarate hydratase deficiency	*FH*	Head & neck PGL; AM	NE	Papillary RCC, uterine fibroids, cutaneous leiomyoma

Abbreviations: AM, adrenal medulla (pheochromocytoma); DA, dopamine; E, epinephrine; GIST, gastrointestinal stromal tumor; NE, norepinephrine; PGL, paraganglioma; RCC, renal cell carcinoma.

18 ANSWER: E) The adrenal tumor increases her risk of cardiovascular events

The evaluation of ACTH-independent hypercortisolism prompted by the incidental discovery of an adrenocortical adenoma is slightly different than screening for Cushing disease based on clinical suspicion. For the adrenal adenoma, the dexamethasone suppression test evaluates the autonomous cortisol production when ACTH is completely suppressed, and its sensitivity is the highest among the conventional tests. Additional tests that interrogate the chronic state of the hypothalamic-pituitary-adrenal axis in these patients are a first-morning plasma ACTH measurement and a random DHEA-S measurement, which is an ACTH-dependent product of the adrenal cortex. Urinary free cortisol excretion is elevated in the minority of patients and is not a very sensitive test for detecting subtle hypercortisolism of any type.

A substantial body of literature now documents the long-term health consequences of even mild degrees of cortisol excess, most commonly derived from autonomous adrenal adenomas. These tumors are typically larger than 2.4 cm in diameter, as in this patient, and although exact minimal criteria for cortisol excess are debated, the 3 main tests (ACTH, DHEA-S, and dexamethasone-suppressed cortisol) are all consistently abnormal. The major morbidity that improves with adrenalectomy is hypertension, which this woman does not have. However, autonomous cortisol excess from adrenal adenomas is associated with a host of other conditions, such as osteoporosis, glucose intolerance, and cardiovascular events (Answer E), including death.

Retrospective and prospective studies have shown that patients without elevated urinary free cortisol excretion might benefit from surgery (thus, Answer A is incorrect), and this degree of cortisol excess can cause morbidities including osteoporosis (thus, Answers B and D are incorrect). The risk of progression in patients with biochemical evidence of hypercortisolism is at least 10% and exceeds 20% in those with tumors larger than 3 cm (thus, Answer C is incorrect).

EDUCATIONAL OBJECTIVE:
Characterize morbidity in patients with autonomous cortisol-producing adenomas.

REFERENCE(S):
Morelli V, Reimondo G, Giordano R, et al. Long-term follow-up in adrenal incidentalomas: an Italian multicenter study. *J Clin Endocrinol Metab.* 2014;99(3):827-834.

Chiodini I, Morelli V, Salcuni AS, et al. Beneficial metabolic effects of prompt surgical treatment in patients with an adrenal incidentaloma causing biochemical hypercortisolism. *J Clin Endocrinol Metab.* 2010;95(6):2736-2745.

Di Dalmazi G, Vicennati V, Garelli S, et al. Cardiovascular events and mortality in patients with adrenal incidentalomas that are either non-secreting or associated with intermediate phenotype or subclinical Cushing's syndrome: a 15-year retrospective study. *Lancet Diabet Endocrinol.* 2014;2(5):396-405.

19 ANSWER: D) Substitute prednisolone, 20 mg daily, for prednisone

Adrenal axis suppression from pharmacologic glucocorticoid dosing is common with doses exceeding 5 mg daily of prednisone or its equivalent when given for 6 or more weeks. The duration of suppression is proportionate to both the dosage and duration of therapy. This woman is clinically cushingoid with laboratory data indicating a suppressed hypothalamic-pituitary-adrenal axis yet preserved renin and aldosterone. Ordinarily, as long as the patient continues the same dosage of glucocorticoid, their physiology will not reflect glucocorticoid deficiency. In this case, however, the patient has developed acute hepatic injury and is taking prednisone, which is a pro-drug that requires conversion by the liver to the active drug prednisolone (via 11β-hydroxysteroid dehydrogenase type 1). In a patient with severely comprised hepatocellular function, this conversion is impaired, and no exposure to active drug results. Switching to an active form of glucocorticoid such as prednisolone (Answer D) will provide drug exposure. Any other active glucocorticoid such as hydrocortisone, methylprednisolone, or dexamethasone at appropriate dosages would also be correct but were not options.

Further testing (Answers A and E) is not necessary given the history, low ACTH and cortisol, and high renin and aldosterone (thus, Answers A and E are incorrect). Fludrocortisone at a dosage of 0.1 mg twice daily (Answer B) adds little to the aldosterone in her circulation and provides negligible glucocorticoid exposure. A higher prednisone dosage (Answer C) is not likely to help given the impaired liver function.

EDUCATIONAL OBJECTIVE:
Choose glucocorticoid drugs in patients with liver failure.

REFERENCE(S):

Tomlinson JW, Walker EA, Bujalska IJ, et al. 11beta-hydroxysteroid dehydrogenase type 1: a tissue-specific regulator of glucocorticoid response. *Endocr Rev*. 2004;25(5):831-866.

Frey BM, Frey FJ. Clinical pharmacokinetics of prednisone and prednisolone. *Clin Pharmacokinet*. 1990;19(2):126-146.

Madsbad S, Bjerregaard B, Henriksen JH, Juhl E, Kehlet H. Impaired conversion of prednisone to prednisolone in patients with liver cirrhosis. *Gut*. 1980;21:52-56.

20 **ANSWER: A) 24-Hour urinary aldosterone and sodium measurement on the third day of a high-salt diet**

For this patient with resistant hypertension, the index of suspicion for primary aldosteronism is high. Nevertheless, the differential diagnosis of resistant hypertension also includes alcohol abuse, medication nonadherence, sleep apnea, and renal insufficiency. Her screening aldosterone-to-renin ratio is at least 23, which is positive; however, this ratio has sensitivity and specificity of only about 80% at a cutoff of 20. For this reason, the guidelines recommend confirmatory testing as the second step in the evaluation, unless the serum aldosterone is greater than 20 ng/dL (554.8 pmol/L) with a suppressed renin and a history of hypokalemia.

An MR-angiogram (Answer B) is appropriate if the renin activity is high, but in this case it is low. Adrenal CT (Answer C) and adrenal venous sampling (Answer E) should be obtained only after the diagnosis is confirmed. While a 1-mg overnight dexamethasone suppression test (Answer D) is sometimes part of the workup, it is not used until the diagnosis is confirmed. The confirmatory tests include:

Saline infusion (2 L over 4 hours); positive = serum aldosterone = >10 ng/dL (>277.4 pmol/L)

24-Hour urinary aldosterone measurement on high-salt diet; positive = urinary aldosterone >12-14 µg/24 h (>33.2-38.8 nmol/d) (Answer A)

Fludrocortisone suppression test; positive = serum aldosterone >6 ng/dL (>166.4 pmol/L)

Captopril challenge test; positive = no fall in serum aldosterone

EDUCATIONAL OBJECTIVE:
Follow the steps in the evaluation of primary aldosteronism.

REFERENCE(S):

Funder JW, Carey RM, Mantero F, et al. The management of primary aldosteronism: case detection, diagnosis, and treatment: an Endocrine Society Clinical Practice Guideline. *J Clin Endocrinol Metab*. 2016;101(5):1889-1916.

Nishizaka MK, Pratt-Ubunama M, Zaman MA, Cofield S, Calhoun DA. Validity of plasma aldosterone-to-renin activity ratio in African American and white subjects with resistant hypertension. *Am J Hypertens*. 2005;18(6): 805-812.

21 **ANSWER: C) Change the hydrocortisone regimen to 20 mg 3 times daily**

Mitotane therapy is typically prescribed for residual adrenal cancer following debulking surgery. Mitotane has a number of adverse effects and alters endocrine laboratory tests through a variety of mechanisms, including direct adrenal cytotoxicity. This patient had Cushing syndrome before surgery, and debulking has left him with adrenal insufficiency and a suppressed hypothalamic-pituitary-adrenal axis, as evidenced by the undetectable plasma ACTH. At the same time, mitotane markedly increases corticosteroid-binding globulin and potently induces expression of P450 3A4, a major enzyme in cortisol catabolism. As a consequence, the dosage requirement and frequency for oral hydrocortisone increases markedly with concomitant mitotane therapy, and this patient's symptoms of adrenal insufficiency are due to inadequate cortisol exposure (thus, Answer C is correct).

Mitotane rarely causes aldosterone deficiency, and fludrocortisone at the dosage of 0.1 mg daily (Answer A) will not provide significant glucocorticoid effect. This patient is at high risk of cancer recurrence, and reducing the mitotane dosage (Answer B) will result in subtherapeutic drug levels, which is unwise. Hypogonadism and gynecomastia can occur with mitotane therapy, due to a rise in sex hormone–binding globulin and some inhibition of testosterone synthesis, but his testosterone and inferred bioavailable testosterone are only slightly reduced and do not account for his symptoms. Thus, both testosterone enanthate (Answer D) and anastrozole (Answer E) are incorrect.

EDUCATIONAL OBJECTIVE:
Adjust the dosage of hydrocortisone during mitotane therapy for adrenal carcinoma.

REFERENCE(S):

Chortis V, Taylor AE, Schneider P, et al. Mitotane therapy in adrenocortical cancer induces CYP3A4 and inhibits 5α-reductase, explaining the need for personalized glucocorticoid and androgen replacement. *J Clin Endocrinol Metab*. 2013;98(1):161-171.

Kroiss M, Quinkler M, Lutz WK, Allolio B, Fassnacht M. Drug interactions with mitotane by induction of CYP3A4 metabolism in the clinical management of adrenocortical carcinoma. *Clin Endocrinol (Oxf)*. 2011;75(5):585-591.

Else T, Kim AC, Sabolch A, et al. Adrenocortical carcinoma. *Endocr Rev*. 2014;35(2):282-326.

22 **ANSWER: D) Normal serum potassium**
Mifepristone is a competitive antagonist for both the glucocorticoid receptor and the progesterone receptor, but it does not block cortisol action on the mineralocorticoid receptor. It is used for the treatment of Cushing syndrome in patients with glucose intolerance or diabetes mellitus. Because mifepristone also antagonizes the feedback inhibition of cortisol on the adenoma, ACTH and cortisol production often rise in Cushing disease on treatment but not enough to offset the beneficial effects of glucocorticoid receptor blockade in peripheral tissues. Consequently, serum cortisol and plasma ACTH tend to rise and exert even greater effects on the mineralocorticoid receptor, which can cause hypokalemia and hypertension. For this reason, serum potassium must be corrected before starting mifepristone (thus, Answer D is correct and Answer E is incorrect). Because of potent progesterone receptor antagonism, menses cease and pregnancy is not possible during mifepristone therapy. Mifepristone will cause abortion in a pregnant woman. Therefore, a negative pregnancy test was documented in this patient before starting therapy, but additional contraception is unnecessary (thus, Answer A is incorrect). In addition, endometrial hypertrophy and vaginal bleeding can occur weeks to months after starting therapy and should be monitored. Blood pressure occasionally rises but more commonly decreases after several weeks of treatment. This patient's degree of blood pressure control is acceptable for starting therapy (thus, Answer B is incorrect). When elevated, serum glucose decreases rapidly with mifepristone treatment, and the improved glycemic control is a reliable indicator of therapeutic effect. In fact, patients treated with insulin and hypoglycemic agents other than metformin should reduce their dosages before commencing mifepristone, and normalizing blood glucose with these agents before starting therapy can lead to dangerous hypoglycemia (thus, Answer C is incorrect). Additional parameters to monitor as indications of therapeutic response include weight loss, improvement in cognition and depression (when present), and regression of cushingoid features, but these changes take much longer than the immediate reduction in glucose.

EDUCATIONAL OBJECTIVE:
Identify contraindications and precautions when using mifepristone therapy for Cushing disease.

REFERENCE(S):

Castinetti F, Fassnacht M, Johanssen S, et al. Merits and pitfalls of mifepristone in Cushing's syndrome. *Eur J Endocrinol*. 2009;160(6):1003-1010.

Fleseriu M, Biller BM, Findling JW, Molitch ME, Schteingart DE, Gross C; SEISMIC Study Investigators. Mifepristone, a glucocorticoid receptor antagonist, produces clinical and metabolic benefits in patients with Cushing's syndrome. *J Clin Endocrinol Metab*. 2012;97(6): 2039-2049.

23 **ANSWER: E) No changes**
Primary aldosteronism elicits more end-organ damage than equivalent degrees of essential hypertension, particularly on the kidney, heart, and vasculature. Proteinuria and renal insufficiency are common complications that improve with targeted treatment, either surgery or mineralocorticoid receptor antagonist therapy. Similar to the early stages of diabetic nephropathy, primary aldosteronism is a state of renal hyperfiltration, and targeted therapy often uncovers occult renal damage, manifest as a rise in serum creatinine. In an older individual with longstanding hypertension and evidence of renal damage, a rise in creatinine is expected with surgical cure or medical treatment of primary aldosteronism with a mineralocorticoid receptor antagonist. The goals of medical therapy are to normalize blood pressure and serum potassium and stabilize renal deterioration. Most authorities also target to increase plasma renin at least to measurable levels, but the increase in renin can take months to years. Consequently, given normal blood pressure and serum potassium on this regimen, the rise in creatinine to a new stable value is expected, and no changes should be made (Answer E).

Reducing the eplerenone dosage to 50 mg daily (Answer A), which did not previously adequately control his blood pressure, is a mistake. It should be noted that dosage adjustments of a mineralocorticoid receptor antagonist should be made slowly, with gradual up-titration, as several weeks are required to observe steady-state changes in blood pressure, as was done in this case. Spironolactone is, if anything, more potent on a milligram-for-milligram basis, and the dosage of 100 mg daily (Answer B) might be excessive and cause hyperkalemia. In addition, there is no reason to change. Given his age and duration of hypertension, he is likely to have a degree of fixed hypertension even with proper treatment of the primary aldosteronism, and his blood pressure would most likely rise if amlodipine is discontinued (Answer C). Eplerenone should not be discontinued (Answer D). A β-adrenergic blocker such as atenolol, which lowers plasma renin, is often used in high-renin hypertension.

EDUCATIONAL OBJECTIVE:
Titrate medical therapy for primary aldosteronism.

REFERENCE(S):
Reincke M, Rump LC, Quinkler M, et al; Participants of German Conn's Registry. Risk factors associated with a low glomerular filtration rate in primary aldosteronism. *J Clin Endocrinol Metab.* 2009;94(3):869-875.

Fourkiotis V, Vonend O, Diederich S, et al; Mephisto Study Group. Effectiveness of eplerenone or spironolactone in preserving renal function in primary aldosteronism. *Eur J Endocrinol.* 2012;168(1):75-81.

Sechi LA, Colussi G, Di Fabio A, Catena C. Cardiovascular and renal damage in primary aldosteronism: outcomes after treatment. *Am J Hypertens.* 2010;23(12):1253-1260.

24 **ANSWER: E) Adrenal CT**
The clinical presentation with hyponatremia, hypokalemia, nausea, and vomiting suggests primary adrenal insufficiency of acute onset. The differential diagnosis for this condition is narrow and includes adrenal infarction or hemorrhage, pituitary apoplexy, and withdrawal of long-term pharmacologic glucocorticoids. Although this patient was treated with prednisone in the past, the course was completed some time ago, and her ACTH is high, not low. Thus, a urine synthetic glucocorticoid screen (Answer C) and pituitary MRI (Answer B) are incorrect. Risk factors for adrenal hemorrhage include the antiphospholipid syndrome, anticoagulation, and sepsis, especially meningococcemia. She has 2 of these risk factors, and adrenal CT (Answer E) will reveal enlarged and poorly enhancing adrenal glands. Serum DHEA-S measurement might be confirmatory but it is unnecessary given the high ACTH and low cortisol. Autoimmune adrenalitis is of gradual onset and is not more common in patients with lupus, so assessment for 21-hydroxylase antibodies (Answer D) is incorrect.

EDUCATIONAL OBJECTIVE:
Identify risk factors for bilateral adrenal hemorrhage.

REFERENCE(S):

Bornstein SR, Allolio B, Arlt W, et al. Diagnosis and treatment of primary adrenal insufficiency: an Endocrine Society Clinical Practice Guideline. *J Clin Endocrinol Metab*. 2016;101(2):364-389.

Charmandari E, Nicolaides NC, Chrousos GP. Adrenal insufficiency. *Lancet*. 2014;383(9935): 2152-2167.

Ramon I, Mathian A, Bachelot A, et al. Primary adrenal insufficiency due to bilateral adrenal hemorrhage-adrenal infarction in the antiphospholipid syndrome: long-term outcome of 16 patients. *J Clin Endocrinol Metab*. 2013;98(8): 3179-3189.

25 ANSWER: D) Decrease in testosterone

This man has ectopic ACTH syndrome, a characteristic paraneoplastic syndrome from small cell lung cancer, which is a type of high-grade neuroendocrine tumor. Ketoconazole inhibits several enzymes in cortisol biosynthesis, primarily P450 17A1 (17-hydroxylase/17,20-lyase), P450 11A1 (cholesterol side-chain cleavage enzyme), and P450 11B1 (11β-hydroxylase). For this reason, ketoconazole is used off-label to treat Cushing syndrome, but it has also been used to treat prostate cancer because inhibition of P450 17A1 and P450 11A1 rapidly and effectively lowers testosterone production at these dosages (Answer D). Consequently, men with hypercortisolemia managed with ketoconazole often require testosterone supplementation.

Metyrapone and osilodrostat primarily inhibit P450 11B1 and thus increase 11-deoxycortisol, but ketoconazole simultaneously inhibits P450 11A1 and P450 17A1, preventing a rise in 11-deoxycortisol (thus, Answer A is incorrect). Although ACTH can rise with medical therapy in Cushing disease, this rise does not occur in ectopic ACTH syndrome due to neuroendocrine carcinomas (thus, Answer B is incorrect). An increase in corticosteroid-binding globulin is seen with mitotane, but no change occurs with ketoconazole per se (thus, Answer E is incorrect). Ketoconazole can cause gynecomastia due to disproportionate reduction in testosterone relative to slight reductions in estradiol, but estradiol does not rise with treatment (thus, Answer C is incorrect).

EDUCATIONAL OBJECTIVE:
Anticipate side effects of ketoconazole therapy for Cushing syndrome.

REFERENCE(S):

Valassi E, Crespo I, Gich I, Rodriguez J, Webb SM. A reappraisal of the medical therapy with steroidogenesis inhibitors in Cushing's syndrome. *Clin Endocrinol (Oxf)*. 2012;77(5):735-742.

Castinetti F, Guignat L, Giraud P, et al. Ketoconazole in Cushing's disease: is it worth a try? *J Clin Endocrinol Metab*. 2014;99(5):1623-1630.

Fleseriu M. Medical treatment of Cushing disease: new targets, new hope. *Endocrinol Metab Clin North Am*. 2015;44(1):51-70.

Ryan CJ, Halabi S, Ou SS, Vogelzang NJ, Kantoff P, Small EJ. Adrenal androgen levels as predictors of outcome in prostate cancer patients treated with ketoconazole plus antiandrogen withdrawal: results from a cancer and leukemia group B study. *Clin Cancer Res*. 2007;13(7):2030-2037.

Calcium and Bone Board Review

Carolyn B. Becker, MD ● Brigham & Women's Hospital

1 ANSWER: C) Genetic testing for a calcium-sensing receptor (*CASR*) mutation

Does this patient have familial hypocalciuric hypercalcemia (FHH) or primary hyperparathyroidism? Answering this question might be easier if she had documentation of previous serum calcium measurements (normal serum calcium values in the past would make FHH unlikely) or relatives in whom serum calcium measurements could be obtained. She is young (<50 years), so surgery would be recommended if she has primary hyperparathyroidism. However, surgery should not be performed until her diagnosis is confirmed (thus, Answer A is incorrect). Similarly, neither imaging with a sestamibi scan (Answer D) nor bone mineral density testing (Answer B) should be done until FHH is ruled out. Continued annual monitoring (Answer E) will not provide any additional information.

The 24-hour urine calcium-to-creatinine clearance ratio is the key to consideration of FHH and came back low at 0.01. The result is calculated as follows: [urine calcium (mg/24 h) × serum creatinine (mg/dL)] / [urine creatinine (mg/24 h) × serum calcium (mg/dL)].

The most common form of FHH, known as FHH type 1, is caused by inactivating mutations in the gene encoding the calcium-sensing receptor (*CASR*). Recently, mutations in the *GNA11* gene have been shown to cause FHH type 2. Additionally, mutations affecting codon 15 in the *AP2S1* gene have been described as FHH type 3.

Persons with FHH continue to secrete PTH because the inactivated calcium-sensing receptor is reading a low serum calcium level. This also occurs in the renal tubular calcium-sensing receptor where it leads to renal calcium conservation (decreased renal calcium excretion). The end result is hypercalcemia and hypocalciuria. A low ratio of calcium clearance to creatinine clearance (<0.01)

is consistent with FHH and should be followed by confirmatory genetic testing.

If the patient has FHH, one of her parents most likely had the same mutation, as transmission is autosomal dominant (although this cannot be confirmed because her parents are deceased). Several different mutations have been described, and a negative result for any of the known mutations would not conclusively exclude FHH. Because primary hyperparathyroidism is much more common than FHH, should the diagnosis still be unclear after genetic testing for a *CASR* mutation, parathyroid surgery should be strongly considered in view of her young age.

EDUCATIONAL OBJECTIVE:
Distinguish familial hypocalciuric hypercalcemia from primary hyperparathyroidism.

REFERENCE(S):

Hovden S, Rejnmark L, Ladefoged SA, Nissen PH. AP2S1 and NA11 mutations – not a common cause of familial hypocalciuric hypercalcemia. *Eur J Endocrinol.* 2017;176(2):177-185.

Christensen SE, Nissen PH, Vestergaard P, Mosekilde L. Familial hypocalciuric hypercalcemia: a review. *Curr Opin Endocrinol Diabetes Obes.* 2011;18(5):359-370.

Eastell R, Arnold A, Brandi ML, et al. Diagnosis of asymptomatic primary hyperparathyroidism: proceedings of the Third International Workshop. *J Clin Endocrinol Metab.* 2009;94(2):340-350.

Shinall MC Jr, Dahir KM, Broome JT. Differentiating familial hypocalciuric hypercalcemia from primary hyperparathyroidism. *Endocr Pract.* 2013;19(4):697-702.

2 **ANSWER: A) Begin alendronate**
This man has an acute vertebral compression fracture at L1 that is symptomatic. This warrants intervention with antiresorptive therapy regardless of the DXA results because vertebral fractures are strong independent predictors of both future vertebral and nonvertebral fractures. Repeating the DXA now (Answer E) is unlikely to be helpful given his degenerative arthritis at the spine and the results will not change recommended therapy. The correct answer is to begin alendronate (Answer A) because it is an approved and effective therapy in this setting.

Teriparatide (Answer C) is contraindicated in a man who has received pelvic irradiation. Invasive procedures, such as bone biopsy and kyphoplasty (Answer D), are not indicated in the acute setting given the absence of clinical or biochemical evidence of recurrent prostate cancer (normal prostate-specific antigen and alkaline phosphatase levels) or other malignancy. Patients with acute vertebral fractures from osteoporosis should generally not be referred for vertebral augmentation (kyphoplasty or vertebroplasty) unless severe pain has not responded to medical therapies.

Because there are no large randomized controlled trials showing antifracture efficacy for testosterone in men with osteoporosis, testosterone therapy (Answer B) should be considered only for hypogonadal men who are symptomatic, have an organic cause for the hypogonadism, have testosterone levels less than 200 ng/dL (<6.9 nmol/L), and/or are not candidates for other therapies. Due to reports of cardiovascular complications, testosterone is not an ideal therapy for an 80-year-old man. In hypogonadal men with benign prostatic hypertrophy, testosterone therapy along with a 5a-reductase inhibitor such as finasteride has been given without exacerbating benign prostatic hypertrophy. However, even men with marked hypogonadism have good skeletal responses to bisphosphonate therapy without correction of the hypogonadism.

EDUCATIONAL OBJECTIVE:
Manage an acute vertebral fracture in an elderly man.

REFERENCE(S):
Watts NB, Adler RA, Bilezikian JP, et al; Endocrine Society. Osteoporosis in men: an Endocrine Society clinical practice guideline. *J Clin Endocrinol Metab.* 2012;97(6):1802-1822.

Cosman F, de Beur SJ, LeBoff MS, et al; National Osteoporosis Foundation. Clinician's guide to prevention and treatment of osteoporosis. *Osteoporos Int.* 2014;25(10):2359-2381.

McConnell CT Jr, Wippold FJ 2nd, Ray CE Jr, et al. ACR appropriateness criteria for management of vertebral compression fractures. *J Am Coll Radiol.* 2014;11(8):757-763.

3 **ANSWER: E) Decrease the cinacalcet dosage**
The PTH level in this patient is lower than the goal in patients undergoing dialysis and may indicate underlying adynamic bone disease. Because of the low PTH and hypocalcemia, the cinacalcet dosage should be decreased (Answer E). Adynamic bone disease, a type of renal osteodystrophy (now called chronic kidney disease–mineral bone disorder [CKD-MBD]), is present in at least one-third of patients receiving dialysis. Adynamic bone disease is characterized by markedly low bone turnover, no accumulation of osteoid, and high fracture risk. Serum PTH levels in adynamic bone disease are relatively low (usually <100 pg/mL [<100 ng/L]) compared with levels in patients undergoing dialysis who have other forms of CKD-MBD.

In patients with end-stage kidney disease, there is resistance to PTH due at least in part to increased N-terminal truncated PTH (7-84), which counteracts the effect of the 1-84 whole molecule on bone. This can be exacerbated by the use of cinacalcet, as well as overly aggressive treatment with calcitriol, both of which reduce PTH secretion. This patient's low alkaline phosphatase level is also consistent with a low bone turnover state.

Increasing the calcitriol dosage (Answer A) would further suppress PTH, which is not a desired outcome. Decreasing the calcitriol dosage (Answer B) may worsen the hypocalcemia. Teriparatide (Answer C) has been used anecdotally in some patients with end-stage renal disease, low bone turnover, and fractures, but it is not an approved therapy in this context. Although denosumab (Answer D) can be used in patients receiving dialysis, it would be inappropriate to administer it now in the face of hypocalcemia, vitamin D deficiency, and probable adynamic bone disease. A potent antiresorptive agent would theoretically worsen the adynamic bone disease and increase fracture risk.

Impaired mineralization, osteitis fibrosa cystica, and mixed renal osteodystrophy are other forms of CKD-MBD, but these diagnoses are unlikely given the laboratory findings (osteitis fibrosa cystica and high bone turnover would be associated with an elevated PTH level; osteomalacia would be associated with a very low 25-hydroxyvitamin D level; and mixed renal osteodystrophy would have both).

EDUCATIONAL OBJECTIVE:
Diagnose and manage adynamic bone disease in a patient undergoing dialysis.

REFERENCE(S):

Cannata-Andía JB, Rodriguez García M, Gómez Alonso C. Osteoporosis and adynamic bone in chronic kidney disease. *J Nephrol.* 2013;26(1):73-80.

Hruska KA, Mathew S. Chronic kidney disease mineral bone disorder (CKD-MBD). In: Rosen CJ, Compston JE, Lian JB, eds. *Primer on the Metabolic Bone Diseases and Disorders of Mineral Metabolism.* Washington, DC: The American Society for Bone and Mineral Research; 2008:343-349.

Brandenburg VM, Floege J. Adynamic bone disease: bone and beyond. *Clin Kidney J.* 2008;1:135-147.

Kidney Disease: Improving Global Outcomes (KDIGO) CKD-MBD Work Group. KDIGO clinical practice guideline for the diagnosis, evaluation, prevention, and treatment of chronic kidney disease-mineral and bone disorder (CKD-MBD). *Kidney Int.* 2009;(Suppl 113): S1-S130.

4 **ANSWER: C) Sestamibi scan**
This patient has mild, asymptomatic primary hyperparathyroidism. Reduced renal function, (estimated glomerular filtration rate <60 mL/min per 1.73 m²), which this patient has, is one of the major criteria for recommending parathyroid surgery in asymptomatic patients. Some studies suggest that parathyroidectomy can halt the deterioration of renal function in primary hyperparathyroidism. Parathyroidectomy with identification of all parathyroid glands (Answer B) would be the best answer if a localizing study such as a sestamibi scan (Answer C) were "nonlocalizing." Otherwise, most patients and surgeons prefer minimally invasive parathyroidectomy, which requires a positive localization study (sestamibi or neck ultrasonography) before surgery. Up to 20% of patients with biochemically proven primary hyperparathyroidism have a nonlocalizing sestamibi scan.

This patient's 1,25-dihydroxyvitamin D level (Answer A) could be low, normal, or high, but determining this value will not help in the management decision. Rechecking calcium, creatinine, and PTH in 6 months (Answer E) is not appropriate because she meets criteria for surgery now. Renal ultrasonography (Answer D) would be useful if her history were positive for nephrolithiasis or nephrocalcinosis, or if her urinary studies were concerning for stones (eg, calcium excretion >400 mg/24 h and abnormal urine stone risk analysis).

Criteria for parathyroid surgery in patients with asymptomatic primary hyperparathyroidism include the following:

- Age <50 years
- Serum calcium >1 mg/dL above upper normal limit
- T score less than –2.5 at any skeletal site on DXA or vertebral compression fracture identified on imaging
- Creatinine clearance <60 mL/min per 1.73 m²
- Kidney stones on imaging or nephrocalcinosis
- Urinary calcium excretion >400 mg/24 h and increased stone risk by biochemical stone risk analysis

EDUCATIONAL OBJECTIVE:
Identify decreased glomerular filtration rate as a criterion for parathyroid surgery in primary hyperparathyroidism and define the role of preoperative imaging.

REFERENCE(S):

Eastell R, Brandi ML, Costa AG, D'Amour P, Shoback DM, Thakker RV. Diagnosis of asymptomatic primary hyperparathyroidism: proceedings of the Fourth International Workshop. *J Clin Endocrinol Metab.* 2014;99(10): 3570-3579.

Tassone F, Guarnieri A, Castellano E, Baffoni C, Attanasio R, Borretta G. Parathyroidectomy halts the deterioration of renal function in primary hyperparathyroidism. *J Clin Endocrinol Metab.* 2015;100(8):3069-3073.

Tassone F, Gianotti L, Baffoni C, Pellegrino M, Castellano E, Borretta G. KDIGO categories of glomerular filtration rate and parathyroid hormone secretion in primary hyperparathyroidism. *Endocr Pract.* 2015;21(6):629-633.

5 ANSWER: B) Decrease calcium supplementation

Patients with hypoparathyroidism cannot stimulate renal tubular reabsorption of filtered calcium due to lack of PTH effect on the kidneys. Therefore, calcium and calcitriol supplementation in the management of chronic hypoparathyroidism can lead to hypercalciuria, nephrolithiasis, nephrocalcinosis, and renal insufficiency. Epidemiologic studies have shown markedly increased relative risks (3- to 6-fold) of renal dysfunction among those with both surgical and nonsurgical hypoparathyroidism. Because of this, it is important to encourage patients to minimize excessive calcium intake, to take the lowest possible calcitriol dosage, and to try to maintain serum calcium in the low-normal or even slightly low range. It is also important to monitor urinary calcium excretion and avoid hypercalciuria. Because this patient has hypercalciuria, continuing the current regimen (Answer A) is not optimal. Sevelamer (Answer C), a phosphate binder, is not indicated for this mild hyperphosphatemia and would not address her hypercalciuria. Her calcium × phosphate product is less than 55, so there is no urgency for a phosphate binder.

The best option is to recommend that she gradually decrease her excessive intake of calcium supplements (Answer B). Hypoparathyroid patients can experience unpleasant symptoms of muscle cramps, spasms, and paresthesias, particularly during or after exercise. So, it is important to work with the patient and gradually try to achieve a lower calcium intake that is both safe and tolerable.

The recent approval of recombinant human PTH(1-84) (Answer D) for management of permanent hypoparathyroidism offers another option, but it is extremely expensive. Moreover, this should be reserved for patients who cannot be managed well on traditional therapies. Guidelines for its use are discussed in the provided references. Thiazide diuretics (Answer E) may be useful adjunctive therapy for some patients with persistent hypercalciuria who are unable to lower calcium intake due to hypocalcemic symptoms. It is reasonable to try a thiazide diuretic in these cases, particularly if serum calcium is on the lower end of normal with persistent hypercalciuria. Often, high dosages (such as 50 mg daily of hydrochlorothiazide or more) are needed to normalize urinary calcium excretion, but some patients respond well to lower dosages. Concomitant potassium-sparing diuretics such as amiloride and low-salt diets may be useful adjunctive therapies. When starting thiazides, serum calcium may rise, allowing reduction in the calcitriol dosage.

Other risks for patients with permanent surgical hypoparathyroidism include neuropsychiatric disease, infections, and seizures. Among those with nonsurgical hypoparathyroidism, there is a higher occurrence of ischemic cardiovascular disease, cataracts, and fractures. The risk of malignancy in patients with nonsurgical hypoparathyroidism is actually decreased (hazard ratio 0.44) compared with that in the general population.

EDUCATIONAL OBJECTIVE:
Manage chronic surgical hypoparathyroidism.

REFERENCE(S):

Bilezikian JP, Khan A, Potts JT Jr, et al. Hypoparathyroidism in the adult: epidemiology, diagnosis, pathophysiology, target-organ involvement, treatment, and challenges for future research. *J Bone Miner Res.* 2011;26(10):2317-2337.

Clarke BL, Brown EM, Collins MT, et al. Epidemiology and diagnosis of hypoparathyroidism. *J Clin Endocrinol Metab.* 2016;101(6):2284-2299.

Bilezikian JP, Brandi ML, Cusano NE, et al. Management of hypoparathyroidism: present and future. *J Clin Endocrinol Metab.* 2016;101(6): 2313-2324.

6 ANSWER: D) Multiple endocrine neoplasia type 1 (*MEN1* gene)

Multiple endocrine neoplasia type 1 (due to mutations in the *MEN1* gene) (Answer D) is inherited as an autosomal dominant disorder, although occasionally de novo mutations occur. It is critical to think about and recommend genetic testing for multiple endocrine neoplasia type 1 in all patients younger than 30 years who present with primary hyperparathyroidism. Up to 10% of all patients with primary hyperparathyroidism have a familial (germline) mutation. Hereditary syndromes should be suspected in patients with a personal history of other endocrine tumors (especially pancreatic-duodenal or pituitary) or a history of parathyroid disease, renal stones, or pancreatic-duodenal/pituitary tumors in first-degree relatives. These syndromes should also be suspected and screened for in patients presenting with atypical or multigland parathyroid adenomas at any age. Only 2% to 4% of all patients with primary hyperparathyroidism present with multigland adenomas.

In addition to multiple endocrine neoplasia type 1, other more rare causes of multiorgan syndromic primary hyperparathyroidism include multiple endocrine neoplasia type 2, multiple endocrine neoplasia type 4, and hyperparathyroidism–jaw tumor syndrome. The latter is caused by mutations in the *CDC73* gene (also known as *HRPT2* or parafibromin) and inheritance is autosomal dominant with variable penetrance. It should be considered in the following clinical situations:

- Familial hyperparathyroidism (at least 2 first- or second-degree relatives have primary hyperparathyroidism)
- Primary hyperparathyroidism in a young person (<35 years)
- Ossifying fibromas of the maxilla or mandible in patient or family member (found in 25%-50%)
- Renal abnormalities such as Wilms tumor, renal cell carcinoma, hamartomas, polycystic kidneys (found in 15%)
- Uterine tumors (benign or malignant) (75% of females with the syndrome)
- Parathyroid carcinoma (found in 15%)

Familial "idiopathic" hyperparathyroidism (Answer A) may be a subtype of hyperparathyroidism–jaw tumor syndrome. It is less likely to be the correct diagnosis because of the father's history of diarrhea and the sibling's history of peptic ulcers (gastrinomas) suggesting a multiple endocrine neoplastic syndrome. Multiple endocrine neoplasia type 2 is associated with primary hyperparathyroidism in about 30% of cases, but it is ruled out in this case by

absence of hypertension, spells, or medullary thyroid carcinoma in any of the affected individuals.

Hereditary "renal leak" hypercalciuria (Answer B) can cause kidney stones and secondary hyperparathyroidism but not primary hyperparathyroidism, and it would not explain the additional family history. Hereditary activation of the calcium-sensing receptor (Answer C) would result in hypocalcemia, not hypercalcemia.

EDUCATIONAL OBJECTIVE:
Pursue the diagnosis of multiple endocrine neoplasia type 1 in young patients presenting with primary hyperparathyroidism.

REFERENCE(S):
Thakker RV, Newey PJ, Walls GV, et al; Endocrine Society. Clinical practice guidelines for multiple endocrine neoplasia 1 (MEN1). *J Clin Endocrinol Metab*. 2012;97(9):2990-3011.

Eastell R, Brandi ML, Costa AG, D'Amour P, Shoback DM, Thakker RV. Diagnosis of asymptomatic primary hyperparathyroidism: proceedings of the Fourth International Workshop. *J Clin Endocrinol Metab*. 2014;99(10):3570-3579.

Lassen T, Friis-Hansen L, Rasmussen AK, Knigge U, Feldt-Rasmussen U. Primary hyperparathyroidism in young people. When should we perform genetic testing for multiple endocrine neoplasia 1 (MEN-1)? *J Clin Endocrinol Metab*. 2014;99(11):3983-3987.

7 ANSWER: E) Biopsy of one of the nodules

This patient has non–PTH-mediated hypercalcemia. In the setting of both hypercalcemia and low PTH, 1,25-dihydroxyvitamin D should be suppressed, not elevated. The inappropriately high 1,25-dihydroxyvitamin D level directs the workup to investigate causes of calcitriol-induced hypercalcemia. Activated vitamin D leads to hypercalcemia primarily by increasing the gut absorption of calcium (and phosphate), and by directly causing osteoclastic bone resorption. Etiologies of calcitriol-induced hypercalcemia include infectious (tuberculosis, fungal), malignant (certain lymphomas and renal cell carcinomas), and other granulomatous disorders (sarcoidosis). The most likely cause of the hypercalcemia in this patient is activation of the 1α-hydroxylase enzyme within activated macrophages in the buttocks and hips due to silicone-induced granulomata. Injections of silicone, methyl methacrylate, and other substances into muscles and soft tissues for cosmetic purposes can result in this syndrome. The best way to confirm the diagnosis is to biopsy one of the nodules (Answer E).

The picture is not consistent with PTHrP-induced hypercalcemia (Answer A) since the calcitriol level would be low, not high. CT of the chest, abdomen, and pelvis (Answer B) would be reasonable if lymphoma or other malignancy were high on the differential list. Similarly, bone marrow aspiration and biopsy (Answer C) could be considered if the workup is negative and particularly if the complete blood cell count is abnormal. An octreotide scan (Answer D) can help locate neuroendocrine tumors or mesenchymal tumors (in tumor-induced osteomalacia), but it has not been used to localize the source of silicone-induced hypercalcemia.

EDUCATIONAL OBJECTIVE:
Diagnose 1,25-dihydroxyvitamin D–mediated hypercalcemia due to foreign-body granulomas.

REFERENCE(S):
Agrawal N, Altiner S, Mezitis NH, Helbig S. Silicone-induced granuloma after injection for cosmetic purposes: a rare entity of calcitriol-mediated hypercalcemia. *Case Rep Med.* 2013; 2013:807292.

Visnyei K, Samuel M, Heacock L, Cortes JA. Hypercalcemia in a male-to-female transgender patient after body contouring injections: a case report. *J Med Case Rep.* 2014;8:71.

Camuzard O, Dumas P, Foissac R, et al. Severe granulomatous reaction associated with hypercalcemia occurring after silicone soft tissue augmentation of the buttocks: a case report. *Aesthetic Plast Surg.* 2014;38(1):95-99.

Negri AL, Rosa Diez G, Del Valle E, et al. Hypercalcemia secondary to granulomatous disease caused by the injection of methacrylate: a case series. *Clin Cases Miner Bone Metab.* 2014;11(1):44-48.

Loke SC, Leow MK. Calcinosis cutis with siliconomas complicated by hypercalcemia. *Endocr Pract.* 2005;11(5):341-345.

8 ANSWER: A) Begin hydrochlorothiazide

In patients with multiple stone episodes—most of whom have already increased their fluid intake—thiazide diuretics (Answer A) and citrate supplements are similarly effective in patients with hypercalciuria, as well as in unselected patients. Hydrochlorothiazide acts to enhance renal calcium reabsorption to reduce urinary calcium excretion. Citrate acts as a stone inhibitor. Reducing dietary calcium (Answer D) is counterproductive since dietary calcium binds with dietary oxalate and helps reduce intestinal oxalate absorption.

Hypercalciuria may be caused by increased sodium intake, which leads to increased sodium excretion and an obligatory loss of calcium in the urine; however, this patient's urinary sodium excretion is normal as is her urinary uric acid level (thus, Answer B is incorrect). Her urinary oxalate level is normal, so there would be no benefit in reducing dietary oxalate (Answer C). Finally, the urine volume of 2.6 L suggests that increased fluid intake (Answer E) would not be helpful. The goal is to aim for urine volume greater than 2.5 L per day.

Other risk factors for recurrent kidney stones include excessive intake of salt and proteins and high dietary acid load. The intake of vegetables and a vegetarian-type diet is encouraged in stone-forming patients. Consumption of sugar-sweetened soda and punch is associated with a higher risk of stone formation, whereas consumption of coffee, tea, beer, wine, and orange juice is associated with a lower risk.

EDUCATIONAL OBJECTIVE:
Recommend a thiazide diuretic as a means to reduce the risk of recurrent kidney stones.

REFERENCE(S):
Fink HA, Wilt TJ, Eldman KE, et al. Medical management to prevent recurrent nephrolithiasis in adults: a systematic review for an American College of Physicians Clinical Guideline [published correction appears in *Ann Intern Med.* 2013;159(3):230-232]. *Ann Intern Med.* 2013; 158(7):535-543.

Vigen R, Weideman RA, Reilly RF. Thiazides diuretics in the treatment of nephrolithiasis: are we using them in an evidence-based fashion? *Int Urol Nephrol.* 2011;43(3):813-819.

Borghi L, Schianchi T, Meschi T, et al. Comparison of two diets for the prevention of recurrent stones in idiopathic hypercalciuria. *N Engl J Med.* 2002; 346(2):77-84.

9 ANSWER: B) Start cinacalcet

This patient has severe primary hyperparathyroidism and is acutely ill with multiple comorbidities that make him a poor surgical candidate. Therefore, urgent surgery (Answer A) is inappropriate. In 2011, the US FDA approved cinacalcet (Answer B) for treatment of severe primary hyperparathyroidism in patients who are poor surgical candidates. The peak action of cinacalcet in lowering serum calcium is observed at 1 week, but significant calcium reduction can be seen in a few days and long-term treatment is effective in maintaining eucalcemia. Cinacalcet may be a useful "bridge" to surgery for patients requiring medical stabilization.

Alendronate (Answer C) is an oral bisphosphonate, which will not improve his hypercalcemia. Nasal calcitonin (Answer E) is not an effective treatment for hypercalcemia. Subcutaneous calcitonin can provide a temporary decrease in calcium levels but is limited by tachyphylaxis within 24 to 48 hours. Amiloride (Answer D), a potassium-sparing diuretic, will not be effective in this setting. Other effective agents for this patient include potent antiresorptive agents such as intravenous bisphosphonates (zoledronic acid or pamidronate) or denosumab, but these do not specifically target PTH excess.

EDUCATIONAL OBJECTIVE:
Recommend cinacalcet as an appropriate treatment for primary hyperparathyroidism in patients with severe hypercalcemia who are poor surgical candidates.

REFERENCE(S):
Khan A, Bilezikian J, Bone H, Gurevich A, Lakatos P, Misiorowski W. Cinacalcet normalizes serum calcium in a double-blind randomized, placebo-controlled study in patients with primary hyperparathyroidism with contraindications to surgery. *Eur J Endocrinol.* 2015;172(5):527-535.

Marcocci C, Bollerslev J, Khan AA, Shoback DM. Medical management of primary hyperparathyroidism: proceedings of the fourth International Workshop on the Management of Asymptomatic Primary Hyperparathyroidism. *J Clin Endocrinol Metab.* 2014;99(10):3607-3618.

10 ANSWER: D) Serum electrolytes, cortisol, and ACTH

This patient has autoimmune polyendocrine syndrome type 1 (APS type 1) due to a mutation of the autoimmune regulator gene (*AIRE*) and presents with symptoms and signs of Addison disease. APS type 1 is also known by the acronym APECED (autoimmune polyendocrinopathy-candidiasis-ectodermal dystrophy). The classic presentation includes at least 2 of the following 3 major clinical components: chronic mucocutaneous candidiasis, primary hypoparathyroidism, and autoimmune adrenal insufficiency. The physical examination notes ectodermal dystrophy of the fingernails. Hyperpigmentation from adrenal insufficiency would also be expected on exam. Primary adrenal insufficiency may be diagnosed before clinical symptoms by checking for antibodies against the 21-hydroxylase enzyme, but in this case, serum electrolytes, cortisol, and ACTH (Answer D) must be measured immediately. Given the physical examination findings, one would expect to find hyponatremia, hyperkalemia, and elevated ACTH along with a low or "normal" serum cortisol (which is being maximally stimulated). Pending the results, a formal ACTH stimulation test should be done.

Serum ceruloplasmin measurement (Answer A) is used to diagnose Wilson disease, a genetic syndrome in which copper accumulates in tissues, including the parathyroid glands. Classic findings include Kayser-Fleischer rings, liver damage, and neuropsychiatric symptoms. Serum ferritin, iron, and total iron-binding capacity (Answer B) can be used to screen for hemochromatosis ("bronze diabetes"), but that would not fit the clinical picture. Serum calcium and magnesium (Answer C) could be checked but are not key to the diagnosis. Severe hypercalcemia from excess calcium and calcitriol could cause his symptoms but would not explain the skin and nail changes.

EDUCATIONAL OBJECTIVE:
Diagnose Addison disease as part of autoimmune polyendocrine syndrome type 1.

REFERENCE(S):

Weiler FG, Dias-da-Silva MR, Lazaretti-Castro M. Autoimmune polyendocrine syndrome type 1: case report and review of literature. *Arq Bras Endocrinol Metabol.* 2012;56(1):54-66.

Akirav EM, Ruddle NH, Herold KC. The role of AIRE in human autoimmune disease. *Nat Rev Endocrinol.* 2011;7(1):25-33.

Eisenbarth GS, Gottlieb PA. Autoimmune polyendocrine syndromes. *N Engl J Med.* 2004;350(20): 2068-2079.

11 ANSWER: A) DXA of the one-third distal radius

This patient most likely has normocalcemic primary hyperparathyroidism. This is defined as persistently normal total and ionized serum calcium levels in the setting of persistently elevated serum intact PTH, along with normal 25-hydroxyvitamin D, serum creatinine, and 24-hour urinary calcium excretion levels. Such patients are often discovered during a workup for low bone mineral density.

It is important to obtain a DXA of the one-third distal radius (Answer A) because this site, rich in cortical bone, is most susceptible to the bone-resorbing effects of sustained hyperparathyroidism. If she has osteoporosis at this site, she would meet criteria for parathyroid imaging and surgery. Longitudinal studies indicate that parathyroidectomy improves bone mineral density in patients with both hypercalcemic and normocalcemic primary hyperparathyroidism.

A sestamibi scan (Answer B) would not be indicated unless parathyroid surgery was planned. Spinal radiographs (Answer C) would be low yield in a patient with normocalcemic hyperparathyroidism without loss of height or kyphosis on examination. Similarly, renal ultrasonography (Answer D) would be low yield without a personal or family history of kidney stones or abnormal urinary calcium excretion. Bone turnover markers (Answer E) are considered ancillary tests and their measurement would not be the most appropriate next step.

Many patients with normocalcemic hyperparathyroidism eventually demonstrate elevated serum calcium levels and at that point, the recommendations for a more complete evaluation may be useful (*see table*).

Table 3. Recommendations for the Evaluation of Patients With Asymptomatic PHPT

Recommended
Biochemistry panel (calcium, phosphate, alkaline phosphatase activity, BUN, creatinine), 25(OH)D
PTH by second- or third-generation immunoassay
BMD by DXA
  Lumbar spine, hip, and distal 1/3 radius
Vertebral spine assessment
  X-ray or VFA by DXA
24-h urine for:
  Calcium, creatinine, creatinine clearance
  Stone risk profile
Abdominal imaging by x-ray, ultrasound, or CT scan
Optional
HRpQCT
TBS by DXA
Bone turnover markers (bone-specific alkaline phosphatase activity, osteocalcin, P1NP [select one]; serum CTX, urinary NTX [select one])
Fractional excretion of calcium on timed urine sample
DNA testing if genetic basis for PHPT is suspected

Abbreviations: BUN, blood urea nitrogen; P1NP, procollagen type 1 N-propeptide; CTX, C-telopeptide cross-linked collagen type I; NTX, N-telopeptide of type I collagen. This evaluation is for PHPT, not to distinguish between PHPT and other causes of hypercalcemia.

Table reprinted from Bilezikian JP, Brandi ML, Eastell R, et al. Guidelines for the management of asymptomatic primary hyperparathyroidism: summary statement from the Fourth International Workshop. *J Clin Endocrinol Metab.* 2014;99(10):3561-3569.

EDUCATIONAL OBJECTIVE:
Evaluate normocalcemic hyperparathyroidism.

REFERENCE(S):

Cusano NE, Maalouf NM, Wang PY, et al. Normocalcemic hyperparathyroidism and hypoparathyroidism in two community-based nonreferral populations. *J Clin Endocrinol Metab.* 2013;98(7):2734-2741.

Rejnmark L, Amstrup AK, Mollerup CL, Heickendorff L, Mosekilde L. Further insights into the pathogenesis of primary hyperparathyroidism: a nested case-control study. *J Clin Endocrinol Metab.* 2013;98(1):87-96.

Lowe H, McMahon DJ, Rubin MR, Bilezikian JP, Silverberg SJ. Normocalcemic primary hyperparathyroidism: further characterization of a new clinical phenotype. *J Clin Endocrinol Metab.* 2007;92(8):3001-3005.

Bilezikian JP, Brandi ML, Eastell R, et al. Guidelines for the management of asymptomatic primary hyperparathyroidism: summary statement from the Fourth International Workshop. *J Clin Endocrinol Metab.* 2014;99(10):3561-3569.

12 ANSWER: C) Stop the calcium supplement

Serum calcium is often slightly (and transiently) elevated in the hours immediately following the day's dose of teriparatide, but it will usually be back within normal limits on samples drawn 16 or more hours after the last dose. Patients who take teriparatide in the morning who need blood work done should be told to delay their teriparatide dose until after samples for lab tests have been drawn, as this patient did. But her serum calcium is still high, suggesting that a change in therapy is needed (thus, Answer E is incorrect).

Due to high bone turnover and calcium flux, some patients do have mild hypercalcemia during the first 3 to 6 months after starting teriparatide. Because she is asymptomatic and the calcium elevation is mild, it is reasonable to first stop her calcium supplement (Answer C) with the understanding that this will be restarted again in the future. There is no indication to stop hydrochlorothiazide (Answer A) or decrease the dosage (Answer B) as she has been on this dosage for many years and she remains mildly hypertensive. Stopping the teriparatide now (Answer D) is not necessary unless she remains persistently hypercalcemic.

EDUCATIONAL OBJECTIVE:
Manage mild hypercalcemia during teriparatide therapy for osteoporosis.

REFERENCE(S):

Satterwhite J, Heathman M, Miller PD, Marin F, Glass EV, Dobnig H. Pharmacokinetics of teriparatide (rhPTH[1-34]) and calcium pharmacodynamics in postmenopausal women with osteoporosis. *Calcif Tiss Int*. 2010;87(6):485-492.

Finkelstein JS, Hayes A, Hunzelman JL, Wyland JJ, Lee H, Neer RM. Effects of parathyroid hormone, alendronate, or both in men with osteoporosis. *N Engl J Med*. 2003;349(13):1216-1226.

Finkelstein JS, Wyland JJ, Leder BZ, et al. Effects of teriparatide retreatment in osteoporotic men and women. *J Clin Endocrinol Metab*. 2009;94(7):2495-2501.

13 ANSWER: D) X-linked hypophosphatemic rickets

X-linked hypophosphatemic rickets (Answer D) is an X-linked dominant form of rickets that is relatively unresponsive to vitamin D. The hypophosphatemia arises as a consequence of a defective *PHEX* gene product (phosphate-regulating gene with homology to endopeptidases on the X chromosome), which ultimately results in elevated fibroblast growth factor 23 levels and impaired renal proximal tubule phosphate reabsorption. In addition, despite severe hypophosphatemia, 1,25-dihydroxyvitamin D_3 production is not appropriately enhanced due to fibroblast growth factor 23–mediated suppression of 1α-hydroxylase activity. Thus, the "normal" level of 1,25-dihydroxyvitamin D_3 is inappropriate in the setting of elevated PTH and low serum phosphate.

Vitamin D–resistant rickets (Answer A) is characterized by low serum calcium, low serum phosphate, high PTH, and normal 25-hydroxyvitamin D levels. The key to distinguishing vitamin D–resistant rickets from other forms of rickets is to measure the 1,25-dihydroxyvitamin D level. There are 2 different types of "vitamin D–resistant rickets." Persons with the first type have inactivating mutations in the gene encoding the 1α-hydroxylase enzyme, are unable to synthesize 1,25-dihydroxyvitamin D, and present with very low or undetectable 1,25-dihydroxyvitamin D levels. These patients respond quite well to treatment with exogenous activated vitamin D metabolites but not as well to the usual vitamin D supplementation (hence, they were considered "resistant" to vitamin D in the era before activated vitamin D supplements were available). In contrast, patients with true vitamin D–resistant rickets have inactivating mutations in the gene encoding the vitamin D receptor, resulting in high 1,25-dihydroxyvitamin D levels and generally poor response to exogenous activated vitamin D metabolites. This patient does not have vitamin D–resistant rickets in view of her normal serum calcium level and lack of an elevated 1,25-dihydroxyvitamin D level.

Oncogenic osteomalacia (Answer B) is highly unlikely given the childhood presentation in this case. In the setting of oncogenic osteomalacia, 1,25-dihydroxyvitamin D levels are severely reduced due to suppression by high fibroblast growth factor 23 levels from these often small mesenchymal tumors. McCune-Albright syndrome (Answer C) can be associated with rickets and osteomalacia due to hyperphosphaturic hypophosphatemia, but one would expect polyostotic fibrous dysplasia, café-au-lait macules, and other endocrine disorders. Finally, this patient's 25-hydroxyvitamin D level of 24 ng/mL (59.9 nmol/L) is not low enough to result in such severe rickets/osteomalacia. In true vitamin D–deficient rickets (Answer E), 25-hydroxyvitamin D levels are often too low to be measured.

EDUCATIONAL OBJECTIVE:
Diagnose X-linked hypophosphatemic rickets.

REFERENCE(S):

Alizadeh Naderi AS, Reilly RF. Hereditary disorders of renal phosphate wasting. *Nat Rev Nephrol.* 2010;2(11):657-665.

Beck-Nielsen SS, Brusgaard K, Rasmussen LM, et al. Phenotype presentation of hypophosphatemic rickets in adults. *Calcif Tissue Int.* 2010;87(2):108-119.

Connor J, Olear EA, Insogna KL, et al. Conventional therapy in adults with X-linked hypophosphatemia: effects on enthesopathy and dental disease. *J Clin Endocrinol Metab.* 2015;100(10):3625-3632.

14 ANSWER: B) Switch to teriparatide

The 2010 guidelines from the American College of Rheumatology recommend some type of pharmacologic treatment for those on supraphysiologic dosages of prednisone (≥7.5 mg daily) for 3 months or longer. The US FDA has approved alendronate, risedronate, zoledronic acid, and teriparatide for management of glucocorticoid-induced osteoporosis. Due to cost, effectiveness, and ease of use, alendronate or risedronate are usually the first-line treatment. However, not many data show persistent efficacy of oral bisphosphonates in glucocorticoid-induced osteoporosis after 2 years. Given this patient's higher prednisone dosage and the spontaneous vertebral fracture while on alendronate, a change in therapy is reasonable. Thus, simply continuing therapy (Answer A) is incorrect.

Zoledronic acid (Answer C) is unlikely to be any more effective in someone who is adherent to oral bisphosphonate therapy. Denosumab (Answer D) is not approved by the US FDA for use in glucocorticoid-induced osteoporosis and raises theoretical concerns about immunosuppression and greater infection risk in this population. Moreover, antiresorptive agents do not address the major defect in glucocorticoid-induced osteoporosis, which is suppression of osteoblastic activity and reduced bone formation.

Teriparatide (Answer B) is currently the only anabolic agent approved for glucocorticoid-induced osteoporosis and in a randomized controlled trial, it was found to be superior to alendronate in terms of bone mineral density and vertebral fracture reduction. In trials not related to glucocorticoid-induced osteoporosis, combination therapy with teriparatide and alendronate (Answer E) blunts the efficacy of the teriparatide, although some dispute this and recommend continuing alendronate when adding teriparatide. Currently, combination therapy is not generally recommended outside of clinical trials or exceptional circumstances.

EDUCATIONAL OBJECTIVE:
Manage a vertebral fracture in a patient with glucocorticoid-induced osteoporosis taking alendronate.

REFERENCE(S):

Grossman JM, Gordon R, Ranganath VK, et al. American College of Rheumatology 2010 recommendations for the prevention and treatment of glucocorticoid-induced osteoporosis. [published correction appears in *Arthritis Care Res (Hoboken).* 2012;64(3):464]. *Arthritis Care Res (Hoboken).* 2010;62(11):1515-1526.

Venuturupalli SR, Sacks W. Review of new guidelines for the management of glucocorticoid induced osteoporosis. *Curr Osteoporos Rep.* 2013;11(4):357-364.

Cosman F, Nieves JW, Dempster DW. Treatment sequence matters: anabolic and antiresorptive therapy for osteoporosis. *J Bone Miner Res.* 2017;32(2):198-202.

Saag KG, Shane E, Boonen S, et al. Teriparatide or alendronate in glucocorticoid-induced osteoporosis. *N Engl J Med.* 2007;357(20):2028-2039.

Saag KG, Zanchetta JR, Devogelaer JP, et al. Effects of teriparatide versus alendronate for treating glucocorticoid-induced osteoporosis: thirty-six-month results of a randomized, double-blind, controlled trial. *Arthritis Rheum.* 2009;60(11):3346-3355.

15 ANSWER: D) Switch to denosumab

A frequent clinical question is when or if to recommend a "bisphosphonate holiday" to patients with osteoporosis who have been on either oral or intravenous bisphosphonates for several years. Because bisphosphonates have a long retention in the skeleton, they may continue to exhibit antifracture effectiveness even after therapy is stopped. The decision to stop bisphosphonate therapy must be individualized. Studies have shown that after 3 years of annual intravenous zoledronic acid or 5 years of oral bisphosphonate therapy, it is reasonable to reassess each patient and determine whether a bisphosphonate holiday should be considered. Patients and physicians worry about the risk of rare but devastating adverse effects (such as osteonecrosis of the jaw and atypical femur fractures) that seem to be correlated with duration of bisphosphonate therapy.

Data from the FLEX and HORIZON extension trials show that many patients can stop bisphosphonate therapy temporarily after 3 to 5 years without loss of bone mineral density or increased fracture risk. However, some subgroups of patients appear to be at higher risk for bone loss or fractures after stopping therapy. For these patients, the options include either continuing the bisphosphonate for up to 10 years with periodic reassessment or stopping the bisphosphonate and switching to a different agent. Patients at highest risk include those with a history of hip or vertebral fractures, multiple fractures, T score of −2.5 or lower at the hip, or other factors placing them "at high risk" for fractures.

This patient has reached a "plateau" on alendronate, has some gait instability and frequent falls, and has persistent osteoporosis at the hip. She is considered to be at high risk for future fractures and needs a change in therapy. Stopping alendronate and reassessing in 1 to 2 years (Answer A) is not acceptable given her risk for falls and fractures. Switching to zoledronic acid (Answer B) (another bisphosphonate) would make sense if she had evidence of treatment nonadherence or malabsorption on the alendronate. But in compliant patients, studies have shown no improvement in bone mineral density (or fracture risk) when patients' regimens are switched from oral to intravenous bisphosphonate.

It might make sense to switch from an antiresorptive agent to the anabolic agent teriparatide (Answer C). This would be especially true if her bone mineral density were very low at the spine or if she had sustained previous vertebral fractures. However, her greatest vulnerability is at the hip and the data for teriparatide reducing hip fractures are not as clear as they are for denosumab (Answer D). Moreover, bone mineral density may actually decline at the hip when patients are switched from alendronate to teriparatide. In contrast, denosumab following bisphosphonate therapy has resulted in further improvements in bone mineral density and is the best next step in this patient's management.

EDUCATIONAL OBJECTIVE:
Manage patients on long-term bisphosphonate therapy with high fracture risk.

REFERENCE(S):
Black DM, Schwartz AV, Ensrud KE, et al; FLEX Research Group. Effects of continuing or stopping alendronate after 5 years of treatment: the Fracture Intervention Trial Long-term Extension (FLEX): a randomized trial. *JAMA.* 2006;296(24):2927-2938.

Black DM, Reid IR, Boonen S, et al. The effect of 3 versus 6 years of zoledronic acid treatment of osteoporosis: a randomized extension to the HORIZON-Pivotal Fracture Trial (PFT) [published correction appears in *J Bone Miner Res.* 2012;27(12):2612]. *J Bone Miner Res.* 2012;27(2):243-254.

Adler RA, Fuleihan GE, Bauer DC, et al. Managing osteoporosis in patients on long-term bisphosphonate treatment: report of a Task force of the American Society for Bone and Mineral Research. *J Bone Miner Res.* 2016;31(1):16-35.

Eiken P, Vestergaard P. Treatment of osteoporosis after alendronate or risedronate. *Osteoporos Int.* 2016;27(1):1-12.

16 ANSWER: A) Nonadherence to treatment

When a patient on potent antiosteoporosis therapy has a poor response, such as a significant decline in bone mineral density, it is important to review the history, physical examination findings, medications, and laboratory results to look for secondary causes that may have been missed or developed in the interim. However, the most common cause for a poor outcome, particularly with self-administered medications, is treatment nonadherence (Answer A). Fifty percent of patients who start oral bisphosphonates are estimated to stop the drugs within 3 to 6 months. Many others take the drugs intermittently or improperly. Consequences of nonadherence include loss of bone mineral density, increased fracture risk, and higher health care costs. Other etiologies of nonresponse include calcium and/or vitamin D deficiencies, poor absorption of oral bisphosphonates, errors in DXA measurements, or underlying diseases that remain undiagnosed or untreated.

Malabsorption (Answer B) is unlikely given the adequate levels of calcium and vitamin D and the normal 24-hour urinary calcium excretion. Although patients who adhere to their treatment regimen may occasionally have inadequate absorption of bisphosphonates, this is much less common than noncompliance. The normal laboratory values, lack of new symptoms, and unchanged physical examination make it highly unlikely that a serious underlying disorder is causing the bone loss (Answer C). Positioning error by the DXA technician (Answer D) is unlikely to result in "bone loss" at both the spine and hip. Finally, all oral bisphosphonates, when taken properly, have been shown to greatly reduce postmenopausal bone loss, although risedronate may be slightly less potent than alendronate (thus, Answer E is incorrect).

EDUCATIONAL OBJECTIVE:
Identify treatment nonadherence as the reason for poor response to osteoporosis therapy.

REFERENCE(S):
Modi A, Siris ES, Tang J, Sen S. Cost and consequences of noncompliance with osteoporosis treatment among women initiating therapy. *Curr Med Res Opin*. 2015;31(4):757-765.

Lewiecki EM, Watts NB. Assessing response to osteoporosis therapy. *Osteoporos Int*. 2008; 19(10):1363-1368.

17 ANSWER: C) Milk-alkali syndrome

This is a classic case of milk-alkali syndrome (Answer C) leading to a hypercalcemic crisis. The triad of hypercalcemia, renal failure, and metabolic alkalosis results from ingestion of excessive amounts of calcium and absorbable alkali over a short period. In this case, the patient was taking very large doses (bottles) of calcium carbonate and aspirin, sodium bicarbonate, and anhydrous citric acid for gastrointestinal distress following an alcohol binge. Recognizing the triad and taking a careful history are keys to making the diagnosis.

In the setting of excess calcium/alkali ingestion, hypercalcemia causes renal vasoconstriction, decreases the glomerular filtration rate, and increases bicarbonate reabsorption. Metabolic alkalosis further increases renal tubular reabsorption of calcium, and hypovolemia from nausea/vomiting further reduces the glomerular filtration rate. A vicious cycle can occur with rapid clinical deterioration and death. Hyperphosphatemia may also be seen with excessive ingestion of milk as the calcium source.

Acute management of a hypercalcemic crisis generally involves saline hydration, subcutaneous calcitonin for 24 to 48 hours, intravenous bisphosphonate (or subcutaneous denosumab in selected cases), and treatment of the underlying disease. Furosemide should be added only when there is clinical evidence of volume overload or congestive heart failure. In cases of vitamin D–mediated hypercalcemia, prednisone, 40 to 60 mg daily, or another glucocorticoid equivalent may be useful, but it should not be given without biochemical evidence of inappropriate vitamin D levels. Finally, in patients with hypercalcemic crisis due to primary hyperparathyroidism, cinacalcet can be a "bridge" to parathyroidectomy.

In milk-alkali syndrome, by simply stopping the exogenous calcium and alkali and providing vigorous saline hydration to increase the glomerular filtration rate and help clear the calcium and bicarbonate, the metabolic disarray can rapidly reverse. In those with acute milk-alkali syndrome, treatment can lead to an acute drop in serum calcium to hypocalcemic levels (with rebound increase in PTH). More chronic cases with nephrocalcinosis take much longer to resolve.

Acute pancreatitis (Answer A) could be a cause of the abdominal pain, but it would not explain the entire picture. The negative abdominal CT also makes this diagnosis less likely. Dehydration (Answer B) certainly contributes to the clinical presentation but would not explain this degree of hypercalcemia and metabolic alkalosis. Neither vitamin D intoxication (Answer D) nor malignancy (Answer E) would respond so quickly to hydration.

EDUCATIONAL OBJECTIVE:
Diagnose milk-alkali syndrome.

REFERENCE(S):
Beall DP, Scofield RH. Milk-alkali syndrome associated with calcium carbonate consumption. Report of 7 patients with parathyroid hormone levels and an estimate of prevalence among patients hospitalized with hypercalcemia. *Medicine (Baltimore).* 1995;74(2):89-96.

Fiorino AS. Hypercalcemia and alkalosis due to the milk-alkali syndrome: a case report and review. *Yale J Biol Med.* 1996;69(6):517-523.

Picolos MK, Lavis VR, Orlander PR. Milk-alkali syndrome is a major cause of hypercalcaemia among non-end-stage renal disease (non-ESRD) inpatients. *Clin Endocrinol (Oxf).* 2005;63(5):566-576.

Bazari H, Palmer WE, Baron JM, Armstrong K. Case records of the Massachusetts General Hospital. Case 24-2016. A 66-year-old man with malaise, weakness, and hypercalcemia. *N Engl J Med.* 2016;375(6):567-574.

18 **ANSWER: E) Albumin**
Fifty percent of circulating calcium is bound to serum proteins, primarily to albumin. In this patient with nephrotic syndrome, serum albumin (Answer E) is almost certainly low. The correction factor is to adjust the serum calcium up or down by 0.8 mg/dL (0.2 mmol/L) for each 1.0 g/dL (10 g/L) deviation of serum albumin below 4 mg/dL (<40 g/L). If her albumin level were 2.6 g/dL (26 g/L) (lower range of normal 3.5 g/dL [35 g/L]), then her adjusted serum calcium level would be 9.0 mg/dL (2.3 mmol/L). Ionized calcium

measurement might also be considered, but false high and low levels are common. She could also have low magnesium (Answer D) in addition to low albumin, but the first step in her evaluation is to determine whether her measured serum calcium is correct by measuring albumin. If she is truly hypocalcemic, with a low corrected calcium, then measuring 25-hydroxyvitamin D (Answer B) and PTH (Answer A) would be appropriate. Measuring 1,25-dihydroxyvitamin D (Answer C) would not be helpful in this situation.

EDUCATIONAL OBJECTIVE:
Investigate the etiology of hypocalcemia and correct for low albumin in this setting.

REFERENCE(S):
Ariyan CE, Sosa JA. Assessment and management of patients with abnormal calcium. *Crit Care Med.* 2004;32(Suppl 4):S146-S154.

Shoback D. Hypocalcemia: definition, etiology, pathogenesis, diagnosis, and management. In: Rosen CJ, Compston JE, Lian JB, eds. *Primer on the Metabolic Bone Diseases and Disorders of Mineral Metabolism.* Washington, DC: The American Society for Bone and Mineral Research; 2008:313-317.

19 **ANSWER: B) Continue calcium and vitamin D and repeat DXA in 2 years**
According to the National Osteoporosis Foundation, osteoporosis can be diagnosed by a T score in the hip or spine of less than –2.5 or by a fracture of the hip or spine. Fractures of fingers or toes do not meet the diagnostic criteria for osteoporosis. Therefore, this patient has low bone mass (osteopenia), and the best tool to determine whether she should be treated pharmacologically is the FRAX calculator. Relying on FRAX results, patients who have an absolute 10-year fracture risk of 20% or higher for any major fracture or 3% or higher for hip fracture should be treated pharmacologically. This patient's fracture risk is well below the treatment threshold, and she should therefore continue with her dietary calcium and vitamin D for now and undergo DXA again in 2 years (Answer B). Treating her with a bisphosphonate (Answer A), the selective estrogen receptor modulator raloxifene (Answer C), or nasal calcitonin (Answer E) is

incorrect. Estrogen replacement therapy (Answer D) is not approved by the US FDA for treatment of osteoporosis, and is only given to postmenopausal women with significant menopausal symptoms.

EDUCATIONAL OBJECTIVE:
Use the FRAX tool to determine treatment of patients with low bone mass.

REFERENCE(S):
Watts NB, Bilezikian JP, Camacho PM, et al. American Association of Clinical Endocrinologists Medical Guidelines for Clinical Practice for the diagnosis and treatment of postmenopausal osteoporosis: executive summary of recommendations. *Endocr Pract.* 2010;16(6):1016-1019.
National Osteoporosis Foundation. *Clinician's Guide to Prevention and Treatment of Osteoporosis.* Washington, DC: National Osteoporosis Foundation; 2014.

20 **ANSWER: D) Fibroblast growth factor 23 measurement**

This patient has tumor-induced osteomalacia caused by a benign mesenchymal tumor that is secreting fibroblast growth factor 23. This causes renal tubular loss of phosphate and inhibits 1α-hydroxylase, resulting in low 1,25-dihydroxyvitamin D levels. These tumors are typically located in the skin, bones, or connective tissue (eg, sinuses) and may be difficult to localize. Imaging to localize the tumor includes nuclear medicine imaging techniques such as bone scan, octreotide scan, or positron emission tomography. In difficult cases, serum fibroblast growth factor 23 on selective venous sampling may be used to localize the extremity from which fibroblast growth factor 23 is being secreted. Tumor removal (if it can be located and removed) normalizes renal phosphate handling within hours to days.

Hypophosphatemia induced by tenofovir (and adefovir) is part of a more generalized syndrome known as Fanconi syndrome in which multiple substances such as bicarbonate, glucose, uric acid, potassium, and phosphate are "wasted" in the urine (Answer E). This patient has no evidence of this syndrome. Measurement of serum and urine protein electrophoresis (Answer A) is used

to diagnose multiple myeloma and would not fit this presentation. Low levels of 24,25-dihydroxyvitamin D (Answer C) can be useful to diagnose patients with hypercalcemia and kidney stones who have mutations in the *CYP24A1* gene. A sestamibi scan (Answer B) is not helpful in diagnosing tumor-induced osteomalacia.

EDUCATIONAL OBJECTIVE:
Diagnose tumor-induced osteomalacia by measuring fibroblast growth factor 23.

REFERENCE(S):
Ruppe MD, Jan de Beur SM. Disorders of phosphate homeostasis. In: Rosen CJ, Compston JE, Lian JB, eds. *Primer on the Metabolic Bone Diseases and Disorders of Mineral Metabolism.* Washington, DC: The American Society for Bone and Mineral Research; 2008:601-612.
Jan de Beur SM. Tumor-induced osteomalacia. *JAMA.* 2005;294(10):1260-1267.
Andreopoulou P, Dumitrescu CE, Kelly MH, et al. Selective venous catheterization for the localization of phosphaturic mesenchymal tumors. *J Bone Miner Res.* 2011;26(6):1295-1302.

21 **ANSWER: C) Worsening arthritis in the hip**

Zoledronic acid should improve the component of pain arising from the pagetic involvement of his left hip, but it is not expected to help the pain due to degenerative arthritis and may not prevent arthritis progression (thus, Answer C is correct and Answer D is incorrect). Paget disease does not extend across joint spaces and has never been reported to develop in new bones not involved at diagnosis (thus, Answer A is incorrect). Since he does not have Paget disease in his skull, it will not cause hearing loss (Answer B). Osteonecrosis of the femoral neck (Answer E) is not more likely after treatment with zoledronic acid or in patients with Paget disease of the hip.

Whether all patients with Paget disease should be treated is controversial. Indications for treatment in asymptomatic patients include the following:

- Involvement of a weight-bearing bone (eg, spine or leg)
- Involvement near a joint

- Involvement of the skull
- Serum alkaline phosphatase level greater than 3 times the upper normal limit

Zoledronic acid is clearly the most effective treatment. It normalizes bone turnover markers and maintains normal values for the longest duration of any medication. Normal turnover markers are associated with the normalization of pagetic woven bone to lamellar bone and can eliminate pain arising from pagetic bone. A single dose of zoledronic acid results in many years of disease inactivity in most patients.

EDUCATIONAL OBJECTIVE:
Counsel patients that treating Paget disease should effectively eliminate pain attributable to the pagetic bone, but it is not expected to resolve pain due to degenerative arthritis.

REFERENCE(S):
Reid IR, Lyles K, Su G, et al. A single infusion of zoledronic acid produces sustained remissions in Paget disease: data to 6.5 years. *J Bone Miner Res.* 2011;26(9):2261-2270.

Langston AL, Campbell MK, Fraser WD, et al; PRISM Trial Group. Randomized trial of intensive bisphosphonate treatment versus symptomatic management in Paget's disease of bone. *J Bone Miner Res.* 2010;25(1):20-31.

Ralston SH. Clinical practice. Paget's disease of bone. *N Engl J Med.* 2013;368(7):644-650.

22 **ANSWER: E) Monitoring only**
This young premenopausal woman has a spinal bone mineral density measurement that is well below the mean for her age group, as indicated by the low Z score. However, this does not define "osteoporosis" since her risk for a fracture is much less than for an older postmenopausal woman with the same bone mineral density. The diagnosis of osteoporosis in premenopausal women is best defined by 1 or more low-trauma (fragility) fractures and requires exclusion of secondary causes such as connective tissue disorders, malabsorption, inflammatory/autoimmune disorders, and many others. Measurement of bone mineral density by DXA should not be used as the sole guide for the diagnosis or treatment of osteoporosis in premenopausal women.

None of the medications used for postmenopausal osteoporosis or for men with osteoporosis 50 years or older are approved for use in premenopausal women, and generally should not be used outside of clinical trials. Therefore, the correct management for this patient is monitoring only (Answer E), and all of the medications listed for osteoporosis (Answers A, B, and C) are incorrect in this clinical setting. There is no advantage to prescribing an oral contraceptive pill (Answer D) for a premenopausal woman with regular menses.

In rare cases, pharmacologic intervention may be considered in premenopausal women. These exceptions include young women with multiple or severe fragility fractures or those with prolonged exposure to illnesses or medications that can cause bone loss and skeletal fragility (eg, high-dosage glucocorticoids or ongoing anorexia nervosa). Special caution is needed before prescribing bisphosphonates to premenopausal women because of their long retention in bone and the ability to cross the placenta during pregnancy.

EDUCATIONAL OBJECTIVE:
Manage low bone mineral density in premenopausal women.

REFERENCE(S):
Cohen A. Premenopausal osteoporosis. *Endocrinol Metab Clin N Am.* 2017;46(1)L117-133.

Ferrari S, Bianchi ML, Eisman JA, et al. Osteoporosis in young adults : pathophysiology, diagnosis, and management. *Osteoporos Int.* 2012;23(12): 2735-2748.

Fazeli PK, Wang IS, Miller KK, et al. Teriparatide increases bone formation and bone mineral density in adult women with anorexia nervosa. *J Clin Endocrinol Metab.* 2014;99(4):1322-1329.

23 **ANSWER: D) Serum estradiol measurement**
This is a prototypical case of a 46,XY male with severe aromatase enzyme deficiency from a mutation in the *CYP19A1* gene. The aromatase enzyme converts androgens to estrogens in both males and females. Males with this syndrome have normal pubertal development but very low or undetectable serum estradiol levels (Answer D). This results in failure to fuse the epiphyses, continued linear

growth, tall stature, and osteoporosis, all due to the lack of estrogen. Since conversion of testosterone to estradiol in the pituitary is important for feedback control of gonadotropins, LH (and FSH) levels are elevated despite the high testosterone levels. The syndrome of aromatase deficiency is very rare but has provided critical insights into the importance of estrogen in male skeletal physiology.

High testosterone and LH could indicate an LH-secreting pituitary tumor, but this would not explain the continued linear growth, tall stature, or osteoporosis, so a pituitary-directed MRI (Answer A) is incorrect. Karyotype analysis (Answer B) would be useful to diagnose Klinefelter syndrome but one would expect low (not high) testosterone, gynecomastia, small firm testes, and other signs that are not present in this vignette. Androgen insensitivity from a mutation in the androgen receptor gene (Answer C) could result in the laboratory findings in this case but would be associated with a female phenotypic appearance (in total androgen insensitivity) or abnormal male virilization (hypospadius and other abnormalities in partial androgen insensitivity). Free testosterone measurement by equilibrium dialysis (Answer E) would not add anything to the diagnosis.

Patients with aromatase deficiency and osteoporosis respond well to estrogen therapy with fusion of epiphyses and marked accrual in bone mass.

EDUCATIONAL OBJECTIVE:
Explain the importance of estrogen in male skeletal physiology and the hallmarks of aromatase deficiency in male patients.

REFERENCE(S):
Bilezikian JP, Morishima A, Bell J, Grumbach MM. Increased bone mass as a result of estrogen therapy in a man with aromatase deficiency. *N Engl J Med.* 1998;339(9):599-603.

Morishima A, Grumbach MM, Simpson ER, Fisher C, Qin K. Aromatase deficiency in male and female siblings caused by a novel mutation and the physiological role of estrogens. *J Clin Endocrinol Metab.* 1995;80(12):3689-3698.

Carani C, Qin K, Simoni M, et al. Effect of testosterone and estradiol in a man with aromatase deficiency. *N Engl J Med.* 1997;337(2):91-95.

24 ANSWER: A) Increased bone mineral density

Osteogenesis imperfecta (or "brittle bone disease") is a rare, inherited disorder of type 1 collagen. Ninety percent of cases result from mutations in the genes encoding type 1 collagen (a1 and a2) (*COL1A1/COL1A2*). The main therapy for osteogenesis imperfecta remains bisphosphonates (intravenous pamidronate and zoledronic acid and oral bisphosphonates). Children with osteogenesis imperfecta who receive bisphosphonate therapy can experience decreased bone pain (Answer B) and decreased fracture risk (Answer E), but these outcomes are not definitive for adults. Improved dentition (Answer C) and more rapid fracture healing (Answer D) are not seen with bisphosphonate therapy in adults with osteogenesis imperfecta. The most consistent benefit in affected adults who receive bisphosphonates is increased bone mineral density (Answer A).

EDUCATIONAL OBJECTIVE:
Describe the role of bisphosphonate therapy for adults with osteogenesis imperfecta.

REFERENCE(S):
Van Dijk FS, Sillence DO. Osteogenesis imperfecta: clinical diagnosis, nomenclature and severity assessment [published correction appears in *Am J Med Genet A.* 2015;167A(5):1178]. *Am J Med Genet A.* 2014;164A(6):1470-1481.

Thomas IH, DiMeglio LA. Advances in the classification and treatment of osteogenesis imperfecta. *Curr Osteoporos Rep.* 2016;14(1):1-9.

Shapiro JR, Thompson CB, Wu Y, Nunes M, Gillen C. Bone mineral density and fracture rate in response to intravenous and oral bisphosphonates in adult osteogenesis imperfecta. *Calcif Tissue Int.* 2010;87(2):120-129.

25 ANSWER: B) Symptomatic hypocalcemia

Denosumab, a human monoclonal antibody against RANK ligand, is approved for treatment of osteoporosis, as well as metastatic solid tumors such as breast cancer. It is a very potent inhibitor of osteoclastic bone resorption. Unlike bisphosphonates, denosumab is not cleared via the kidneys and has no effect on renal function (thus, Answer A is incorrect). Although cases of osteonecrosis of the jaw

(Answer C) have been reported with both bisphosphonates and denosumab, this is very unlikely after only 1 dose of the drug. Severe flulike syndromes (Answer D) (also known as "acute-phase reactions") are much more common with intravenous bisphosphonates than with denosumab. Potent antiresorptive agents such as denosumab have not been shown to impair fracture healing (Answer E).

The major adverse effect to be expected in this setting is profound, symptomatic hypocalcemia (Answer B) within 7 to 10 days following denosumab administration. Patients at greatest risk for this complication are those with significantly impaired renal function. At highest risk are those with impaired renal function coupled with high bone turnover and elevated alkaline phosphatase. The potent inhibition of osteoclastic bone resorption by denosumab stops the efflux of calcium from bone and can lower serum calcium dramatically. The usual physiologic responses to hypocalcemia, such as a rise in PTH and calcitriol production, that would normally lead to increased renal tubular reabsorption of calcium and increased gut absorption of calcium, will not work in the setting of renal failure.

EDUCATIONAL OBJECTIVE:
Anticipate the risk of symptomatic hypocalcemia following denosumab in the setting of renal failure.

REFERENCE(S):

Dave V, Chiang CY, Booth J, Mount PF. Hypocalcemia post denosumab in patients with chronic kidney disease stage 4-5. *Am J Nephrol.* 2015;41(2):129-137.

Body JJ, Bone HG, de Boer RH, et al. Hypocalcaemia in patients with metastatic bone disease treated with denosumab. *Eur J Cancer.* 2015;51(13):1812-1821.

Kinoshita Y, Arai M, Ito N, et al. High serum ALP level is associated with increased risk of denosumab-related hypocalcemia in patients with bone metastases from solid tumors. *Endocr J.* 2016;63(5):479-484.

Stopeck AT, Lipton A, Body JJ, et al. Denosumab compared with zoledronic acid for the treatment of bone metastases in patients with advanced breast cancer: a randomized, double-blind study. *J Clin Oncol.* 2010;28(35):5132-5139.

26 ANSWER: C) Obesity

The average serum 25-hydroxyvitamin D response to 1000 IU of vitamin D daily for 8 to 12 weeks is an increase of about 12 ng/mL (30.0 nmol/L). In this vignette, the patient's level would be expected to increase from 15 ng/mL to 27 ng/mL (37.4 nmol/L to 67.4 nmol/L) over a period of 2 to 3 months. Instead, her 25-hydroxyvitamin D level only increased by 3 ng/mL (7.5 nmol/L). The most likely cause for this blunted response is class 3 obesity (Answer C). A number of studies have shown that patients who are overweight or obese require much higher dosages of vitamin D than normal-weight participants to achieve adequate levels. Obese patients are estimated to require 2 to 3 times the usual daily dose of cholecalciferol to achieve adequate levels. The mechanism is not well understood.

Occult malabsorption (Answer A) from celiac disease or some other gastrointestinal illness could certainly cause this pattern, but it is unlikely in the setting of obesity and a normal complete blood cell count, iron, and vitamin B_{12} levels. Low vitamin D–binding protein (Answer B) has been reported to occur in some African American patients with low 25-hydroxyvitamin D levels, but these individuals also tend to have normal PTH levels. An activating mutation in the gene encoding the 24,25-hydroxylase enzyme (Answer D) could increase the metabolism of 25-hydroxyvitamin D to the inactive 24,25-hydroxyvitamin D form and such mutations have been reported in patients with variable responses to vitamin D supplementation. However, this would be a much more unusual cause for the phenomenon seen in this patient. Finally, treatment nonadherence (Answer E) is always a possibility, but it is less likely in this patient with excellent blood pressure and glycemic control.

EDUCATIONAL OBJECTIVE:
Recommend appropriate vitamin D supplementation for obese patients.

REFERENCE(S):

Heaney RP, Davies KM, Chen TC, Holick MF, Barger-Lux MJ. Human serum 25-hydroxychole-calciferol response to extended oral dosing with cholecalciferol [published correction appears in *Am J Clin Nutr.* 2003;78(5):1047]. *Am J Clin Nutr.* 2003;77(1):204-210.

Ekwaru JP, Zwicker JD, Holick MF, Giovannucci E, Veugelers PJ. The importance of body weight for the dose response relationship of oral vitamin D supplementation and 25-hydroxyvitamin D in healthy volunteers. *PLoS One.* 2014;9(11):e111265.

Holick MF, Binkley NC, Bischoff-Ferrari HA, et al; Endocrine Society. Evaluation, treatment, and prevention of vitamin D deficiency: an Endocrine Society clinical practice guideline. *J Clin Endocrinol Metab.* 2011;96(7):1911-1930.

27 ANSWER: E) Serum magnesium

This elderly man presents with symptoms of tetany and biochemical evidence of hypoparathyroidism. In the setting of severe hypocalcemia, an intact PTH within the normal range is inappropriate as it should be frankly elevated. The most likely etiology for the subacute hypoparathyroidism is magnesium deficiency (Answer E) due to proton-pump inhibitor therapy.

The association between proton-pump inhibitor therapy and hypomagnesemic hypoparathyroidism was first reported in 2006. Although it is still a relatively rare syndrome, the patients at highest risk appear to be those on proton-pump inhibitor therapy for 1 year or longer, elderly patients, and those on concurrent diuretics. It also appears to be a class effect that can occur with any of the available proton-pump inhibitors. The underlying mechanism is unclear, but it is most likely an effect on gastrointestinal absorption of magnesium.

The phenomenon of hypocalcemia secondary to hypomagnesemia is due to functional hypoparathyroidism as PTH release is a magnesium-dependent process. This type of hypocalcemia is typically refractory to correction until the magnesium deficit has been corrected. A second mechanism of hypocalcemia in the setting of proton-pump inhibitor use relates to the decrease in calcium bioavailability in the presence of gastric achlorhydria, given that calcium absorption is a pH-dependent process.

Measurement of 25-hydroxyvitamin D (Answer A) or 24-hour urinary calcium excretion (Answer D) would be useful in cases of hypocalcemia and secondary hyperparathyroidism where deficiencies of vitamin D and low urinary calcium excretion would be expected. A search for causes of malabsorption such as occult celiac disease with assessment for tissue transglutaminase antibodies (Answer C) would be appropriate in secondary hyperparathyroidism. Levels of 1,25-dihydroxyvitamin D (Answer B) can be normal, low, or high in hypocalcemic patients depending on the substrate, renal function, and PTH levels, so its measurement is not helpful.

Finally, it should be noted that proton-pump inhibitors have been associated with an increased risk of falls, bone loss, and fractures.

EDUCATIONAL OBJECTIVE:
Recognize hypomagnesemic hypoparathyroidism associated with proton-pump inhibitor use.

REFERENCE(S):

Epstein M, McGrath S, Law F. Proton-pump inhibitors and hypomagnesemic hypoparathyroidism. *N Engl J Med.* 2006;355(17):1834-1836.

Fatuzzo P, Portale G, Scollo V, Zanoli L, Granata A. Proton pump inhibitors and symptomatic hypomagnesemic hypoparathyroidism. *J Nephrol.* 2017;30(2):297-301.

28 ANSWER: A) Radionuclide bone scan

Atypical femur fractures after long-term bisphosphonate treatment for osteoporosis occur in up to 1 in 500 patients and have a number of common features. In approximately 50% of cases, they are bilateral, and since this patient has bilateral groin pain, her right femur should be evaluated. A nuclear bone scan (Answer A) (*see image*) is a more sensitive way to evaluate her right femur than another radiograph (Answer C). Bilateral femur MRIs would be an alternative way to evaluate her. Serum CTX measurement (Answer B), bone mineral density test (Answer D), and iliac crest bone biopsy after double-tetracycline labeling (Answer E) are not diagnostic for this complication.

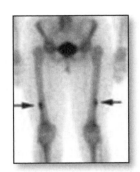

A task force of the American Society for Bone and Mineral Research released new case definitions for atypical femur fractures that are located on the femoral diaphysis and include 4 of 5 major features:

- Fracture is associated with minimal or no trauma (eg, fall from standing height)
- Fracture line originates at the lateral cortex and is substantially transverse in orientation although it may become oblique as it traverses medially across the femur
- Complete fractures extend through both cortices and may be associated with a medial spike; incomplete fractures include only the lateral cortex
- Fractures are noncomminuted or only minimally comminuted
- Localized periosteal or endosteal thickening of the lateral cortex is present at the fracture site ("beaking" or "flaring")

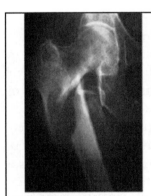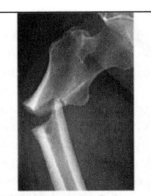

TYPICAL Subtrochanteric Fracture
- Spiral pattern
- Substantial comminution
- Thin cortices

ATYPICAL Subtrochanteric Fracture
- Transverse or short oblique orientation
- No comminution
- Thick cortices – focal or generalized

FIG. 5. Radiographic appearance and characteristics of a typical vs. atypical subtrochanteric fracture (courtesy of Dr. Melvin Rosenwasser, Columbia University, New York, NY).

The two images above illustrate the differences between "typical" and "atypical" femur fractures very well (reference: Khosla S, Bilezikian JP, Dempster DW, et al. Benefits and risks of bisphosphonate therapy for osteoporosis. *J Clin Endocrinol Metab.* 2012;97:2272-2282.).

EDUCATIONAL OBJECTIVE:
Evaluate an impending atypical femur fracture and assess for bilaterality.

REFERENCE(S):
Shane E, Burr D, Ebeling PR, et al; American Society for Bone and Mineral Research. Atypical subtrochanteric and diaphyseal femoral fractures: report of a task force of the American Society for Bone and Mineral Research [published correction appears in *J Bone Miner Res*;26(8):1987]. *J Bone Miner Res.* 2010;25(11):2267-2294.

Shaikh W 3rd, Morris D, Morris S 4th. Signs of insufficiency fractures overlooked in a patient receiving chronic bisphosphonate therapy. *J Am Board Fam Med.* 2016;29(3):404-407.

Selga J, Nuñez JH, Minguell J, Lalanza M, Garrido M. Simultaneous bilateral atypical femoral fracture in a patient receiving denosumab: case report and literature review. *Osteoporos Int.* 2016;27(2):827-832.

29 ANSWER: D) Referral for wide surgical resection

This patient with severe hypercalcemia, very elevated PTH, and a neck mass has parathyroid carcinoma. Parathyroid carcinoma is rare, occurring in less than 0.5% of cases of primary hyperparathyroidism, but it can be highly aggressive. With the exception of the hyperparathyroidism–jaw tumor syndrome (caused by mutations in the *CDC73* gene), parathyroid carcinoma does not seem to evolve through a benign intermediate, such as a parathyroid adenoma, but rather occurs de novo. Women and men are affected equally and patients usually present with very symptomatic hypercalcemia and a neck mass. Occasionally, parathyroid carcinoma is found incidentally and is nonsecretory. When parathyroid carcinoma is suspected, FNAB (Answer B) should be avoided as both bleeding and tumor seeding along the needle track have been reported. Optimal treatment is surgical resection of the entire tumor with negative margins, as well as resection of the ipsilateral thyroid lobe and any other involved structures (Answer D). Bisphosphonates and high-dosage cinacalcet have been used for management of hypercalcemia when surgery is not curative.

A sestamibi scan (Answer A) will not be particularly useful in a patient with a palpable, obvious neck mass and hyperparathyroidism. Genetic testing for *RET* proto-oncogene mutations (Answer C) would be useful in patients with other features suggestive of multiple endocrine neoplasia type 2 in addition to primary hyperparathyroidism (eg, medullary carcinoma and pheochromocytoma), which this patient does not have. Additionally, one would expect patients with this syndrome to have a positive family history and to present earlier in life.

Parafibromin is a tumor suppressor protein encoded by the *CDC73* gene, and mutations in this gene are associated with the autosomal dominant hyperparathyroidism–jaw tumor syndrome. Recently, patients with apparent sporadic, non-familial parathyroid carcinomas were found to have loss of parafibromin staining on immunohistochemistry. Loss of parafibromin staining in the parathyroid tissue is associated with greater likelihood of local recurrence and metastatic disease. However, serum parafibromin measurement (Answer E) is not clinically useful or available.

EDUCATIONAL OBJECTIVE:
Recognize and manage parathyroid carcinoma.

REFERENCE(S):

Cao J, Chen C, Wang QL, Xu JJ, Ge MH. Parathyroid carcinoma: a report of six cases with a brief review of the literature. *Oncol Lett.* 2015;10(6):3363-3368.

Cetani F, Banti C, Pardi E, et al. CDC73 mutational status and loss of parafibromin in the outcome of parathyroid cancer. *Endocr Connect.* 2013;2(4):186-195.

Cetani F, Pardi E, Marcocci C. Update on parathyroid carcinoma. *J Endocrinol Invest.* 2016;39(6):595-606.

30 **ANSWER: E) Her spine bone mineral density was measured incorrectly**

It is always important to look at the images and numbers of a DXA study, particularly when the results do not make sense. Although gains in bone mineral density at one site and loss at another are possible, this situation is very uncommon. In this patient's images, the placement of the spine analysis bars is incorrect, one level higher up than the previous study (ie, L4 on the current study is actually L3) (Answer E). After correct reanalysis, the difference in her spine bone mineral density was not significant.

Her hip images are correct (thus, Answer D is incorrect). She appears to be responding to alendronate (thus, Answer B is incorrect) and therefore she is most likely taking it correctly (thus, Answer A is incorrect); the gains seen in the hip are higher than the least significant change, assumed to be 2.8% for total hip and 5% for femoral neck in clinical DXA studies. There is no reason to suspect that she has an undiagnosed secondary cause of osteoporosis (Answer C).

EDUCATIONAL OBJECTIVE:
Carefully review DXA images and identify common technical errors.

REFERENCE(S):

Watts NB. Fundamentals and pitfalls of bone densitometry using dual-energy X-ray absorptiometry (DXA). *Osteoporos Int.* 2004;15(11):847-854.

Schousboe JT, Shepherd JA, Bilezikian JP, Baim S. Executive summary of the 2013 international society for clinical densitometry position development conference on bone densitometry. *J Clin Densitom.* 2013;16(4):455-466.

Obesity/Lipids Board Review

Andrea D. Coviello, MD ● Duke University

1 ANSWER: B) Orlistat

Orlistat (Answer B) is a pancreatic lipase inhibitor that works by blocking fat metabolism and consequently fat absorption in the gut causing excretion of approximately 30% of ingested fats in the stool. All the other US FDA-approved medications work through appetite suppression.

Phentermine (Answer A) is a sympathomimetic agent that stimulates satiety through central nervous system pathways in the hypothalamus; phentermine stimulates noradrenergic and GABA receptors suppressing appetite. The drug combination of phentermine and topiramate (Answer C) also suppresses appetite through signaling in the central nervous system. Topiramate blocks the AMPA glutamate receptor, which suppresses appetite. Topiramate is approved for use in patients with seizure disorders and chronic migraines to reduce the frequency of both; the weight-loss effect occurs at lower dosages, generally less than 100 mg daily. Lorcaserin (Answer D) is a serotonin reuptake inhibitor that works at the 5-HT2C receptor subclass to suppress appetite. The combination medication naltrexone/bupropion (Answer E) acts jointly to suppress appetite and promote satiety through 2 different pathways. Naltrexone is an opioid antagonist that works on the reward pathways in the hypothalamus. Bupropion is an inhibitor of dopamine and noradrenaline uptake and is used as an antidepressant and to help patients stop smoking cigarettes. Liraglutide is another weight-loss medication choice, but it was not a listed option. Liraglutide is a glucagonlike peptide 1 receptor agonist that acts directly at glucagonlike peptide 1 receptors on POMC-CART neurons to stimulate satiety and indirectly suppress hunger signaling through AgRP-NPY neuronal pathways in the hypothalamus. None of the currently FDA-approved weight-loss medications improve energy expenditure by changing the resting metabolic rate.

EDUCATIONAL OBJECTIVE:
Explain the mechanism of action behind the weight-loss medications currently approved by the US FDA.

REFERENCE(S):

Apovian CM, Aronne LJ, Bessesen DH, et al; Endocrine Society. Pharmacological management of obesity: an Endocrine Society clinical practice guideline. *J Clin Endocrinol Metab.* 2015;100(2): 342-362.

Jensen MD, Ryan DH, Apovian CM, et al; American College of Cardiology/American Heart Association Task Force on Practice Guidelines; Obesity Society. 2013 AHA/ACC/TOS guideline for the management of overweight and obesity in adults: a report of the American College of Cardiology/American Heart Association Task Force on Practice Guidelines and The Obesity Society. *J Am Coll Cardiol.* 2014;63(25 Pt B): 2985-3023.

Yanovski SZ, Yanovski JA. Long-term drug treatment for obesity: a systematic and clinical review. *JAMA.* 2014;311(1):74-86.

2 ANSWER: A) Phentermine/topiramate titrated to 15 mg/92 mg daily

The 2015 Endocrine Society's clinical practice guideline on the pharmacologic management of obesity and the 2013 AHA/TOS guidelines recommend consideration of a weight-loss medication for obese individuals (BMI >30 kg/m²) or overweight individuals (BMI >27 kg/m²) who also have a weight-related comorbidity such as type 2 diabetes, hypertension, or dyslipidemia. Most weight-loss medications are associated with a 3% to 10% weight loss over 6 to 12 months. Long-term data defined as longer than 1 year are available only for orlistat (4 years of follow-up) and liraglutide (3 years of follow-up). The reported average percentage weight loss from baseline in the literature is presented in the table. Phentermine/topiramate (Answer A) has the greatest reported weight loss in shorter studies: 6% to 9% at 1 year and 10.5% at 2 years.

Medication	Data at ~1 year	Longer-Term Data (1-4 years)
Phentermine/topiramate titrated to 15 mg/92 mg daily	6%-9%	10.5% at 2 years
Lorcaserin, 10 mg twice daily	3%-4%	6.8% at 2 years
Naltrexone/bupropion ER	4%-5%	…
Liraglutide, 3.0 mg daily	5%-6%	6.1% at 3 years

EDUCATIONAL OBJECTIVE:
Counsel patients on the expected range of weight loss with the use of US FDA-approved weight-loss medications in conjunction with a diet and exercise program.

REFERENCE(S):

Apovian CM, Aronne LJ, Bessesen DH, et al; Endocrine Society. Pharmacological management of obesity: an Endocrine Society clinical practice guideline. *J Clin Endocrinol Metab.* 2015;100(2): 342-362.

Jensen MD, Ryan DH, Apovian CM, et al; American College of Cardiology/American Heart Association Task Force on Practice Guidelines; Obesity Society. 2013 AHA/ACC/TOS guideline for the management of overweight and obesity in adults: a report of the American College of Cardiology/American Heart Association Task Force on Practice Guidelines and The Obesity Society. *J Am Coll Cardiol.* 2014;63(25 Pt B): 2985-3023.

Yanovski SZ, Yanovski JA. Long-term drug treatment for obesity: a systematic and clinical review. *JAMA.* 2014;311(1):74-86.

le Roux CW, Astrup A, Fujioka K, et al; SCALE Obesity Prediabetes NN8022-1839 Study Group. 3 years of liraglutide versus placebo for type 2 diabetes risk reduction and weight management in individuals with prediabetes: a randomised, double-blind trial. *Lancet.* 2017;389(10077): 1399-1409.

Pi-Sunyer X, Astrup A, Fujioka K, et al; SCALE Obesity and Prediabetes NN8022-1839 Study Group. A randomized, controlled trial of 3.0 mg of liraglutide in weight management. *N Engl J Med.* 2015;373(1):11-22.

Yanovski SZ, Yanovski JA. Naltrexone extended-release plus bupropion extended-release for treatment of obesity. *JAMA.* 2015;313(12): 1213-1214.

Garvey WT, Ryan DH, Look M, et al. Two-year sustained weight loss and metabolic benefits with controlled-release phentermine/topiramate in obese and overweight adults (SEQUEL): a randomized, placebo-controlled, phase 3 extension study. *Am J Clin Nutr.* 2012;95(2):297-308.

Smith SR, Weissman NJ, Anderson CM, et al; Behavioral Modification and Lorcaserin for Overweight and Obesity Management (BLOOM) Study Group. Multicenter, placebo-controlled trial of lorcaserin for weight management. *N Engl J Med.* 2010;363(3):245-256.

3 ANSWER: C) Ghrelin ↑, glucagonlike peptide 1 ↓, peptide YY ↓, cholecystokinin ↓
Multiple peptide hormones secreted by the gastrointestinal tract regulate appetite through signaling primarily in the arcuate nucleus of the hypothalamus. Ghrelin is a peptide hormone secreted by cells lining the stomach that acts in the hypothalamus to stimulate hunger. Ghrelin production is suppressed after eating and rises again several hours later in the fasting state to stimulate hunger and food intake. Glucagonlike peptide 1, peptide YY, and cholecystokinin are peptide hormones secreted by the intestines in response to the presence of nutrients after food ingestion that stimulate satiety pathways in the central nervous system and meal cessation. After a weight loss of approximately 10%, this hormonal profile shifts to favor weight regain. Ghrelin levels increase and glucagonlike peptide 1, peptide YY, and cholecystokinin are suppressed (Answer C), which causes the individual to feel hungrier and less satiated after food intake. This pattern promotes weight regain and correlates with the experience that weight maintenance or continued weight loss are progressively harder after initial weight loss.

EDUCATIONAL OBJECTIVE:
Identify the changes in gut hormones that occur after 10% weight loss.

REFERENCE(S):

Sumithran P, Prendergast LA, Delbridge E, et al. Long-term persistence of hormonal adaptations to weight loss. *N Engl J Med.* 2011;365(17): 1597-1604.

4 ANSWER: D) Phentermine/topiramate

Selection of weight-loss medications should be based on a patient's individual characteristics and clinical profile. Polycystic ovary syndrome is associated with overweight and obesity and significant metabolic dysfunction, including insulin resistance, type 2 diabetes mellitus, metabolic syndrome, and fatty liver disease. Weight loss will improve this patient's metabolic and reproductive dysfunction. There are no data to suggest one medication works better than another for weight loss in patients with polycystic ovary syndrome specifically. However, her clinical picture should guide selection of a weight-loss medication, particularly her history of migraines and gallbladder disease.

Phentermine/topiramate (Answer D) is a combination medication containing phentermine (increasing doses up to 15 mg daily) and topiramate (increasing doses up to 92 mg daily). Topiramate is approved by the US FDA for use in patients with chronic migraines to reduce the frequency of migraines and for patients with seizure disorders to reduce the frequency of seizures. Although topiramate itself is not approved for weight loss, topiramate in combination with phentermine is in the combination medication phentermine/topiramate. Given this patient's chronic migraines, phentermine/topiramate is a good choice for her.

One of the most common adverse effects of naltrexone/bupropion (Answer A) is headache, which would make it a poor choice in a patient with chronic migraines. Lorcaserin (Answer B) is a serotonin reuptake inhibitor (blocking 5-HT2C receptors) that increases serotonergic activity. Use of lorcaserin in patients who are already taking a selective serotonin reuptake inhibitor, as this patient is for depression, increases the risk of serotonin syndrome. Liraglutide, 3.0 mg daily, (Answer C) is associated with gallbladder disease, including cholecystitis and gallstone pancreatitis. Over 3 years, treatment with liraglutide, 3.0 mg daily, for weight loss was associated with gallbladder disease in 4.9% of patients with consistent risk of gallbladder problems throughout the 3-year observation period. Given this patient's recurrent abdominal pain and known gallstones, liraglutide is not a good choice for her, although it would most likely improve her insulin resistance. Weight loss itself is associated with increased gallbladder dysfunction believed to be due to decreased gallbladder contractility, and glucagonlike peptide 1 receptor agonists are associated with added risk of gallbladder disease irrespective of the degree of weight loss.

EDUCATIONAL OBJECTIVE:
Select appropriate medical therapy for weight loss based on a patient's individual characteristics and risk profile.

REFERENCE(S):

Apovian CM, Aronne LJ, Bessesen DH, et al; Endocrine Society. Pharmacological management of obesity: an endocrine Society clinical practice guideline. *J Clin Endocrinol Metab.* 2015;100(2): 342-362.

Yanovski SZ, Yanovski JA. Long-term drug treatment for obesity: a systematic and clinical review. *JAMA.* 2014;311(1):74-86.

Garvey WT, Ryan DH, Look M, et al. Two-year sustained weight loss and metabolic benefits with controlled-release phentermine/topiramate in obese and overweight adults (SEQUEL): a randomized, placebo-controlled, phase 3 extension study. *Am J Clin Nutr.* 2012;95(2):297-308.

Smith SR, Weissman NJ, Anderson CM, et al; Behavioral Modification and Lorcaserin for Overweight and Obesity Management (BLOOM) Study Group. Multicenter, placebo-controlled trial of lorcaserin for weight management. *N Engl J Med.* 2010;363(3):245-256.

le Roux CW, Astrup A, Fujioka K, et al; SCALE Obesity Prediabetes NN8022-1839 Study Group. 3 years of liraglutide versus placebo for type 2 diabetes risk reduction and weight management in individuals with prediabetes: a randomised, double-blind trial. *Lancet.* 2017;389(10077): 1399-1409.

Pi-Sunyer X, Astrup A, Fujioka K, et al; SCALE Obesity and Prediabetes NN8022-1839 Study Group. A randomized, controlled trial of 3.0 mg of liraglutide in weight management. *N Engl J Med.* 2015;373(1):11-22.

Yanovski SZ, Yanovski JA. Naltrexone extended-release plus bupropion extended-release for treatment of obesity. *JAMA.* 2015;313(12): 1213-1214.

Huang G, Coviello A. Clinical update on screening, diagnosis and management of metabolic disorders and cardiovascular risk factors associated with polycystic ovary syndrome. *Curr Opin Endocrinol Diabetes Obes.* 2012;19(6):512-519.

5 ANSWER: A) Melanocortin 4 receptor (*MC4R*) mutation

Although knowledge of the monogenic forms of severe childhood obesity is most relevant for pediatric endocrinologists, adult endocrinologists will on occasion encounter a patient with one of these syndromes, and genetic forms of obesity provide insights into important pathways that regulate body weight.

The most common monogenic form of early-onset obesity is caused by mutations in the gene than encodes the melanocortin 4 receptor (*MC4R*) (Answer A). The melanocortin 4 receptor is involved in hypothalamic signaling along the neural pathway that responds to leptin. The hypothalamus has a central role in the regulation of food intake. Leptin and insulin act on proopiomelanocortin (POMC) neurons in the arcuate nucleus to increase the expression and release of α-melanocyte–stimulating hormone, which then binds to melanocortin 4 receptors (*MC4R*) on postsynaptic cells to reduce food intake. A mutation blocking receptor function would lead to the loss of satiety and unblocked hunger leading to hyperphagia. These patients present with childhood obesity.

Individuals who have mutations in the genes encoding leptin (Answer B) or the leptin receptor (Answer C) have hypothalamic hypogonadism and subtle impairments in GH and immune function. A mutation in the gene encoding proopiomelanocortin (Answer D) causes a rare form of early-onset, childhood obesity due to hyperphagia. POMC has an important role in regulating satiety and energy expenditure. POMC is cleaved into melanocyte-stimulating hormone and ACTH, which is necessary for normal adrenal function.

Affected patients present with childhood obesity, as well as adrenal insufficiency, which may present with hypoglycemia in the neonatal period. The adrenal insufficiency is treated with glucocorticoid replacement, but the obesity is difficult to treatment. Two affected individuals were treated with setmelanotide, a melanocortin 4 receptor agonist that reduced hunger and induced weight loss of 44 to 110 lb (20-50 kg) over 12 to 42 weeks.

EDUCATIONAL OBJECTIVE:
Identify monogenic forms of early-onset obesity.

REFERENCE(S):
Kuhnen P, Clement K, Wiegand S, et al. Proopiomelanocortin deficiency treated with a melanocortin-4 receptor agonist. *N Engl J Med.* 2016;375(3):240-246.

Farooqi S, O'Rahilly S. Genetics of obesity in humans. *Endocr Rev.* 2006;27(7):710-718.

Ranadive SA, Vaisse C. Lessons from extreme human obesity: monogenic disorders. *Endocrinol Metab Clin North Am.* 2008;37(3):733-751.

Schwartz MW, Woods SC, Porte D Jr, Seeley RJ, Baskin DG. Central nervous system control of food intake. *Nature.* 2000;404(6778):661-671.

6 ANSWER: A) *FTO*

While lifestyle and environmental factors are extremely important in weight gain, genetic factors are also important. Genome-wide association studies have identified many gene loci that are important determinates of BMI. The single gene most commonly associated with typical human obesity is *FTO* (Answer A). This association has been documented in different populations. Individuals with the at-risk allele weigh 4.4 to 6.6 lb (2 to 3 kg) more than those without the allele. Many studies have tried to determine the mechanisms by which the at-risk alleles in the *FTO* gene produce increased BMI. Most of the physiologic data suggest this occurs through a predisposition for increased food intake.

Genetic variants in the *MCR4* gene (Answer D) are associated with severe, early-onset childhood obesity, but these cases are very rare compared with the prevalence of the *FTO* gene variant. This patient did not have early-onset obesity as a child, which makes a monogenic form of obesity unlikely.

The other 3 genes listed have been associated with obesity, but the effect sizes are smaller than that of the *FTO* gene. *IRS1* (Answer B) is associated with a higher BMI but also lower risk of coronary artery disease, lower triglycerides, higher HDL cholesterol, higher adiponectin, and lower insulin levels. *TLR4* (Answer C) is associated with higher BMI and is hypothesized to influence weight through the microbiome. Variations in the *HHIP* gene (Answer E) are associated with increased BMI but paradoxically a decreased risk of type 2 diabetes and higher HDL cholesterol.

A recent study using the most definitive methods applied to date provides strong evidence that DNA near the *FTO* gene interacts with other genes at a distance to foster the development of adipocyte precursors to either white or brown/beige adipocytes. More than 100 genetic mutations have been identified that are associated with BMI, but together they explain less than 5% of the variation in BMI. This suggests that while genetic susceptibility has a role in common adult-onset obesity, common obesity is a complex disorder with many contributing factors.

EDUCATIONAL OBJECTIVE:
Identify the most common gene variant associated with obesity.

REFERENCE(S):
Locke AE, Kahali B, Berndt SI, et al. Genetic studies of body mass index yield new insights for obesity biology. *Nature.* 2015;518(7538):197-206.

Loos RJ, Yeo GS. The bigger picture of FTO--the first GWAS-identified obesity gene. *Nat Rev Endocrinol.* 2014;10(1):51-61.

Qi Q, Downer MK, Kilpelainen TO, et al. Dietary intake, FTO genetic variants, and adiposity: a combined analysis of over 16,000 children and adolescents. *Diabetes.* 2015;64(7):2467-2476.

Claussnitzer M, Dankel SN, Kim KH, et al. FTO obesity variant circuitry and adipocyte browning in humans. *N Engl J Med.* 2015;373(10):895-907.

7 **ANSWER: C) Decrease the glipizide dosage**
Glucagonlike peptide 1 receptor agonists are now used extensively to treat type 2 diabetes. Liraglutide at a dosage of 1.8 mg daily improves glycemic control in patients with type 2 diabetes, but it is used for weight loss as an adjunct to diet and exercise at a dosage of 3.0 mg daily. Hypoglycemia is very uncommon in obese patients without type 2 diabetes who take liraglutide. Only 1.6% of patients on liraglutide experience symptoms of hypoglycemia compared with 1.1% on placebo.

If the higher dosage of liraglutide is used for weight loss in individuals with type 2 diabetes who take other medications to lower blood glucose, one must be aware of the risk of hypoglycemia and adjust medications appropriately. In a randomized controlled trial of liraglutide, 3.0 mg daily, or placebo given to obese patients taking 1 of 3 oral agents (metformin, pioglitazone, or a sulfonylurea), the rates of hypoglycemia in patients on metformin or pioglitazone was 25.7% compared with 7.6% in the placebo group. The rate of hypoglycemia was 43.6% in those taking liraglutide plus a sulfonylurea compared with 27.3% in those taking placebo plus a sulfonylurea. It is recommended that the dosage of sulfonylureas be lowered at least 50% or stopped with the initiation of liraglutide and that blood glucose be monitored closely during dosage escalation to 3.0 mg daily (thus, Answer C is correct). One would not increase the dosage of sulfonylurea (Answer B) when initiating liraglutide. His hemoglobin A_{1c} is above target at 7.6% (60 mmol/mol), and treatment with liraglutide will most likely lower his hemoglobin A_{1c} by more than 0.5%.

Similarly, despite his hemoglobin A_{1c} level of 7.6%, the risk of hypoglycemia when adding liraglutide, 3.0 mg daily, to metformin is still high (25.7%), but lower than when adding liraglutide to a sulfonylurea (43.6%). One would not want to increase the metformin dosage (Answer A) at the same time as adding liraglutide due to increased risk of hypoglycemia. According to the 2013 American College of Cardiology/American Heart Association Cholesterol Lowering Guidelines, this patient would benefit the most from a high-intensity statin (which he is currently taking—atorvastatin, 40 mg daily). Lowering his dosage into the moderate-intensity statin range would be inappropriate. Statins are associated with incident diabetes. Raising or lowering his statin dosage (Answers D and E) would not affect his weight or significantly alter his glycemic control compared with a glucagonlike peptide 1 receptor agonist.

EDUCATIONAL OBJECTIVE:
Manage oral diabetes medications in patients with type 2 diabetes mellitus when starting liraglutide for weight loss.

REFERENCE(S):

Davies MJ, Bergenstal R, Bode B, et al; NN8022-1922 Study Group. Efficacy of liraglutide for weight loss among patients with type 2 diabetes: the SCALE Diabetes Randomized Clinical Trial. *JAMA.* 2015;314(7):687-699.

Pi-Sunyer X, Astrup A, Fujioka K, et al; SCALE Obesity and Prediabetes NN8022-1839 Study Group. A randomized, controlled trial of 3.0 mg of liraglutide in weight management. *N Engl J Med.* 2015;373(1):11-22.

8   ANSWER: B) Roux-en-Y gastric bypass

Patients commonly ask their endocrinologists for advice about the risks and benefits of bariatric surgery. It is important, therefore, to have a sense of both the amount of weight loss that a patient might expect from the commonly performed bariatric surgical procedures, as well as the potential problems associated with each.

The laparoscopic banding procedure (Answer C) was popular for many years because it was relatively easy for the surgeon to perform and had low perioperative risk. Because it was potentially reversible, it satisfied many patients' desire to not have their "plumbing changed." However, it is now clear that the weight loss with the banding procedure is less (18%-22% of baseline weight) than that of other procedures and that mechanical problems are more common with this procedure over the long term. Sleeve gastrectomy (Answer A) is gaining in popularity because it does not require ongoing adjustment (as does the band), results in better weight loss (22%-25%), and is relatively easy for the surgeon to perform. Despite these advantages, recent studies have shown that the sleeve gastrectomy is not as effective as gastric bypass in either producing weight loss or improving glucose control in patients with type 2 diabetes. Roux-en-Y gastric bypass (Answer B) provides the most weight loss (25%-28%) of the 3 operations listed and often dramatically improves glucose levels in patients with type 2 diabetes. However, it results in a lifelong need for vitamin supplementation and most likely puts patients at risk for metabolic bone disease. Biliopancreatic diversion, which is not listed as a choice, is a more extensive operation that is not often performed currently. It is important for endocrinologists to be aware of this procedure, however, as they may see patients who are thinking of having it or who have had it in the past. It is associated with the greatest degree of weight loss (32%-35%) and has the greatest effect on glucose levels, but it is not widely used because of more frequent complications and adverse effects, including severe and potentially difficult-to-treat vitamin deficiencies.

The endoscopically placed duodenal sleeve (Answer D) is an experimental device that mimics the duodenal bypass that is part of the gastric bypass procedure. In animal studies done in rodent models of diabetes, it appears to have beneficial effects on glucose control. The limited data available in humans suggest about a 13% weight loss 6 months after placement.

EDUCATIONAL OBJECTIVE:
Describe the expected weight loss associated with different bariatric surgical procedures.

REFERENCE(S):

Dumon KR, Murayama KM. Bariatric surgery outcomes. *Surg Clin North Am.* 2011;91(6): 1313-1338.

Chang SH, Stoll CR, Song J, Varela JE, Eagon CJ, Colditz GA. The effectiveness and risks of bariatric surgery: an updated systematic review and meta-analysis, 2003-2012. *JAMA Surg.* 2014; 149(3):275-287.

Padwal R, Klarenbach S, Wiebe N, et al. Bariatric surgery: a systematic review and network meta-analysis of randomized trials. *Obes Rev.* 2011; 12(8):602-621.

9   ANSWER: D) 80%

Glucagonlike peptide 1 receptor agonists are now widely used in the treatment of type 2 diabetes to improve glycemic control. While all formulations are delivered by subcutaneous injection, the duration of action varies with twice-daily, once-daily, and now weekly formulations. Only one glucagonlike peptide 1 receptor agonist is currently approved for the treatment of overweight and obesity—liraglutide at a dosage of 3.0 mg daily (Saxenda). It is important to note that liraglutide is also the active ingredient in Victoza, which is US FDA-approved for treatment of type 2 diabetes at a maximum dosage of 1.8 mg daily, but it is not approved to treat obesity.

The SCALE trial examined the safety and efficacy of liraglutide, 3 mg daily. There was a 9.2% weight loss in the liraglutide group compared with a 3.5% weight loss in the placebo group by the end of the first year (intention-to-treat analysis: weight loss of 7.4% vs 3.0% from baseline, $P<.0001$). Participants with prediabetes randomly assigned to liraglutide or placebo were followed for an additional 2 years. For patients with prediabetes who participated in the extension trial for a total of 160 weeks of drug therapy, the liraglutide group lost about 7.1% of their baseline weight compared with 2.7% in the placebo group ($P<.0001$). At the end of 3 years of treatment, 6% of the placebo group progressed from prediabetes to type 2 diabetes compared with 2% of the liraglutide group, with a hazard ratio of 0.21 (95% confidence interval, 0.13-0.34) for a 79% reduction in risk of developing type 2 diabetes (thus, Answer D is correct and Answers A, B, C, and E are incorrect). Additionally, two-thirds of patients who had prediabetes and were taking liraglutide reverted to normoglycemia at 160 weeks compared with about one-third of patients on placebo.

EDUCATIONAL OBJECTIVE:
Counsel patients on the reduced risk for progression from prediabetes to type 2 diabetes with weight loss achieved with use of the glucagonlike peptide 1 receptor agonist liraglutide.

REFERENCE(S):
le Roux CW, Astrup A, Fujioka K, et al; SCALE Obesity Prediabetes NN8022-1839 Study Group. 3 years of liraglutide versus placebo for type 2 diabetes risk reduction and weight management in individuals with prediabetes: a randomised, double-blind trial. *Lancet.* 2017;389(10077): 1399-1409.

Pi-Sunyer X, Astrup A, Fujioka K, et al; SCALE Obesity and Prediabetes NN8022-1839 Study Group. A randomized, controlled trial of 3.0 mg of liraglutide in weight management. *N Engl J Med.* 2015;373(1):11-22.

Apovian CM, Aronne LJ, Bessesen DH, et al; Endocrine Society. Pharmacological management of obesity: an endocrine Society clinical practice guideline. *J Clin Endocrinol Metab.* 2015;100(2): 342-362.

10 ANSWER: C) 20%
Over the last 5 years, an increasing body of data has emerged on the benefits of bariatric surgery on glucose control in patients with type 2 diabetes. Early studies were simply case series—not randomized controlled trials—that suggested high rates of remission. However, these studies did not always define remission rigorously. The STAMPEDE trial (Surgical Therapy and Medications Potentially Eradicate Diabetes Efficiently) is one of the first prospective randomized controlled trials to compare traditional medical therapy for type 2 diabetes with either gastric bypass surgery or sleeve gastrectomy compared to intensive medical therapy. The patients enrolled had a BMI of 27 to 43 kg/m² at baseline complicated by type 2 diabetes. These investigators defined remission a priori as a hemoglobin A_{1c} level less than 6.0% on no glucose-lowering medications. Five-year follow-up data are now available (released February 2017) on 134 of the 150 participants with type 2 diabetes in the original cohort. Fourteen patients who underwent Roux-en-Y gastric bypass (29%) and 11 who underwent sleeve gastrectomy (23%) remained in remission from type 2 diabetes compared with 2 (5%) in the medical therapy group. In the surgical groups, 89% remained off insulin with an average hemoglobin A_{1c} level of 7.0% compared with 61% of patients in the medical therapy group with an average hemoglobin A_{1c} level of 8.5%.

EDUCATIONAL OBJECTIVE:
Describe the data from randomized controlled trials documenting the remission of diabetes after gastric bypass surgery.

REFERENCE(S):
Schauer PR, Bhatt DL, Kirwan JP, et al. Bariatric surgery versus intensive medical therapy for diabetes - 5-year outcomes. *N Engl J Med.* 2017;376(7):641-651.

Schauer PR, Kashyap SR, Wolski K, et al. Bariatric surgery versus intensive medical therapy in obese patients with diabetes. *N Engl J Med*. 2012; 366(17):1567-1576.

Schauer PR, Bhatt DL, Kirwan JP, et al; STAMPEDE Investigators. Bariatric surgery versus intensive medical therapy for diabetes--3-year outcomes. *N Engl J Med*. 2014;370(21):2002-2013.

11 ANSWER: A) Lorcaserin

Obesity is an independent risk factor for cardiovascular disease and can adversely affect other risk factors for cardiovascular disease, including hypertension, type 2 diabetes, and dyslipidemia. Weight loss can lower cardiovascular risk for both primary and secondary prevention. Care must be taken when selecting a weight-loss medication for use in patients with a recent coronary heart disease event or who are at risk for tachyarrhythmias, as most of the currently approved weight-loss medications can affect blood pressure and heart rate. Furthermore, resting tachycardia is commonly present in obese patients, even in the absence of known heart disease.

Phentermine (Answer B) and diethylpropion (Answer E) are sympathomimetic agents, or stimulants, that suppress appetite and are known to increase both blood pressure and heart rate and would thus be contraindicated in this patient. Phentermine/topiramate (Answer C) is a combination medication containing topiramate and phentermine, which makes it a poor choice for weight loss in this patient. Glucagonlike peptide 1 receptor agonists, including liraglutide (Answer D), are known to increase resting heart rate although they are not associated with increases in blood pressure. Liraglutide, 3.0 mg daily, is associated with an average 2 to 3 beat/min increase in heart rate, but a proportion of patients may experience an increase in resting heart rate of greater than 10 beats/min (34% compared with 19% on placebo) or greater than 20 beat/min (5% compared with 2% on placebo), but only 0.9% develop a resting heart rate higher than 100 beats/min compared with 0.3% on placebo. Thus, liraglutide, 3.0 mg daily, would not be a good choice for this patient.

Lorcaserin (Answer A) is a serotonin receptor reuptake inhibitor that is selective for the 5-HT2C receptors. Lorcaserin does not significantly increase blood pressure or heart rate. Fenfluramine was used in combination with phentermine in the weight-loss medication phen-fen or Redux, which was associated with valvular heart disease due to stimulation of a different subclass of serotonin receptors (the 5-HT2B receptors), and it was removed from the market in 1997. Lorcaserin has not been associated with valvular heart disease or other forms of heart disease and would be a reasonable selection for this patient given its safety profile.

EDUCATIONAL OBJECTIVE:
Select weight-loss medications for a patient with a history of cardiovascular disease and arrhythmic potential.

REFERENCE(S):
Apovian CM, Aronne LJ, Bessesen DH, et al; Endocrine Society. Pharmacological management of obesity: an Endocrine Society clinical practice guideline. *J Clin Endocrinol Metab*. 2015;100(2): 342-362.

Yanovski SZ, Yanovski JA. Long-term drug treatment for obesity: a systematic and clinical review. *JAMA*. 2014;311(1):74-86.

Pi-Sunyer X, Astrup A, Fujioka K, et al; SCALE Obesity and Prediabetes NN8022-1839 Study Group. A randomized, controlled trial of 3.0 mg of liraglutide in weight management. *N Engl J Med*. 2015;373(1):11-22.

le Roux CW, Astrup A, Fujioka K, et al; SCALE Obesity Prediabetes NN8022-1839 Study Group. 3 years of liraglutide versus placebo for type 2 diabetes risk reduction and weight management in individuals with prediabetes: a randomised, double-blind trial. *Lancet*. 2017;389(10077): 1399-1409.

Smith SR, Weissman NJ, Anderson CM, et al; Behavioral Modification and Lorcaserin for Overweight and Obesity Management (BLOOM) Study Group. Multicenter, placebo-controlled trial of lorcaserin for weight management. *N Engl J Med*. 2010;363(3):245-256.

Lorcaserin [package insert]. Woodcliff Lake, NJ: Eisai Inc; 2012.

12 ANSWER: C) Cholelithiasis

The most effective treatment currently available for weight loss is bariatric surgery. However, aggressive energy restriction with a very low-calorie diet is almost as effective as gastric banding. Very low-calorie diets are restricted to fewer than 800 kcal per day. Very low-calorie diets are high in protein to maximally preserve lean body mass. Very low-calorie diets produce, on average, 17% to 18% weight loss over 3 months. However, 25% of patients on such a diet for 2 months develop gallbladder disease, particularly acute cholecystitis due to cholelithiasis, frequently requiring surgery (6%). The increase in gallbladder disease is believed to be due to decreased gallbladder contractility. The greater the rate and magnitude of weight loss, the greater the risk of gallbladder disease. This patient already has known gallstones, which would put her at even higher risk for cholecystitis and potentially gallstone pancreatitis (thus, Answer C is correct).

Very low-calorie diets have also been shown to produce dramatic improvements in glucose levels in persons with type 2 diabetes (thus, Answer E is incorrect). Fatty liver disease is generally improved with weight loss, particularly with diets lower in fats (thus, Answer A is incorrect), which can also effectively lower triglycerides and improve dyslipidemia (thus, Answer B is incorrect). Weight loss is associated with depression and suicidal ideation, although the latter is very rare. Depression and suicidality are more common after bariatric surgery than after weight loss through dietary measures, which makes this complication less concerning than acute gallbladder disease, assuming there is appropriate medical supervision (thus, Answer D is incorrect). Concerns remain about the long-term maintenance of weight loss with this strategy. Long-term weight loss with very low-calorie diets tends to be the same as that for low-calorie diets.

EDUCATIONAL OBJECTIVE:
Counsel patients about the benefits and risks of very low-calorie diets.

REFERENCE(S):
Tsai AG, Wadden TA. The evolution of very-low-calorie diets: an update and meta-analysis. *Obesity*. 2006;14(8):1283-1293.

13 ANSWER: E) Fluoxetine

Patients suffering from depression can experience fluctuations in their weight, particularly weight gain but also weight loss. According to the Centers for Disease Control, 11% of the US population older than 12 years is taking an antidepressant and more than 60% have taken an antidepressant for more than 2 years (https://www.cdc.gov/nchs/data/databriefs/db76.htm). Antidepressants can also affect a patient's weight, making selection of an antidepressant an important decision. The selective serotonin reuptake inhibitor paroxetine is associated with the most weight gain, which can be dramatic with long-term use. Amitriptyline (Answer A) is also associated with the most weight gain of the tricyclic antidepressants, followed by nortriptyline (although imipramine is weight neutral). Mirtazapine (Answer B), a noradrenergic and serotonergic receptor blocking antidepressant, is weight promoting. The combination serotonin and norepinephrine reuptake inhibitors venlafaxine (Answer C) and duloxetine are weight promoting. The selective serotonin reuptake inhibitor sertraline (Answer D) is weight neutral as are citalopram and escitalopram. However, fluoxetine (Answer E) promotes weight loss and is the best choice for this patient. Bupropion, a selective dopamine and norepinephrine reuptake inhibitor, promotes weight loss and is combined with naltrexone in a combination weight-loss medication, but this was not presented as an answer choice.

EDUCATIONAL OBJECTIVE:
Describe the effects of various antidepressant agents on weight and identify those that are weight neutral or promote weight loss.

REFERENCE(S):
Apovian CM, Aronne LJ, Bessesen DH, et al; Endocrine Society. Pharmacological management of obesity: an Endocrine Society clinical practice guideline. *J Clin Endocrinol Metab*. 2015;100(2): 342-362.

Serretti A, Mandelli L. Antidepressants and body weight: a comprehensive review and meta-analysis. *J Clin Psychiatry*. 2010;71(10):1259-1272.

Rosenzweig-Lipson S, Beyer CE, Hughes ZA, et al. Differentiating antidepressants of the future: efficacy and safety. *Pharmacol Ther.* 2007; 113(1):134-153.

Himmerich H, Minkwitz J, Kirkby KC. Weight gain and metabolic changes during treatment with antipsychotics and antidepressants. *Endocr Metab Immune Disord Drug Targets.* 2015;15(4):252-260.

Gadde KM, Xiong GL. Bupropion for weight reduction. *Expert Rev Neurother.* 2007;7(1):17-24.

14 ANSWER: D) Atorvastatin

Many commonly prescribed medications are associated with weight gain. Of the available antihypertensive medications, β-adrenergic blockers (Answer A) are associated with weight gain, while ACE inhibitors, angiotensin receptor blockers, calcium channel blockers, and diuretics are not. Many diabetes medications are associated with weight gain, up to 10 to 20 lb (4.5-9.1 kg) in the first 6 to 12 months, including the anabolic hormone insulin, insulin secretagogues (eg, sulfonylureas, meglitinides), and thiazolidinediones (Answer B). Metformin is weight neutral in general, although it is associated with mild weight loss in some. Dipeptidyl-peptidase 4 inhibitors and α-glucosidase inhibitors are weight neutral and glucagonlike peptide 1 receptor agonists promote weight loss in addition to blood glucose control. Sodium-glucose cotransporter 2 inhibitors are associated with mild weight loss in the context of glucosuria and water loss. More recently, antihistamines (Answer C) have been recognized as weight promoting. The more potent the antihistamine, the more likely the patient is to gain weight with long-term use. The H1-antihistamines such as cetirizine are the most likely to be associated with weight gain. Inhaled glucocorticoids (Answer E) are associated with weight gain. Other medication classes that can lead to weight gain include glucocorticoids, antidepressants, antipsychotic agents, and hormonal contraceptives. The statin class of medications (Answer D) is not associated with significant weight gain.

EDUCATIONAL OBJECTIVE:
Identify weight-promoting and weight-neutral medications among commonly prescribed medications for adults.

REFERENCE(S):

Apovian CM, Aronne LJ, Bessesen DH, et al; Endocrine Society. Pharmacological management of obesity: an Endocrine Society clinical practice guideline. *J Clin Endocrinol Metab.* 2015;100(2): 342-362.

15 ANSWER: C) Gastric band erosion

Patients who had gastric banding procedures many years ago often fail to follow-up with their surgeon. Endocrinologists who follow these patients for diabetes or other comorbid illnesses may be the only physicians who see them in long-term follow-up. For this reason, it is important for endocrinologists to recognize some of the long-term complications of gastric banding and gastric bypass operations. In particular, endocrinologists should be aware of the anatomy produced by the different bariatric surgical procedures and consider the possibility of a mechanical or anatomic problem when they see patients with new symptoms who have had bariatric surgical procedures.

The symptoms that this patient describes are typical for a gastric band erosion (Answer C). In this complication, the gastric band erodes through the stomach wall. Band erosion may present as unexplained weight regain with abdominal pain, or may present with signs of infection and inflammation as the gastric wall is perforated at the site of the erosion, with gastric contents tracking along the filling catheter to the subcutaneous port site. Gastric band erosion typically occurs in the first year after surgery, but can present 2 to 5 years after implantation.

Staple line dehiscence (Answer B) and anastomotic leaks (Answer D) are complications of gastric bypass operations, thus they could not occur in the described patient because a gastric banding procedure does not have any staple lines or intestinal anastomoses. Food impaction in a band (Answer E) typically occurs shortly after a band adjustment and subsequent solid food intake without adequate chewing. Affected patients present to the emergency department with abdominal pain and the inability to keep anything down, including saliva. The condition can be treated endoscopically. While a patient could conceivably manipulate the injection port (Answer A), there is no incentive to do this and the patient would not have the symptoms described.

REFERENCE(S):

Levine MS, Carucci LR. Imaging of bariatric surgery: normal anatomy and postoperative complications. *Radiology.* 2014;270(2):327-341.

Aarts EO, van Wageningen B, Berends F, Janssen I, Wahab P, Groenen M. Intragastric band erosion: experiences with gastrointestinal endoscopic removal. *World J Gastroenterol.* 2015;21(5): 1567-1572.

O'Brien PE, MacDonald L, Anderson M, Brennan L, Brown WA. Long-term outcomes after bariatric surgery: fifteen-year follow-up of adjustable gastric banding and a systematic review of the bariatric surgical literature. *Ann Surg.* 2013; 257(1):87-94.

16 ANSWER: B) Achilles tendon xanthomas

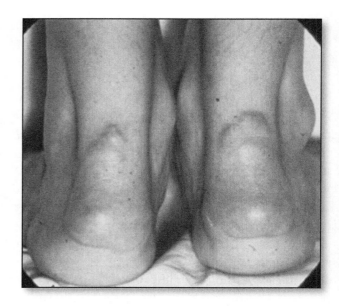

Familial hypercholesterolemia is relatively common with a prevalence of 1 in 250 to 500 persons depending on geographic region and race/ethnicity. Persons with familial hypercholesterolemia commonly have a heterozygous mutation in the gene encoding the LDL receptor. Defective apolipoprotein B, the ligand for the receptor, and a defect in an intracellular adaptor protein cause a similar phenotype. Persons who are heterozygous have total cholesterol levels of 350 to 600 mg/dL (9.06 to 15.54 mmol/L), LDL-cholesterol levels greater than 250 mg/dL (>6.48 mmol/L), and premature coronary artery disease. The homozygous form of familial hypercholesterolemia leads to atherosclerosis before age 20 to 30 years (sometimes in childhood). Liver transplant is sometimes used to treat homozygous familial hypercholesterolemia. Genetic testing does not alter therapy and is not usually performed. Patients are diagnosed based on their clinical phenotype with pathognomonic physical findings and a characteristic lipid profile. Patients with familial hypercholesterolemia develop cholesterol deposits in the soft tissues, specifically tendon sheaths leading to thickened tendons over the knuckles of the hands and particularly thickened Achilles tendons (Answer B) (*see image*).

It is not clear why lipid accumulates in the tendons, but it is thought to be secondary to recurrent inflammation and macrophage recruitment to where the tendon interacts with its overlying sheath. Cholesterol also deposits in the cornea around the iris giving a blue-grey ring–like appearance around the iris of the eye (arcus cornealis) at an early age. This appearance can also occur with aging, so it becomes less specific in older patients (arcus senilis).

High-dosage statin treatment is the first-line therapy. Documenting the physical manifestations of familial hyperlipidemia will become increasingly important when considering adding a PCSK9 inhibitor, as some insurance groups are following the Dutch Lipid Criteria that use family history, including high cholesterol (>95th percentile in the patient's children), in addition to physical signs (eg, tendinous xanthoma and early-onset arcus cornealis) and genetic analysis if available (eg, mutations in the *LDLR, APOB,* or *PCSK9* genes).

Lipemia retinalis (Answer A) is the milky appearance of the retina and retinal vessels that accompanies severe hypertriglyceridemia, which this patient does not have. Eruptive xanthomas (Answer C) are acnelike papules found on extensor surfaces of the arms and on the back and buttocks that present in the setting of severe hypertriglyceridemia. Palmar xanthomas (Answer D) are lipid depositions in the creases of the palms that occur with dysbetalipoproteinemia (formerly called type 3 hyperlipoproteinemia).

Orange tonsils (Answer E) are the hallmark of Tangier disease, which is characterized by extremely low HDL-cholesterol levels, not high LDL-cholesterol levels.

Current indications for PCSK9 inhibitor therapy include heterozygous familial hyperlipidemia and clinical atherosclerotic cardiovascular disease such as acute coronary syndromes, stable and unstable angina, myocardial infarction, peripheral vascular disease, history of coronary of other arterial revascularization, transient ischemic attack, and stroke for secondary prevention.

EDUCATIONAL OBJECTIVE:
Identify typical physical findings of familial hyperlipidemia to aid in diagnosis.

REFERENCE(S):
Semenkovich CF, Goldberg AC, Goldberg IJ. Disorders of lipid metabolism. In: Melmed S, Polonsky KS, Larsen PR, Kronenberg HM, eds. *Williams Textbook of Endocrinology.* 12th ed. Philadelphia, PA: Elsevier Saunders; 2011: 1633-1674.

17 **ANSWER: D) Add evolocumab**
Given that this patient had progressive coronary disease while on high-intensity statin therapy (atorvastatin, 80 mg daily), with an LDL-cholesterol level of 68 mg/dL (1.76 mmol/L) (which is less than the commonly used threshold of less than 70 mg/dL [<1.81 mmol/L] for patients with type 2 diabetes), he would benefit from the addition of a PCSK9 inhibitor (Answer D). PCSK9 is a hepatic-produced protease that is secreted, binds to cell-surface LDL receptors, and mediates their intracellular degradation. Antibodies to PCSK9 prevent this and lead to increased LDL-receptor levels, which in turn reduce circulating LDL levels. Up-regulation of LDL receptors is also the mechanism for statin-mediating LDL-cholesterol reductions because inhibition of de novo cholesterol biosynthesis increases sterol-responsive element–binding protein (SREBP)–mediated transcription of the LDL receptor. Oligonucleotide inhibition of apolipoprotein B and inhibition of microsomal triglyceride transfer protein are therapies recently approved for treatment of the rare homozygous form of familial hypercholesterolemia.

Current indications for PCSK9 inhibitors include heterozygous familial hyperlipidemia and clinical atherosclerotic cardiovascular disease such as acute coronary syndromes, stable and unstable angina, myocardial infarction, peripheral vascular disease, history of coronary of other arterial revascularization, transient ischemic attack, and stroke for secondary prevention.

EDUCATIONAL OBJECTIVE:
List the indications for addition of PCSK9 inhibitors to statin therapy to reduce risk of cardiovascular disease events.

REFERENCE(S):
Sabatine MS, Giugliano RP, Keech AC, et al; FOURIER Steering Committee and Investigators. Evolocumab and clinical outcomes in patients with cardiovascular disease. *N Engl J Med.* 2017;376(18):1713-1722.
Sabatine MS, Giugliano RP, Wiviott SD, et al; Open-Label Study of Long-Term Evaluation against LDL Cholesterol (OSLER) Investigators. Efficacy and safety of evolocumab in reducing lipids and cardiovascular events. *N Engl J Med.* 2015;372(16):1500-1509.
Ajufo E, Rader DJ. Recent advances in the pharmacological management of hypercholesterolaemia. *Lancet Diabetes Endocrinol.* 2016;4(5):436-446.

18 **ANSWER: A) Familial hypertriglyceridemia**
This patient presented with very high triglyceride levels at a young age on a screening test. Her history of estrogen exposure with oral contraceptive pill use before the development of severe hypertriglyceridemia is consistent with an underlying genetic disorder in lipid metabolism. Estrogen can increase triglycerides but usually not above 1000 mg/dL (>11.30 mmol/L) unless there is an underlying disorder. She then had moderately elevated triglyceride levels of 300 to 400 mg/dL (3.39-4.52 mmol/L) while off oral contraceptives.

Polycystic ovary syndrome (Answer B) is associated with a 2-fold increased risk for metabolic syndrome with high triglycerides and low HDL cholesterol, but triglycerides in that setting are not this high (usually <300 mg/dL [<3.39 mmol/L]). Lipoprotein lipase deficiency (Answer C) and apolipoprotein C1 deficiency (Answer D) are both associated with extremely high triglycerides (>1000 mg/dL [>11.30 mmol/L]), which this patient does not have at her baseline off oral contraceptives. Although the estrogen in the oral contraceptive pills did most likely increase her triglycerides into the range of 2000 mg/dL (22.60 mmol/L), she still had moderately elevated triglycerides when off estrogen. This patient probably has familial hypertriglyceridemia, an autosomal dominant disorder that she most likely inherited from her father.

Familial hypertriglyceridemia usually presents in adulthood with the introduction of a second insult that drives triglycerides even higher, such as estrogen in hormonal contraceptives or fertility treatment, alcohol use, certain medications, obesity, or hyperglycemia from poorly controlled diabetes. Baseline triglycerides are usually moderately elevated. Her second episode of severe hypertriglyceridemia was most likely caused by a poor diet rich in carbohydrates that drove her blood glucose values greater than 300 mg/dL (>16.65 mmol/L) and her triglyceride values greater than 1000 mg/dL (>11.30 mmol/L), leading to her first episode of pancreatitis.

EDUCATIONAL OBJECTIVE:
Identify primary and secondary disorders of hypertriglyceridemia.

REFERENCE(S):
Austin MA, Edwards KL, Monks SA, et al. Genome-wide scan for quantitative trait loci influencing LDL size and plasma triglyceride in familial hypertriglyceridemia. *J Lipid Res.* 2003;44(11): 2161-2168.

Brunzell JD. Clinical practice. Hypertriglyceridemia. *N Engl J Med.* 2007;357(10):1009-1017.

Brunzell JD, Schrott HG. The interaction of familial and secondary causes of hypertriglyceridemia: role in pancreatitis. *J Clin Lipidol.* 2012;6(5): 409-412.

Chait A, Brunzell JD. Severe hypertriglyceridemia: role of familial and acquired disorders. *Metabolism.* 1983;32(3):209-214.

Semenkovich CF, Goldberg AC, Goldberg IJ. Disorders of lipid metabolism. In: Melmed S, Polonsky KS, Larsen PR, Kronenberg HM, eds. *Williams Textbook of Endocrinology.* 12th ed. Philadelphia, PA: Elsevier Saunders; 2011: 1633-1674.

Huang G, Coviello A. Clinical update on screening, diagnosis and management of metabolic disorders and cardiovascular risk factors associated with polycystic ovary syndrome. *Curr Opin Endocrinol Diabetes Obes.* 2012;19(6):512-519.

19 ANSWER: B) Cholesteryl ester transfer protein deficiency

The patient's presentation is classic for cholesterol ester transfer protein (CETP) deficiency (Answer B). CETP catalyzes the exchange of triglyceride and cholesterol ester between triglyceride-rich lipoprotein particles and HDL particles. In normal individuals, the result is a net transfer of triglyceride to HDL, which leads to increased catabolism and reduced HDL-cholesterol levels. Persons with CETP deficiency have very high levels of HDL cholesterol. This condition is more common in individuals of Asian ancestry. Given this underlying physiology, pharmaceutical companies have developed CETP inhibitors. However, these medications to date have not been shown to reduce cardiovascular disease risk despite raising HDL levels significantly.

Alcohol use (Answer A) can raise HDL-cholesterol levels mildly, but typically not to this degree, and alcohol use is often associated with increases in triglycerides. Several medical conditions, including multiple myeloma and other paraproteinemias, can result in problems with the laboratory measurement of HDL cholesterol (Answer C), but in these cases, HDL cholesterol is low, not high. Apolipoprotein A1 is a major protein component and its deficiency (Answer D) can lead to low HDL cholesterol. Lipoprotein lipase deficiency (Answer E) is associated with low, not high, HDL-cholesterol levels and very high triglycerides.

EDUCATIONAL OBJECTIVE:
Differentiate among the causes of high HDL cholesterol and describe the clinical features of cholesterol ester transfer protein deficiency.

REFERENCE(S):
de Grooth GJ, Klerkx AH, Stroes ES, Stalenhoef AF, Kastelein JJ, Kuivenhoven JA. A review of CETP and its relation to atherosclerosis. *J Lipid Res.* 2004;45(11):1967-1974.

Niesor EJ. Different effects of compounds decreasing cholesteryl ester transfer protein activity on lipoprotein metabolism. *Curr Opin Lipidol.* 2011;22(4):288-295.

Pownall HJ. Alcohol: lipid metabolism and cardio-protection. *Curr Atheroscler Rep.* 2002;4(2): 107-112.

Rader DJ, Hovingh GK. HDL and cardiovascular disease. *Lancet.* 2014;384(9943):618-625.

20 ANSWER: D) No further testing

According to the 2013 American College of Cardiology/American Heart Association Cholesterol Lowering Guidelines, this patient does not meet criteria for obligate high-dosage statin therapy (no known atherosclerotic cardiovascular disease, no diabetes, LDL cholesterol less than 190 mg/dL [<4.92 mmol/L], and 10-year cardiovascular disease risk less than 7.5%). He is in an intermediate cardiovascular disease risk group.

Other biomarkers of elevated cardiovascular risk have been used to further quantify risk of cardiovascular disease in patients without known coronary disease, including apolipoprotein B (Answer A), lipoprotein (a) (Answer B), and high-sensitivity C-reactive protein (Answer C). In the absence of genetic testing, an elevated apolipoprotein B value potentially supports the diagnosis of familial hypercholesterolemia and is associated with high risk of cardiovascular disease. Lipoprotein (a) is highly atherogenic and is associated with increased risk of cardiovascular disease. Lipoprotein (a) is an LDL particle with a large protein (apo [a]) attached. Lipoprotein (a) can be modestly elevated in the setting of familial hyperlipidemia as well, but it is not part of the Dutch Lipid Clinic Network Diagnostic Criteria for Familial Hypercholesterolemia algorithm that is currently being used by insurers to determine the likelihood of an accurate diagnosis of familial hyperlipidemia. Elevated high-sensitivity C-reactive protein is also associated with increased cardiovascular disease risk, particularly related to insulin resistance, but it is not related to familial hyperlipidemia directly.

The 2013 American College of Cardiology/ American Heart Association Cholesterol Lowering Guidelines do not currently recommend measurement of biomarkers such as apolipoprotein B, lipoprotein (a), and high-sensitivity C-reactive protein for the purpose of risk stratification in addition to the lipid profile. This patient is at intermediate risk for cardiovascular disease and he is a viable candidate for a moderate-intensity statin. Thus, no further testing is needed (Answer D).

Myalgias occur in approximately 5% to 10% of patients who are prescribed statin therapy. This occurs at a much higher prevalence than statin-induced myopathy, which the US FDA defines as a creatine phosphokinase level greater than 10 times the upper normal limit or rhabdomyolysis, defined as a creatine phosphokinase level greater than 10,000 U/L. A statin trial is reasonable in this patient.

EDUCATIONAL OBJECTIVE:
Apply the 2013 American College of Cardiology/American Heart Association Cholesterol Lowering Guideline recommendations for the use of additional biomarkers beyond the lipid profile for further cardiovascular risk stratification.

REFERENCE(S):
Stone NJ, Robinson JG, Lichtenstein AH, et al; American College of Cardiology/American Heart Association Task Force on Practice Guidelines. 2013 ACC/AHA guideline on the treatment of blood cholesterol to reduce atherosclerotic cardiovascular risk in adults: a report of the American College of Cardiology/American Heart Association Task Force on Practice Guidelines [published correction appears in *Circulation*. 2014;129(25 Suppl 2):S46-S48]. *Circulation*. 2014;129(25 Suppl 2):S1-S45.

21 ANSWER: A) Low-dosage rosuvastatin

Myalgias occur in approximately 5% to 10% of patients who are prescribed statin therapy. This occurs at a much greater prevalence than statin-induced myopathy, which the US FDA defines as a creatine phosphokinase level greater than 10 times the upper normal limit or rhabdomyolysis, defined as a creatine phosphokinase level greater than 10,000 U/L. Rhabdomyolysis is an emergent condition that warrants the immediate cessation of statin therapy to prevent renal failure. However, this condition occurs in only 3 per 100,000 person-years.

Deciding what to do when patients have muscle pain, weakness, or cramps when taking a statin is a difficult clinical problem. Several options are available and no clear clinical trial data define the best approach. Statins are currently the single best class of medications for cardiovascular disease prevention. As a result, the first goal is to try to keep a patient such as this one on the highest tolerated statin dosage possible. The best first approach is to prescribe a lower dosage of a statin that the patient has not tried before. For the described patient, that would be rosuvastatin (Answer A). Another option is to try alternate day or weekly statin use. However, no clinical trials show cardiovascular event reduction using this approach.

While fenofibrate (Answer B), niacin (Answer E), and ezetimibe (Answer C) can all have favorable effects on serum lipid levels, none has been shown to produce reductions in cardiovascular end points when used as a single agent, so prescribing any one of them would not be the next step until various approaches to prescribing statins have failed.

Both current PCSK9 inhibitors evolocumab (Answer D) and alirocumab are approved by the US FDA for use in patients with clinical atherosclerotic cardiovascular disease and heterozygous familial hyperlipidemia, which this patient does not have. PCSK9 inhibitors have been studied in statin-intolerant patients with LDL-cholesterol levels in this patient's range (GAUSS-1 and GAUSS-2 studies), but statin intolerance alone is not currently an approved indication in the United States in the absence of clinical atherosclerotic cardiovascular disease or familial hyperlipidemia.

EDUCATIONAL OBJECTIVE:
Recommend options for managing statin-associated muscle pain.

REFERENCE(S):

Joy TR, Hegele RA. Narrative review: statin-related myopathy. *Ann Intern Med.* 2009;150(12):858-868.

Cornier MA, Eckel RH. Non-traditional dosing of statins in statin-intolerant patients-is it worth a try? *Curr Atheroscler Rep.* 2015;17(2):475.

Ahmad Z. Statin intolerance. *Am J Cardiol.* 2014;113(10):1765-1771.

Stroes E, Colquhoun D, Sullivan D, et al. Anti-PCSK9 antibody effectively lowers cholesterol in patients with statin intolerance: the GAUSS-2 randomized, placebo-controlled phase 3 clinical trial of evolocumab. *J Am Coll Cardiol.* 2014; 63(23):2541-2548.

Sullivan D, Olsson AG, Scott R, et al. Effect of a monoclonal antibody to PCSK9 on low-density lipoprotein cholesterol levels in statin-intolerant patients: the GAUSS randomized trial. *JAMA.* 2012;308(23):2497-2506.

22 ANSWER: B) Add ezetimibe

This patient is at high risk for a cardiovascular event given his known coronary disease in addition to type 2 diabetes mellitus and hypertension, and he would benefit from aggressive lowering of his LDL cholesterol (>50%), according to the 2013 American College of Cardiology/American Heart Association Cholesterol Lowering Guidelines. On the basis of the IMPROVE-IT trial, the addition of ezetimibe (Answer B) to simvastatin, 40 mg daily, would lower LDL cholesterol, as well as the risk of future cardiovascular events by approximately 6.4%. Although the 2013 American College of Cardiology/American Heart Association Guidelines focus on moderate- vs high-intensity statins as a class, the IMPROVE-IT trial and now the FOURIER study, which assessed the addition of the PCSK9 inhibitor evolocumab to the highest-dosage statin tolerated, have shown additional reduction of cardiovascular events with lower LDL-cholesterol levels beyond current targets (thus, Answer E is incorrect). In the future, there will most likely be renewed focus on lowering LDL cholesterol to the lowest extent possible for cardiovascular disease risk reduction.

Niacin (Answer A) (AIM-HIGH Study) and fenofibrate (Answer C) (ACCORD and FIELD Studies) have not been shown to lower cardiovascualr event risk. Pitavastatin (Answer D) is considered a moderate-intensity statin, so switching from simvastatin to pitavastatin is not as likely to further reduce cardiovascular risk as adding ezetimibe to simavastatin.

EDUCATIONAL OBJECTIVE:
Explain the benefits of adding ezetimibe to simvastatin for LDL-cholesterol lowering and reducing the risk of cardiovascular disease events.

REFERENCE(S):

Stone NJ, Robinson JG, Lichtenstein AH, et al; American College of Cardiology/American Heart Association Task Force on Practice Guidelines. 2013 ACC/AHA guideline on the treatment of blood cholesterol to reduce atherosclerotic cardiovascular risk in adults: a report of the American College of Cardiology/American Heart Association Task Force on Practice Guidelines [published correction appears in *Circulation*. 2014;129(25 Suppl 2):S46-S48]. *Circulation*. 2014;129(25 Suppl 2):S1-S45.

Cannon CP, Blazing MA, Giugliano RP, et al; IMPROVE-IT Investigators. Ezetimibe added to statin therapy after acute coronary syndromes. *N Engl J Med.* 2015;372(25):2387-2397.

Murphy SA, Cannon CP, Blazing MA, et al. Reduction in total cardiovascular events with ezetimibe/simvastatin post-acute coronary syndrome: the IMPROVE-IT trial. *J Am Coll Cardiol.* 2016;67(4):353-361.

Sabatine MS, Giugliano RP, Keech AC, et al; FOURIER Steering Committee and Investigators. Evolocumab and clinical outcomes in patients with cardiovascular disease. *N Engl J Med.* 2017;376(18):1713-1722.

Cholesterol Treatment Trialists' (CTT) Collaboration, Baigent C, Blackwell L, et al. Efficacy and safety of more intensive lowering of LDL cholesterol: a meta-analysis of data from 170,000 participants in 26 randomized trials. *Lancet.* 2010;376(9753):1670-1681.

ACCORD Study Group, Ginsberg HN, Elam MB, et al. Effects of combination lipid therapy in type 2 diabetes mellitus [published correction appears in *N Engl J Med.* 2010;362(18):1748]. *N Engl J Med.* 2010;362(17):1563-1574.

Jun M, Foote C, Lv J, et al. Effects of fibrates on cardiovascular outcomes: a systematic review and meta-analysis. *Lancet.* 2010;375(9729):1875-1884.

Nordestgaard BG, Varbo A. Triglycerides and cardiovascular disease. *Lancet.* 2014;384(9943):626-635.

23 ANSWER: A) Continue fenofibrate

Serum total cholesterol, HDL-cholesterol, LDL-cholesterol, and triglyceride levels increase during pregnancy (in normal women, the increases are by 75%, 40%, 70%, and 330%, respectively). The mean values for total cholesterol and triglycerides during pregnancy are 317 mg/dL (8.21 mmol/L) and 300 mg/dL (3.39 mmol/L), respectively. After delivery, lipid levels slowly return to prepartum levels. In women with underlying disorders of triglyceride metabolism, levels may rise during pregnancy to a degree that puts the mother at risk for pancreatitis, which could have serious implications for both the mother and the fetus. In addition, the development of gestational diabetes could increase the risk of marked hypertriglyceridemia.

Drugs used for the treatment of lipid disorders should generally be stopped before conception. Statins are teratogenic and contraindicated in pregnancy (thus, Answer B is incorrect). Ideally, all medications should be avoided during pregnancy, particularly during the first trimester when embryogenesis and tissue differentiation occur. This patient continued fenofibrate during the critical first trimester. Few data are available on the treatment of hypertriglyceridemia during pregnancy. Omega-3 fatty acids (Answer D) have been used to treat hypertriglyceridemia during pregnancy, but the available data suggest that they are not very effective. However, omega-3 fatty acids may be the treatment of choice in the first trimester.

Observational studies and case reports suggest that fibrates may be used safely and effectively during pregnancy. Fenofibrate (Answer A) is more potent than omega-3 fatty acids, so it is most likely the best choice in the second and third trimesters and it should be continued in this patient. Nicotinic acid (Answer C) is less effective than fenofibrate in reducing triglyceride levels.

When pancreatitis due to hypertriglyceridemia develops during pregnancy, a number of treatment approaches have been used. The standard approach of fasting, fluid administration, and pain control is the best first step. If hyperglycemia is present, then intravenous insulin can be administered. Other treatments that have been tried include intravenous heparin, plasma exchange, lipoprotein apheresis, and cesarean delivery if the pregnancy is far enough along.

EDUCATIONAL OBJECTIVE:
Develop an approach to treating severe hypertriglyceridemia during pregnancy.

REFERENCE(S):

Amin T, Poon LC, Teoh TG, et al. Management of hypertriglyceridaemia-induced acute pancreatitis in pregnancy. *J Matern Fetal Neonatal Med.* 2014:1-5.

Crisan LS, Steidl ET, Rivera-Alsina ME. Acute hyperlipidemic pancreatitis in pregnancy. *Am J Obstet Gynecol.* 2008;198(5):e57-e59.

Whitten AE, Lorenz RP, Smith JM. Hyperlipidemia-associated pancreatitis in pregnancy managed with fenofibrate. *Obstet Gynecol.* 2011;117(2 Pt 2): 517-519.

Nakao J, Ohba T, Takaishi K, Katabuchi H. Omega-3 fatty acids for the treatment of hypertriglyceridemia during the second trimester. *Nutrition.* 2015;31(2):409-412.

24 ANSWER: B) Colesevelam

Of the listed options, only colesevelam (Answer B), a bile acid–binding resin, has been shown to improve diabetes control, either due to reduced absorption of glucose from the gut or suppression of gluconeogenesis. Niacin and extended-release niacin (Answer A) worsen glucose control and can precipitate the need for diabetes therapies in patients with impaired glucose tolerance. Pitavastatin (Answer C) is a newer statin with a wider catabolic pathway; it has no known effect on glucose. However, high dosages of stronger statins such as atorvastatin and rosuvastatin may increase the incidence of diabetes. Ezetimibe (Answer D) inhibits the NPCL1 (Niemann-Pick disease, type C1, gene like 1) cholesterol uptake receptor in the gut and has no known effect on glucose. Anacetrapib (Answer E) is a cholesteryl ester transfer protein inhibitor that is currently in clinical trials. It has no known effect on glucose control.

EDUCATIONAL OBJECTIVE:
Treat hypercholesterolemia in the setting of diabetes mellitus.

REFERENCE(S):

Potthoff MJ, Potts A, He T, et al. Colesevelam suppresses hepatic glycogenolysis by TGR5-mediated induction of GLP-1 action in DIO mice. *Am J Physiol Gastrointest Liver Physiol.* 2013; 304(4):G371-G380.

Bays HE. Colesevelam hydrochloride added to background metformin therapy in patients with type 2 diabetes mellitus: a pooled analysis from 3 clinical studies. *Endocr Pract.* 2011;17(6):933-938.

Navarese EP, Buffon A, Andreotti F, et al. Meta-analysis of impact of different types and doses of statins on new-onset diabetes mellitus. *Am J Cardiol.* 2013;111(8):1123-1130.

Cannon CP, Shah S, Dansky HM, et al. Determining the efficacy and tolerability investigators. Safety of anacetrapib in patients with or a high risk for coronary heart disease. *N Engl J Med.* 2010; 363(25):2406-2415.

25 ANSWER: D) Lipoprotein lipase deficiency

This patient has homozygous lipoprotein lipase deficiency (Answer D) and has a classic presentation with feeding difficulty beginning in childhood. Patients with lipoprotein lipase deficiency cannot breakdown triglycerides and have levels generally greater than 1000 mg/dL (>11.30 mmol/L). Triglyceride levels in this range are associated with abnormal lipid deposits in the skin (eruptive xanthomas as seen in the picture), and high circulating levels give a white-yellow "milky" appearance to the blood vessels in the retina.

This episode of severe hypertriglyceridemia and pancreatitis was probably precipitated by alcohol ingestion. Alcohol can severely elevate triglyceride levels in persons who have an underlying disorder in lipid metabolism. Alcohol has several effects on liver triglyceride metabolism, including reducing fatty acid oxidation and increasing de novo triglyceride production. Other factors that can significantly elevate triglycerides in genetically predisposed individuals include type 2 diabetes, use of estrogen-containing medications, and pregnancy.

This genetic disorder is especially common in French Canada because of a founder effect; the defect is thought to occur in 1 in 40 persons of French Canadian descent (compared with 1 in 1 million in the general population). Heterozygous forms of this enzyme deficiency are sometimes associated with hyperchylomicronemia and pancreatitis when superimposed on a second triglyceride-elevating stress, such as diabetes, pregnancy, or alcohol ingestion. Several other very rare causes of lipoprotein lipase inactivity have been discovered recently, and they lead to a similar hyperchylomicronemia phenotype.

Adipose triglyceride lipase is an intracellular enzyme that does not modulate plasma triglyceride levels (thus, Answer B is incorrect). This enzyme is required to release stored triglyceride from adipose and muscles. Hepatic lipase mediates removal of triglyceride from remnant lipoproteins and modulates HDL-cholesterol levels. Patients with hepatic lipase deficiency (Answer C) present with increased triglyceride and cholesterol levels without HDL-cholesterol reductions, but are not at risk of pancreatitis. Apolipoprotein B is a protein associated with increased LDL cholesterol and increased cardiovascular risk but not elevated triglycerides and pancreatitis (thus, Answer A is incorrect).

Pancreatic lipase is an enzyme secreted by the pancreas into the pancreatic ducts draining into the small intestine where it breaks down lipids emulsified by bile salts into fatty acids and glycerol for absorption into the circulation through the gut. Lipase is also secreted by oral and gastric mucosa. Lack of pancreatic lipase, sometimes from pancreatic insufficiency in patients with damage from chronic pancreatitis or in those with cystic fibrosis, leads to excessive amounts of fat in the stool and steatorrhea. Pancreatic lipase deficiency (Answer E) does not lead to elevated triglycerides or cause pancreatitis.

EDUCATIONAL OBJECTIVE:
Recognize primary and secondary causes of severe hypertriglyceridemia.

REFERENCE(S):

Berglund L, Brunzell JD, Goldberg AC, et al; Endocrine Society. Evaluation and treatment of hypertriglyceridemia: an Endocrine Society clinical practice guideline. *J Clin Endocrinol Metab*. 2012;97(9):2969-2989.

Johansen CT, Kathiresan S, Hegele RA. Genetic determinants of plasma triglycerides. *J Lipid Res*. 2011;52(2):189-206.

Johansen CT, Wang J, McIntyre AD, et al. Excess of rare variants in non-genome-wide association study candidate genes in patients with hypertriglyceridemia. *Circ Cardiovasc Genet*. 2012;5(1):66-72.

26 ANSWER: B) Lecithin-cholesterol acyltransferase (LCAT) deficiency

The most striking feature of this patient's clinical presentation is his very low HDL-cholesterol level. His phenotype is typical for lecithin-cholesterol acyltransferase (LCAT) deficiency (Answer B). The enzyme LCAT is responsible for converting the relatively polar free cholesterol in the developing HDL particle into nonpolar cholesterol esters. Cholesterol esters are then "trapped" in the HDL particle to be taken back to the liver.

When LCAT is deficient, free cholesterol does not stay associated with the HDL particle, resulting in low circulating levels of HDL. This condition is associated with cholesterol accumulation in the eyes resulting in corneal clouding. Affected patients also have proteinuria that develops in childhood, progressive renal dysfunction leading eventually to end-stage renal disease, and anemia due to red cell fragility secondary to abnormal membrane lipids.

ATP-binding cassette A1 (ABCA1) deficiency, or Tangier disease (Answer A), is also a cause of very low HDL cholesterol, but it is not associated with abnormal renal function. Tangier disease is associated with accumulation of cholesterol in lymphoid tissue giving a classic physical finding: orange tonsils. Defective apolipoprotein B (Answer C) looks clinically like familial hypercholesterolemia with very high levels of LDL cholesterol and tendinous xanthomas. Lipoprotein lipase deficiency (Answer D) results in very high triglyceride levels (>1000 mg/dL [>11.3 mmol/L]) and a more modest decrease in HDL cholesterol. Surreptitious anabolic steroid use (Answer E) can lower HDL-cholesterol levels but generally modestly. However, individuals abusing testosterone would be expected to exhibit findings of excess androgens (increased muscle mass, acne) that are not described here, and such individuals would not have the eye or kidney problems described in this patient.

EDUCATIONAL OBJECTIVE:
Describe the clinical features of conditions that cause very low HDL-cholesterol levels.

REFERENCE(S):
Rader DJ, deGoma EM. Approach to the patient with extremely low HDL-cholesterol. *J Clin Endocrinol Metab*. 2012;97(10):3399-3407.

Schaefer EJ, Anthanont P, Asztalos BF. High-density lipoprotein metabolism, composition, function, and deficiency. *Curr Opin Lipidol*. 2014;25(3): 194-199.

Rader DJ, Hovingh GK. HDL and cardiovascular disease. *Lancet*. 2014;384(9943):618-625.

27 ANSWER: C) Apolipoprotein E genotyping

This patient has dysbetalipoproteinemia, which is diagnosed with apolipoprotein E genotyping (Answer C). Increased triglycerides commensurate with increased cholesterol occur in 2 situations: familial combined hyperlipidemia and dysbetalipoproteinemia. The former is due to an increase in both VLDL and LDL and is a relatively common dyslipidemia, especially in patients with diabetes mellitus. However, this patient's cholesterol concentration and her lack of obesity or thyroid disorder suggest that she has a primary genetic abnormality. She has palmar xanthomas and cholesterol and triglyceride levels greater than 600 mg/dL that are approximately equal. This finding occurs in dysbetalipoproteinemia, a disorder that is usually associated with an *APOE*E2*/*APOE*E2* genotype. This molecular defect is autosomal recessive, but it occurs in 1% of the population. However, only 1 in 10,000 patients presents with the phenotype of this disease. Therefore, it is assumed that there must be an additional underlying factor that leads to its manifestation. Apolipoprotein E is needed to clear many lipoprotein particles by the liver, and presumably a high-fat diet leads to large numbers of circulating remnant lipoproteins that are not efficiently cleared. Unlike LDL, the shortened apolipoprotein B_{48} in chylomicrons is unable to serve as a ligand for liver lipoprotein receptors, and remnant lipoproteins produced in the intestine use apolipoprotein E as the primary ligand for receptor-mediated uptake by the liver. As an alternative to genotyping, centrifugation analysis of VLDL particles should show that they are cholesterol enriched. Patients with dysbetalipoproteinemia respond well to fibric acids. Untreated, the disorder is associated with a marked increase in both cardiovascular and peripheral vascular disease. Of note, this is the same genetic locus that is associated with risk for Alzheimer disease (*APOE*E4*/*APOE*E4* genotype).

Apolipoprotein A1 is a structural lipoprotein associated with HDL cholesterol. Measuring this patient's circulating apolipoprotein A1 (Answer A) would not help to identify the correct disorder. Measurement of LDL particle size (Answer B) would not inform the diagnosis of a disorder also characterized by high triglycerides. Lipoprotein (a) is associated with increased risk of cardiovascular disease, but it is not associated with elevated triglycerides and palmar xanthoma. Thus, genetic analysis of lipoprotein (a) (Answer D) would not yield the correct diagnosis.

EDUCATIONAL OBJECTIVE:
Evaluate mixed hyperlipidemia and diagnose dysbetalipoproteinemia.

REFERENCE(S):
Chahil TJ, Ginsberg HN. Diabetic dyslipidemia. *Endocrinol Metab Clin North Am*. 2006;35(3): 491-510.

Mahley RW, Huang Y, Rall SC Jr. Pathogenesis of type III hyperlipoproteinemia (dysbetalipoproteinemia). Questions, quandaries, and paradoxes. *J Lipid Res*. 1999;40(11):1933-1949.

Berglund L, Brunzell JD, Goldberg AC, et al; Endocrine Society. Evaluation and treatment of hypertriglyceridemia: an Endocrine Society clinical practice guideline. *J Clin Endocrinol Metab*. 2012;97(9):2969-2989.

28 ANSWER: E) Accumulation of lipoprotein X

Primary biliary cirrhosis is a progressive liver disease that most commonly presents in older women and can be associated with marked elevation of serum lipid levels. Elevated total cholesterol levels in these patients are most often due to the presence of an abnormal LDL-like particle called lipoprotein X (Answer E). Lipoprotein X is made up in part by biliary lipids that are not being excreted by the liver. There is evidence that unlike LDL, lipoprotein X is not atherogenic. Several clinical studies do not show an increased risk of coronary artery disease in these patients, despite high levels of what would be LDL cholesterol if the Friedewald formula were used to estimate LDL-cholesterol levels. Individuals with high levels of lipoprotein X can develop coronary artery disease, and they do have a reduction in cholesterol levels with statins, but they just do not appear to have a level of risk for coronary artery disease that would be expected given the high level of "LDL-like" lipoprotein particles.

Lecithin-cholesterol acyltransferase (LCAT) is the enzyme that converts free cholesterol to cholesterol esters, thereby trapping the cholesterol in HDL to be taken to the liver. LCAT deficiency (Answer C) is a genetic disorder that is associated with very low levels of HDL cholesterol, hemolytic anemia, corneal opacities, renal insufficiency, and, uncommonly, atherosclerosis. While LCAT deficiency may be part of the pathogenesis of lipoprotein X production, it is not the only mechanism at work. Lipoprotein (a) (Answer A) is an LDL particle that has apolipoprotein (a) covalently attached to the apolipoprotein B, which is the structural backbone of LDL. It is not associated with primary biliary cirrhosis. Ursodeoxycholic acid treatment (Answer B) does not worsen serum lipids in patients with primary biliary cirrhosis; in fact, data suggest that cholesterol levels fall with the use of this medication. Liver disease is a secondary cause of hyperlipidemia that should routinely be screened for when caring for a patient with hyperlipidemia. Increased production of apolipoprotein B is the underlying cause of hyperlipidemia in familial combined hyperlipidemia. However, increased production of apolipoprotein B (Answer D) is not typical in primary biliary cirrhosis and would not be expected to increase total cholesterol levels to the degree seen in this patient.

EDUCATIONAL OBJECTIVE:
Identify the lipid abnormalities associated with primary biliary cirrhosis.

REFERENCE(S):
Sorokin A, Brown JL, Thompson PD. Primary biliary cirrhosis, hyperlipidemia, and atherosclerotic risk: a systematic review. *Atherosclerosis.* 2007;194(2):293-299.

Longo M, Crosignani A, Battezzati PM, et al. Hyperlipidaemic state and cardiovascular risk in primary biliary cirrhosis. *Gut.* 2002;51(2):265-269.

29 ANSWER: D) Familial combined hyperlipidemia

This patient's clinical picture is typical of a person with familial combined hyperlipidemia (Answer D), the most common lipid abnormality among patients with coronary artery disease. Familial combined hyperlipidemia was discovered from studies of families that had many individuals afflicted with coronary artery disease and high serum lipid levels. In a large percentage of patients, it is also associated with insulin resistance and the metabolic syndrome. Although familial, the phenotype is typically not expressed until the third or later decades of life. Affected family members can have 1 of 3 lipid abnormalities: hypercholesterolemia, hypertriglyceridemia, or both. The lipid abnormality may change and vary from time to time in each patient, probably because of nutritional factors (weight gain/weight loss). Familial combined hyperlipidemia is caused by overproduction of apolipoprotein B by the liver. The variable serum lipid phenotype reflects individual differences in the metabolism of VLDL depending on diet composition and other genes present in an individual.

Individuals with lipoprotein lipase deficiency (Answer B) have very high triglyceride levels, often greater than 1000 mg/dL (>11.30 mmol/L). Familial hypercholesterolemia (Answer A) and familial defective apolipoprotein B (Answer C) are characterized by very high LDL cholesterol levels (200-300 mg/dL [5.18-7.77 mmol/L]) and specific physical features, including tendinous xanthomas. Apolipoprotein A1 is the structural lipoprotein associated with HDL. Patients with apolipoprotein A1 deficiency (Answer E), also known as hypoalphalipoproteinemia, have very low HDL-cholesterol levels.

EDUCATIONAL OBJECTIVE:
Identify the features of familial combined hyperlipidemia.

REFERENCE(S):
Brunzell JD, Albers JJ, Chait A, Grundy SM, Groszek E, McDonald GB. Plasma lipoproteins in familial combined hyperlipidemia and monogenic familial hypertriglyceridemia. *J Lipid Res.* 1983;24(2):147-155.

Hopkins PN, Heiss G, Ellison RC, et al. Coronary artery disease risk in familial combined hyperlipidemia and familial hypertriglyceridemia: a case-control comparison from the National Heart, Lung, and Blood Institute Family Heart Study. *Circulation.* 2003;108(5):519-523.

30 ANSWER: A) Hypobetalipoproteinemia
This patient has hypobetalipoproteinemia (Answer A) with a reduction in production of both LDL (cholesterol) and VLDL (triglyceride). This condition is most often due to a defect in liver production of apolipoprotein B–containing lipoproteins because of defective production of apolipoprotein B or microsomal triglyceride transfer protein. With apolipoprotein B, a defective protein is associated with lower than one-half normal LDL-cholesterol levels. In hypobetalipoproteinemia, inability to efficiently secrete lipoproteins from the liver can lead to nonalcoholic fatty liver disease.

Hypobetalipoproteinemia should be distinguished from abetalipoproteinemia (Answer B), a rare autosomal recessive disorder caused by a mutation in the gene encoding the microsomal transfer protein causing low levels of apolipoproteins used in the synthesis and export of chylomicrons and VLDL. LDL-cholesterol and triglyceride levels are much lower in this setting, and affected patients develop deficiencies of fat-soluble vitamins with neurologic symptoms, including weakness and balance problems as adults. This profile can also be the result of drugs that inhibit microsomal triglyceride transfer protein or antisense therapies to reduce apolipoprotein B secretion. Dysbetalipoproteinemia (Answer C) is an autosomal recessive disorder associated with an *APOE*E2/APOE*E2* genotype and clinically characterized by palmar xanthomas with roughly equal and significant elevations in both total cholesterol and triglycerides, not low levels. This is the same genetic locus that is associated with risk for Alzheimer disease (*APOE*E4/APOE*E4* genotype). Persons with hypoalphalipoproteinemia (Answer D), also known as apolipoproteinemia A1 deficiency, lack a structural protein associated with HDL and consequently have very low HDL-cholesterol levels but the other lipid fractions are not as low as in this vignette.

EDUCATIONAL OBJECTIVE:
Identify conditions characterized by very low cholesterol levels and associated health risks.

REFERENCE(S):
Musunuru K, Pirruccello JP, Do R, et al. Exome sequencing, ANGPTL3 mutations, and familial combined hypolipidemia. *N Engl J Med.* 2010;363(23):2220-2227.

Cuchel M, Bloedon LT, Szapary PO, et al. Inhibition of microsomal triglyceride transfer protein in familial hypercholesterolemia. *N Engl J Med.* 2007;356(2):148-156.

Tanoli T, Yue P, Yablonskiy D, Schonfeld G. Fatty liver in familial hypobetalipoproteinemia: roles of the APOB defects, intra-abdominal adipose tissue, and insulin sensitivity. *J Lipid Res.* 2004;45(5):941- 947.

Mahley RW, Huang Y, Rall SC Jr. Pathogenesis of type III hyperlipoproteinemia (dysbetalipoproteinemia). Questions, quandaries, and paradoxes. *J Lipid Res.* 1999;40(11):1933-1949.

Berglund L, Brunzell JD, Goldberg AC, et al; Endocrine Society. Evaluation and treatment of hypertriglyceridemia: an Endocrine Society clinical practice guideline. *J Clin Endocrinol Metab.* 2012;97(9):2969-2989.

Brunzell JD, Albers JJ, Chait A, Grundy SM, Groszek E, McDonald GB. Plasma lipoproteins in familial combined hyperlipidemia and monogenic familial hypertriglyceridemia. *J Lipid Research.* 1983;24(2):147-155.

Pituitary Board Review
Mark E. Molitch, MD ● Northwestern University

1 ANSWER: C) Measurement of HAMA (human anti-mouse antibodies)

The typical patient with hyperthyroidism, including Graves disease, has autonomous production of thyroid hormone by the thyroid with resultant suppression of TSH levels. In a hyperthyroid patient, when TSH levels are normal or elevated in the setting of elevated T_4 and T_3 levels, the most common cause is a TSH-producing tumor. Therefore, MRI is often done next. In this case, the MRI was normal. In patients with TSH-secreting tumors, there is commonly an imbalance in the secretion of α-subunit, resulting in a relative increase in α-subunit disproportionate to the TSH level (not β subunit [Answer A]). The free α-subunit test was not an answer choice in this vignette.

An alternative explanation for the elevated TSH level in a patient such as this one is that the TSH measurement is artifactually elevated due to the presence of heterophile antibodies. These antibodies are directed against specific animal immunoglobulins, usually human anti-mouse antibodies (HAMA) (Answer C). In this case, a commercial laboratory detected the presence of HAMA antibodies. When specific HAMA-blocking reagents were added, the TSH concentration was documented to be <0.01 mIU/L.

A T_3 suppression test (Answer B) is now rarely done in patients with toxic nodular goiters. Petrosal sinus sampling (Answer D) is done primarily to distinguish between pituitary vs ectopic ACTH secretion in patients with Cushing syndrome. However, ectopic TSH secretion outside the cranium has actually never been reported in TSH-dependent hyperthyroidism.

EDUCATIONAL OBJECTIVE:
Evaluate patients with hyperthyroidism who have nonsuppressed TSH levels.

REFERENCE(S):

Beck-Peccoz P, Lania A, Beckers A, Chatterjee K, Werneau JL. 2013 European Thyroid Association Guidelines for the diagnosis and treatment of thyrotropin-secreting pituitary tumours. *Eur Thyroid J.* 2013;2(2):76-82.

Després N, Grant AM. Antibody interference in thyroid assays: a potential for clinical misinformation. *Clin Chem.* 1998;44(3):440-454.

2 ANSWER: A) Measure GH during an oral glucose tolerance test

There is a discrepancy in this case between the degree of prolactin elevation and the size of the tumor, implying that this is not a simple prolactin-secreting macroadenoma. However, the tumor is not so large that one would assume the prolactin levels would be very high (>10,000 ng/mL [>434.8 nmol/L]) requiring a 1:100 dilution to rule out the "hook effect" (Answer B). Testing was done appropriately to rule out hypopituitarism in this patient with a macroadenoma, and her IGF-1 level was elevated—a surprising finding given that she has no clinical evidence of acromegaly. The possibility of subclinical GH hypersecretion should be evaluated further by measuring GH after hyperglycemia is induced during an oral glucose tolerance test (Answer A). There is no urgency for surgery before determining tumor type, and medication (Answers C and D) should not be started before determining whether indeed this is a GH-secreting tumor. In fact, the patient did have a GH-secreting tumor that was removed surgically and she remarked 3 months later how much finer her facial features appeared, how much looser her rings felt, how she stopped snoring, how her skin seemed less oily, and how much better she felt overall.

REFERENCE(S):
Katznelson L, Laws ER Jr, Melmed S, et al; Endocrine Society. Acromegaly: an Endocrine Society clinical practice guideline. *J Clin Endocrinol Metab.* 2014;99(11):3933-3951.
Cooper O, Melmed S. Subclinical hyperfunctioning pituitary adenomas: the silent tumors. *Best Pract Res Clin Endocrinol Metab.* 2012;26(4):447-460.

3 ANSWER: E) Measure β2-transferrin in the nasal discharge

Cerebrospinal fluid rhinorrhea can occur when there is a large, invasive, skull-based prolactinoma that serves as a "cork" in the base of the skull. When the tumor size is reduced substantially through dopamine agonist use, cerebrospinal fluid can leak around the tumor into the sphenoid sinus and nasal passages. The development of profuse rhinorrhea in this patient suggests that this is what is happening. To distinguish between cerebrospinal fluid and simple nasal mucus, the fluid should be sent to the laboratory for measurement of β2-transferrin (Answer E), which is an asialotransferrin isoform found only in cerebrospinal fluid, ocular fluids, and perilymph and is an accepted marker of cerebrospinal fluid leakage. The major concern with such leaks is the risk of meningitis, and surgical repair is needed.

Although reducing the cabergoline dosage (Answer C) may cause the tumor size to increase, thus plugging the leak, judging the exact dosage and the change in tumor size is difficult and not reliable and surgery is the best course once cerebrospinal fluid rhinorrhea is diagnosed. Increasing the cabergoline dosage (Answer B) would not help, and an MRI (Answer A) would only show that the tumor is smaller, but would not demonstrate the leak. Pseudoephedrine (Answer D) may decrease nasal congestion, but it will not affect cerebrospinal fluid leakage.

REFERENCE(S):
Suliman SG, Gurlek A, Byrne JV, et al. Nonsurgical cerebrospinal fluid rhinorrhea in invasive macro-prolactinoma: incidence, radiological, and clinicopathological features. *J Clin Endocrinol Metab.* 2007;92(10):3829-3835.
Warnecke A, Averbeck T, Wurster U, Harmening M, Lenarz T, Stover T. Diagnostic relevance of beta2-transferrin for the detection of cerebrospinal fluid fistulas. *Arch Otolaryngol Head Neck Surg.* 2004;130(10):1178-1184.

4 ANSWER: B) Continue the mifepristone dosage at 600 mg daily

Mifepristone is a glucocorticoid receptor blocker that is effective in the treatment of patients with all forms of Cushing syndrome. Because it blocks the glucocorticoid receptor, cortisol and ACTH levels may actually rise during treatment, but these higher levels are biologically unimportant because of the receptor blockade. Therefore, it is not recommended that cortisol and ACTH measurements be used for dosage adjustment during mifepristone treatment; the dosage should be adjusted solely based on clinical parameters of the activity of Cushing syndrome while avoiding symptoms of adrenal insufficiency. Thus, this patient is doing very well clinically and no dosage adjustment is needed (thus, Answer B is correct and Answers A and C are incorrect). There is no need to add pasireotide (Answer D) or to do radiotherapy (Answer E). Incidentally, pasireotide is approved by the US FDA for Cushing disease only in the subcutaneous form and for acromegaly only in the long-acting release (LAR) form.

REFERENCE(S):
Fleseriu M, Molitch ME, Gross C, Schteingart DE, Vaughan TB 3rd, Biller BM. A new therapeutic approach in the medical treatment of Cushing's

syndrome: glucocorticoid receptor blockade with mifepristone. *Endocr Pract.* 2013;19(2):313-326.

5 ANSWER: E) Measure 8-AM cortisol and ACTH levels

Mistakenly, this patient's hypercortisolism was assumed to be due to an adrenal adenoma. About 10% of adrenal incidentalomas are bilateral. Bilateral macronodular hyperplasia can occur in patients with Cushing disease (ie, from excessive pituitary secretion of ACTH). In studies in which abdominal CT scans were performed in all patients with Cushing disease, 5% to 17% of patients have bilateral macronodular hyperplasia and several cases have been reported in which there was marked asymmetry with a large nodule on one side and questionable activity on the other side. In patients with Cushing syndrome, an ACTH level should always be measured (Answer E). This patient's ACTH level was elevated and her Cushing disease was cured by resection of a pituitary adenoma with resultant improvement in her symptoms and hirsutism and a reduction in the adrenal nodule size.

An ACTH stimulation test with measurement of 17-hydroxyprogesterone (Answer A) is sometimes helpful when diagnosing 21-hydroxylase deficiency but not Cushing syndrome. Adrenal-directed evaluations/treatment (Answers B and D) should be done only if the ACTH level is suppressed. Petrosal sinus sampling for ACTH (Answer C) is done in patients in whom it is difficult to distinguish between a pituitary or an ectopic source of ACTH.

EDUCATIONAL OBJECTIVE:
Evaluate patients with Cushing syndrome.

REFERENCE(S):
Nieman LK, Biller BM, Findling JW, et al. The diagnosis of Cushing's syndrome: an Endocrine Society Clinical Practice Guideline. *J Clin Endocrinol Metab.* 2008;93(5):1526-1540.

Imaki T, Naruse M, Takano K. Adrenocortical hyperplasia associated with ACTH-dependent Cushing's syndrome: comparison of the size of adrenal glands with clinical and endocrinological data. *Endocrine J.* 2004;51(1):89-95.

6 ANSWER: D) No assessment for GH deficiency is indicated as she is not a candidate for GH therapy

This patient has a history of a sarcoma resection just 1 year ago. Although there are no conclusive data that GH therapy will make a malignant neoplasm grow, an active malignancy is one of the absolute contraindications to GH therapy based on the idea that growth factors could promote growth of such a neoplasm. Thus, she is not a candidate for GH treatment and no assessment for GH deficiency should be done (Answer D).

An insulin tolerance test (Answer A) remains the gold standard for assessment of GH reserve, but caution is needed in a patient with previous cranial surgery because of concerns regarding possible seizure induction by hypoglycemia. In that case, a glucagon stimulation test (Answer B) would be a reasonable alternative stimulation test. However, she has 3 pituitary hormone axes that are deficient, indicating that she has about a 96% chance of being GH deficient by any stimulation test, so no stimulation test is really necessary. Thus, even if she were a candidate for GH treatment, which she is not, a repeated IGF-1 measurement (Answer C) would also not be necessary.

EDUCATIONAL OBJECTIVE:
List the contraindications for GH replacement therapy.

REFERENCE(S):
Molitch ME, Clemmons DR, Malozowski S, Merriam GR, Vance ML; Endocrine Society. Evaluation and treatment of adult growth hormone deficiency: an Endocrine Society clinical practice guideline. *J Clin Endocrinol Metab.* 2011;96(6):1587-1609.

7 ANSWER: B) Ipilimumab

Ipilimumab (Answer B) is a monoclonal antibody used in the treatment of metastatic melanoma. Hypophysitis has been reported in 10% to 15% of treated patients; pituitary enlargement can occur within 2 months of treatment initiation, and corticotrophs and thyrotrophs are the most common cell types affected. This form of hypophysitis is different from lymphocytic hypophysitis that occurs peripartum in women.

Bevacizumab (Answer A) is a vascular endothelial growth factor inhibitor that has been used to treat proliferative diabetic retinopathy but does not cause hypophysitis. Temozolomide (Answer C) is an alkylating agent used in the treatment of gliomas that has been useful in the treatment of some patients with pituitary carcinomas and very aggressive macroadenomas. Sunitinib (Answer D) is a tyrosine kinase inhibitor that has been used to treat thyroid cancer, among other cancers, but it has not been implicated as a cause of hypophysitis.

EDUCATIONAL OBJECTIVE:
Identify medications that can cause hypophysitis.

REFERENCE(S):
Corsello SM, Barnabei A, Marchetti P, De Vecchis L, Salvatori R, Torino F. Endocrine side effects Induced by immune checkpoint inhibitors. *J Clin Endocrinol Metab.* 2013;98(4):1361-1375.

Faje AT, Sullivan R, Lawrence D, et al. Ipilimumab-induced hypophysitis: a detailed longitudinal analysis in a large cohort of patients with metastatic melanoma. *J Clin Endocrinol Metab.* 2014;99(11):4078-4085.

Albarel F, Gaudy C, Castinetti F, et al. Long-term follow-up of ipilimumab-induced hypophysitis, a common adverse event of the anti-CTLA-4 antibody in melanoma. *Eur J Endocrinol.* 2015;172(2):195-204.

8 ANSWER: C) An adverse effect of cabergoline

Several studies have shown that dopamine agonists, both cabergoline and bromocriptine, can cause compulsive behavior in 15% to 20% of treated patients. This may take the form of hypersexuality or, as in this case, compulsive gambling (thus, Answer C is correct). The effect appears to be somewhat dosage dependent, so lowering the dosage may be helpful in some circumstances.

This patient's tumor is probably not large enough to cause substantial hypothalamic damage, (Answer B). There are no reports substantiating that normalizing testosterone levels unmasks obsessive behavior (Answer A). While a behavior change unrelated to this tumor or treatment (Answer D) is possible, an adverse effect of cabergoline is the most likely explanation.

EDUCATIONAL OBJECTIVE:
Describe potential adverse effects of dopamine agonist treatment in patients with prolactinomas.

REFERENCE(S):
Bancos I, Nannenga MR, Bostwick JM, Silber MH, Erickson D, Nippoldt TB. Impulse control disorders in patients with dopamine agonist-treated prolactinomas and nonfunctioning pituitary adenomas: a case-control study. *Clin Endocrinol (Oxf).* 2014;80(6):863-868.

Noronha S, Stokes V, Karavitaki N, Grossman A. Treating prolactinomas with dopamine agonists: always worth the gamble? *Endocrine.* 2016;51(2):205-210.

9 ANSWER: E) Perform pituitary-directed MRI

This patient responded nicely to cabergoline and stopped it appropriately when she became pregnant. However, now at 7 months' gestation, she is having increasingly frequent and severe headaches. This could be due to an increase in tumor size, pre-eclampsia, pregnancy-induced hypertension, anxiety, etc. In other words, the headaches themselves are nonspecific. A good first step in determining whether the headaches are caused by tumor growth is to perform formal visual field testing, which, in this patient, was normal. Before instituting a specific treatment (restarting cabergoline [Answer A], which would be the correct treatment; starting bromocriptine [Answer B]; or performing surgery [Answer C]), it would be important to determine whether, in fact, the tumor has substantially increased in size. MRI with or without contrast (Answer E) is safe during pregnancy, although there is reluctance on the part of radiologists to perform such scans. Delivering the baby (Answer D) is a reasonable option later in gestation, but it is not recommended at 7 months' gestation.

EDUCATIONAL OBJECTIVE:
Manage prolactinoma during pregnancy.

REFERENCE(S):

Molitch ME. Endocrinology in pregnancy: Management of the pregnant patient with prolactinoma. *Eur J Endocrinol.* 2015;172(5):R205-R213.

De Wilde JP, Rivers AW, Price DL. A review of the current use of magnetic resonance imaging in pregnancy and safety implications for the fetus. *Prog Biophys Mol Biol.* 2005;87(2-3):335-353.

10 ANSWER: E) Pasireotide

Somatostatin analogues such as octreotide (Answer A), lanreotide (Answer B), and pasireotide (Answer E) decrease GH and IGF-1 and therefore improve insulin resistance. However, all 3 also inhibit insulin secretion to some extent, and when large groups of patients treated with octreotide and lanreotide have been analyzed, some were found to have improvement in diabetes status, some to have worsening, and some to have no change. The situation is much worse with pasireotide (Answer E) because it decreases glucagon-like peptide 1 and glucose insulinotropic peptide and worsens glucose tolerance in many patients. Pegvisomant (Answer C) works entirely by blocking the GH receptor, thereby decreasing insulin resistance, and it has no effect on insulin. Therefore, an improvement in glycemic status occurs in virtually everyone. Cabergoline (Answer D) is generally much less effective than pegvisomant, and the improvement that can be expected in glycemic status is therefore also less.

EDUCATIONAL OBJECTIVE:
Identify adverse effects of medications used in the treatment of acromegaly.

REFERENCE(S):

Barkan AL, Burman P, Clemmons DR, et al. Glucose homeostasis and safety in patients with acromegaly converted from long-acting octreotide to pegvisomant. *J Clin Endocrinol Metab.* 2005;90(10):5684-5691.

Colao A, Bronstein MD, Freda P, et al; Pasireotide C2305 Study Group. Pasireotide versus octreotide in acromegaly: a head-to-head superiority study. *J Clin Endocrinol Metab.* 2014;99(3):791-799.

Katznelson L, Laws ER Jr, Murad MH, et al; Endocrine Society. Acromegaly: an Endocrine Society Clinical Practice Guideline. *J Clin Endocrinol Metab.* 2014;99(11):3933-3951.

11 ANSWER: B) Mifepristone

All of these treatment modalities can improve Cushing disease, and treatment during pregnancy is advocated because it results in better fetal outcomes. Transsphenoidal surgery (Answer C) has a cure rate of 80% to 90% in expert neurosurgical hands with very low complication and fetal loss rates when done in the second trimester. Ketoconazole (Answer A) now has a black box warning regarding liver function abnormalities; it has never been approved for use during pregnancy and is only modestly successful. Mifepristone (Answer B) was originally developed as a progesterone receptor blocker and is a potent abortifacient (RU486); therefore, its use in pregnancy is absolutely contraindicated. There is experience with only about 50 cases in which somatostatin analogues have been used to treat acromegaly during pregnancy, with relatively minor adverse effects. However, somatostatin analogues cross the placenta and have unknown effects on the fetus. There is no experience with pasireotide (Answer D) during pregnancy, and it would be expected to worsen glucose tolerance in this population susceptible to gestational diabetes. Although cabergoline (Answer E) is safe when stopped after conception, there is little experience when used throughout pregnancy, and its ability to normalize cortisol levels in Cushing disease is only modest. Neither pasireotide nor cabergoline is absolutely contraindicated during pregnancy.

EDUCATIONAL OBJECTIVE:
Guide treatment of Cushing disease during pregnancy.

REFERENCE(S):

Marions L. Mifepristone dose in the regimen with misoprostol for medical abortion. *Contraception.* 2006;74(1):21-25.

Lindsay JR, Jonklaas J, Oldfield EH, Nieman LK. Cushing's syndrome during pregnancy: personal experience and review of the literature. *J Clin Endocrinol Metab.* 2005;90(5):3077-3083.

Cohen-Kerem R, Railton C, Oren D, Lishner M, Koren G. Pregnancy outcome following non-obstetric surgical intervention. *Am J Surgery*. 2005;190(3):467-473.

12 ANSWER: D) Oral contraceptives

Because this woman does not desire pregnancy in the near future, there is no critical need to restore ovulation. However, she has been amenorrheic for 4 years, implying hypoestrogenemia and an increased risk for osteoporosis. Oral contraceptives (Answer D) will supply needed estrogen and simultaneously provide contraception. Studies have shown that oral contraceptive use is safe in women with microadenomas and there is minimal risk of tumor enlargement. If the patient's course were followed with observation only (Answer E), her hypoestrogenemic state would persist, putting her at even higher risk of osteoporosis. The dopamine agonists bromocriptine (Answer B) and cabergoline (Answer C) can restore ovulatory cycles in more than 80% of women, but an additional mode of contraception would be needed. Furthermore, oral contraceptives are much cheaper than either bromocriptine or cabergoline, an important consideration in this woman with uncertain insurance coverage. A dopamine agonist would be indicated if pregnancy were desired and/or if the galactorrhea were bothersome. In this clinical setting, transsphenoidal surgery (Answer A) is less effective than dopamine agonists and carries with it considerably higher risk and cost.

EDUCATIONAL OBJECTIVE:
Recommend treatment options for women with prolactin-secreting microadenomas.

REFERENCE(S):
Melmed S, Casanueva FF, Hoffman AR, et al; Endocrine Society. Diagnosis and treatment of hyperprolactinemia: an Endocrine Society clinical practice guideline. *J Clin Endocrinol Metab*. 2011;96(2):273-288.

Glezer A, Bronstein MD. Prolactinomas. *Endocrinol Metab Clin North Am*. 2015;44(1):71-78.

13 ANSWER: A) He may need another transsphenoidal operation performed by an experienced pituitary surgeon in the next few years

In patients truly cured of Cushing disease, ACTH and cortisol levels are very low because the normal corticotropes have been suppressed by the previously high cortisol levels. If the postoperative cortisol level is greater than 10 μg/dL (275.9 nmol/L), the chance that the patient has been cured is less than 10% and it is rare to need steroid support postoperatively. He will most likely need another operation (Answer A) sometime in the next few years.

This patient does not currently truly have hypercortisolism, as demonstrated by his normal 24-hour urinary free cortisol, so medical therapy (Answer C) is not indicated now. Radiotherapy (Answer D) would be indicated only if repeated surgery, and perhaps medical therapy, has failed. Cortisol levels are usually less than 5 μg/dL (<137.9 nmol/L) when patients are cured and hydrocortisone is generally needed for several months initially for both maintenance and stress and then later just for stress (thus, Answer B is incorrect). Petrosal sinus sampling (Answer E) is not generally reliable for localization of a tumor within the pituitary.

EDUCATIONAL OBJECTIVE:
Assess patients with Cushing disease postoperatively.

REFERENCE(S):
Esposito F, Dusick JR, Cohan P, et al. Clinical review: early morning cortisol levels as a predictor of remission after transsphenoidal surgery for Cushing's disease. *J Clin Endocrinol Metab*. 2006;91(1):7-13.

Hameed N, Yedinak CG, Brzana J, et al. Remission rate after transsphenoidal surgery in patients with pathologically confirmed Cushing's disease, the role of cortisol, ACTH assessment and immediate reoperation: a large single center experience. *Pituitary*. 2013;16(4):452-458.

14 ANSWER: C) Give hypertonic saline to raise the serum sodium by 6 mEq/L (6 mmol/L) over 6 hours

Even a standard dose of DDAVP can cause hyponatremia if a person continues to drink; usually progressive nausea limits the intake. Unfortunately in this case, the patient has lost her thirst mechanism, so she continued to drink despite her marked hyponatremia. The treatment at this point is tricky. She is having significant mental symptoms from the hyponatremia and is thus developing brain edema and is at risk for seizures and brain herniation. Therefore, hypertonic saline at a rate of 1 mL/kg per h should be given over a few hours to raise her serum sodium about 4 to 6 mEq/L (4 to 6 mmol/L) to remove her from acute danger (Answer C). Simply restricting fluids (Answer A and B), giving normal saline with furosemide (Answer D), or giving the vasopressin receptor blocker conivaptan (Answer E) will not result in a fast-enough correction. Although DDAVP should be held initially, the urine output must be observed very carefully; when it wears off, she will start to excrete high volumes of dilute urine and might experience an overly rapid correction of the hyponatremia. Correcting the hyponatremia at rates higher than about 12 mEq/L (12 mmol/L) over 24 hours could put her at risk for central pontine myelinolysis. Therefore, her urine output and serum sodium must be monitored every 2 to 4 hours to avoid a correction that is too rapid. Reinstitution of DDAVP at a lower dosage when urine output increases may then be indicated.

EDUCATIONAL OBJECTIVE:
Treat the acute development of severe hyponatremia.

REFERENCE(S):
Verbalis JG, Goldsmith SR, Greenberg A, et al. Diagnosis, evaluation, and treatment of hyponatremia: expert panel recommendations. *Am J Med*. 2013;126(10 Suppl 1):S1-S42.

Ball SG, Iqbal Z. Diagnosis and treatment of hyponatraemia. *Best Pract Res Clin Endocrinol Metab*. 2016;30(2):161-173.

15 ANSWER: A) Deferral of further workup until after delivery

Acromegaly can be very difficult to diagnose during pregnancy because of the production of a GH variant by the placenta that is biologically active and stimulates IGF-1 production. Thus, IGF-1 levels may be elevated normally in the second half of pregnancy. The GH variant is measured as GH in most standard GH assays and its production does not suppress with hyperglycemia, so performing an oral glucose tolerance test and measuring the GH response (Answer C) is not helpful. Given the generally slow course of acromegaly and the difficulty in making the diagnosis during pregnancy, the best course in this patient is to defer the definitive workup until after delivery (Answer A). A pituitary-directed MRI (Answer D) can then be done if there is biochemical confirmation of acromegaly. There is no urgency to begin treatment with a somatostatin analogue (Answer E). Gonadal function in acromegalic women is impaired for a variety of reasons (hyperprolactinemia, hypopituitarism, the elevated GH and IGF-1 levels themselves), so it is uncommon for a woman with acromegaly to become pregnant. Measuring IGF-1 again (Answer B) will most likely document that it is still elevated and this would not distinguish between stimulation by the GH variant or pituitary GH.

EDUCATIONAL OBJECTIVE:
In a pregnant woman, delay the definitive workup of acromegaly until after delivery and review the changes in GH physiology during pregnancy.

REFERENCE(S):
Grynberg M, Salenave S, Young J, Chanson P. Female gonadal function before and after treatment of acromegaly. *J Clin Endocrinol Metab*. 2010;95(10):4518-4525.

Cheng V, Faiman C, Kennedy L, et al. Pregnancy and acromegaly: a review. *Pituitary*. 2012; 15(1):59-63.

Cheng S, Grasso L, Martinez-Orozco JA, et al. Pregnancy in acromegaly: experience from two referral centers and systematic review of the literature. *Clin Endocrinol (Oxf)*. 2012;76(2): 264-271.

16 **ANSWER: E) Temozolomide**
This patient has a rapidly enlarging macroprolactinoma that is unresponsive to cabergoline, 2 operations, and gamma-knife radiotherapy. The tumor is certainly acting in a malignant fashion. However, distant metastases would have to be demonstrated for this to qualify as a true malignancy. Some of these very aggressive tumors and some true pituitary carcinomas respond to temozolomide (Answer E), an alkylating agent used primarily for the treatment of glioblastomas. However, even those who respond for a while to this agent may have, over time, a bad outcome. Additional radiotherapy (Answer A) or surgery (Answer B) is unlikely to help. It is extremely rare for a patient with a prolactinoma to respond to a somatostatin analogue, such as lanreotide (Answer C). Ipilimumab (Answer D) can cause hypophysitis and is a monoclonal antibody used in the treatment of some cancers.

EDUCATIONAL OBJECTIVE:
Recommend a treatment strategy for aggressive pituitary tumors and pituitary carcinomas.

REFERENCE(S):
Whitelaw BC, Dworakowska D, Thomas NW, et al. Temozolomide in the management of dopamine agonist-resistant prolactinomas. *Clin Endocrinol (Oxf)*. 2012;76(6):877-886.
Chatzellis E, Alexandraki KI, Androulakis II, Kaltsas G. Aggressive pituitary tumors. *Neuroendocrinology*. 2015;101(2):87-104.

17 **ANSWER: B) Increased peak bone mass**
The *transition period* refers to the time of life between the end of puberty and full maturation of bone, muscle, and body fat composition. Peak bone mass usually occurs by age 25 years, and GH deficiency during the transition period results in a failure to attain this peak bone mass, but continuing GH will allow this to occur (Answer B). His epiphyses have completely closed, so a further increase in height (Answer A) cannot be expected. GH therapy has not been demonstrated to have an effect on memory (Answer D). No data yet prove that GH treatment reduces the risk of mortality (Answer C) in patients with hypopituitarism, although findings from some recent studies suggest that this may be true. GH therapy may improve overall quality of life, but it does not increase libido (Answer E).

EDUCATIONAL OBJECTIVE:
Explain the effects of GH therapy in the transition period (between the end of puberty and full maturation of bone, muscle, and body fat composition).

REFERENCE(S):
Clayton PE, Cuneo RC, Juul A, Monson JP, Shalet SM, Tauber M; European Society of Paediatric Endocrinology. Consensus statement on the management of the GH-treated adolescent in the transition to adult care. *Eur J Endocrinol*. 2005;152(2):165-170.
Radovick S, DiVall S. Approach to the growth hormone-deficient child during transition to adulthood. *J Clin Endocrinol Metab*. 2007; 92(4):1195-1200.
Gaillard RC, Mattsson AF, Akerblad AC, et al. Overall and cause-specific mortality in GH-deficient adults on GH replacement. *Eur J Endocrinol*. 2012;166(6):1069-1077.
Hartman ML, Xu R, Crowe BJ, et al; International HypoCCS Advisory Board. Prospective safety surveillance of GH-deficient adults: comparison of GH-treated vs untreated patients. *J Clin Endocrinol Metab*. 2013;98(3):980-988.

18 **ANSWER: C) Assessment for macroprolactin**
Macroprolactin is a large-molecular-weight form of prolactin in which prolactin is either complexed with IgG or with itself to form heteromers. Overall, the macroprolactin complex has less bioactivity than monomeric prolactin. Macroprolactin comprises about 10% to 20% of prolactin in the serum of normal individuals, but it may occasionally be considerably higher. When it is present in higher amounts, it is read as being high in standard assays. Thus, this patient's modestly elevated prolactin level could easily be due to the presence of macroprolactin, especially because she has no symptoms suggestive of hyperprolactinemia such as amenorrhea or galactorrhea. In the context of normal menses and no galactorrhea, her decreased libido is more likely related to her depression than

to the elevated prolactin. Thus, the correct step is to assess for macroprolactin (Answer C). Many laboratories can perform this by precipitating the large-molecular-weight forms with polyethylene glycol and then re-assaying the monomeric form. If the monomeric level is normal, no further evaluation is needed. Measurement of macroprolactin is much less expensive than performing an MRI (Answer A) and should be done first. If menses are normal, there is no additional knowledge to be gained by measuring gonadotropins or estradiol (Answers B and E). There is no suspicion of a large tumor in this patient and assessment of prolactin with dilution (Answer D) is not indicated.

EDUCATIONAL OBJECTIVE:
Describe the entity of macroprolactin and appropriately assess for it.

REFERENCE(S):
Fahie-Wilson M, Smith TP. Determination of prolactin: the macroprolactin problem. *Best Pract Res Clin Endocrinol Metab.* 2013;27(5):725-742.

Samson SL, Hamrahian AH, Ezzat S; AACE Neuroendocrine and Pituitary Scientific Committee; American College of Endocrinology (ACE). American Association of Clinical Endocrinologists, American College of Endocrinology Disease State Clinical Review: Clinical relevance of macroprolactin in the absence or presence of true hyperprolactinemia. *Endocr Pract.* 2015;21(12):1427-1435.

19 ANSWER: D) *AIP* (aryl hydrocarbon receptor interacting protein)

A small number of germline mutations are implicated in somatotroph tumorigenesis. These include mutations in *AIP* (associated with familial isolated pituitary adenomas), *MEN1*, (associated with multiple endocrine neoplasia type 1), and *PRKAR1A* (associated with the Carney complex). Germline inactivating mutations in *AIP* (aryl hydrocarbon receptor interacting protein) predispose individuals to pituitary tumors, especially somatotropinomas. Overall, approximately one-third of families with familial acromegaly harbor a germline *AIP* mutation. Furthermore, as many as 20% of individuals younger than 18 years who have apparently sporadic pituitary macroadenomas harbor a pathogenic germline *AIP* mutation. Tumors associated with *AIP* mutations are large and are often diagnosed in childhood or early adulthood, hence the typical presentation with gigantism.

Pituitary adenomas occur in a subset of individuals with multiple endocrine neoplasia type 1 (Answer E); however, hyperparathyroidism is the most frequent and usually the earliest presenting manifestation of this syndrome. Even in the unlikely event that this patient is a de novo case, the absence of parathyroid or a second endocrine neoplasia renders this diagnosis even more unlikely. Postzygotic activating mutations in the *GNAS* gene (Answer A) are responsible for the rare entity known as McCune-Albright syndrome, which consists of polyostotic fibrous dysplasia, cutaneous pigmentation ("coast of Maine"), precocious pseudopuberty in girls, hyperthyroidism, Cushing syndrome, and/or acromegaly due to somatotroph hyperplasia. Somatic activating point mutations in *GNAS*, referred to as the *Gsp* oncogene, however, represent one of the most common molecular alterations identified in sporadic somatotroph adenomas and are present in about 30% of sporadic GH-secreting tumors. The protein encoded by *PROP1* (Answer C) is a transcription factor important in the differentiation of the GH and prolactin cell line. Germline mutations in the *TBX19* gene (Answer B), which encodes a transcription factor that is important for terminal differentiation of pituitary pro-opiomelanocortin–expressing cells, do not cause pituitary adenomas, but instead cause a neonatal-onset form of congenital isolated ACTH deficiency.

EDUCATIONAL OBJECTIVE:
Identify the genes associated with familial pituitary adenoma syndromes.

REFERENCE(S):
Vandeva S, Jaffrain-Rea ML, Daly AF, Tichomirowa M, Zacharieva S, Beckers A. The genetics of pituitary adenomas. *Best Pract Res Clin Endocrinol Metab.* 2010;24(3):461-476.

Schöfl C, Honegger J, Droste M, et al. Frequency of AIP gene mutations in young patients with acromegaly. *J Clin Endocrinol Metab.* 2014;99(12):E2789-E2793.

Rostomyan L, Beckers A. Screening for genetic causes of growth hormone hypersecretion. *Growth Horm IGF Res.* 2016;30-31:52-57.

20 ANSWER: A) Another MRI in 6 to 12 months

This 78-year-old patient has known coronary artery disease and a 1.2-cm incidental macroadenoma. He may have mild hypopituitarism, as evidenced by his low testosterone level with normal gonadotropin levels, but those measurements could also be unrelated. His morning cortisol and free T_4 levels are normal. Thus, there is no indication for surgery (Answer B) or irradiation (Answers D and E). Appropriate management would simply be to assess for a change in tumor size in up to 1 year with another MRI (Answer A). Tumors such as this one grow quite slowly (0.6 mm/year on average), so he is in no imminent danger from tumor growth. At age 78 years, with known coronary artery disease, he is at greater risk of an adverse effect of surgery or irradiation than an adverse effect of tumor growth. If the MRI had shown significant suprasellar extension with abutment of the optic chiasm, then visual field testing (Answer C) should be performed; otherwise, it should not.

EDUCATIONAL OBJECTIVE:
Manage pituitary incidentaloma.

REFERENCE(S):
Freda PU, Beckers AM, Katznelson L, et al; Endocrine Society. Pituitary incidentalomas: an Endocrine Society clinical practice guideline. *J Clin Endocrinol Metab.* 2011;96(4):894-904.

Vasilev V, Rostomyan L, Daly AF, et al. Management of endocrine disease: pituitary 'incidentaloma': neuroradiological assessment and differential diagnosis. *Eur J Endocrinol.* 2016;175(4): R171-R184.

21 ANSWER: D) Hydrocortisone replacement

This pregnant woman has a pituitary mass presenting near term that is most likely lymphocytic hypophysitis. Her prepregnancy history, indicating that she was well and had no problems conceiving, makes it very unlikely that this mass is a prolactinoma. MRI shows diffuse pituitary enlargement, which is more compatible with hypophysitis than with a tumor, and, had gadolinium been given, there would have been diffuse enhancement rather than focal enhancement. (No data show adverse effects of performing MRI scans or giving gadolinium during pregnancy.) One of the striking features of hypophysitis occurring during pregnancy is the high risk of ACTH deficiency. This patient had a morning serum cortisol level of 6.0 µg/dL (165.5 nmol/L), which does not seem very low. However, it should be remembered that cortisol production increases 3-fold during pregnancy and cortisol-binding globulin levels are also very high, resulting in normal morning cortisol levels well above 20 µg/dL (>551.8 nmol/L). Therefore, her cortisol level of 6.0 µg/dL is fairly low, and giving hydrocortisone (Answer D) is the correct answer.

As previously mentioned, she is very unlikely to have a prolactinoma, and instituting bromocriptine (Answer A) or cabergoline (Answer B) is not indicated. Unless her headaches become uncontrollable with pain medication or she develops a visual field defect, there is no indication for surgery (Answer C). Although in hypophysitis the pituitary size often decreases after delivery, it is a relatively gradual reduction and there is no indication for urgent cesarean delivery (Answer E).

EDUCATIONAL OBJECTIVE:
Diagnose and treat lymphocytic hypophysitis in a pregnant woman.

REFERENCE(S):
Carmichael JD. Update on the diagnosis and management of hypophysitis. *Curr Opin Endocrinol. Diabetes Obes.* 2012;19(4):314-321.

22 **ANSWER: A) Pituitary-directed MRI**
This older woman with fatigue, weight gain, and decreased libido has a low free T_4 level but a normal TSH level. A normal TSH level does not by itself exclude hypothyroidism because the hypothyroidism may be secondary. Her LH and FSH levels are low, but they should be elevated in menopause. This combination of central hypothyroidism and hypogonadism makes it important to exclude a mass in the pituitary/hypothalamic area with an MRI (Answer A). In this context, measuring the serum estradiol level (Answer B) would not add much to the evaluation. Although an evaluation for hemochromatosis (Answer C) is reasonable, hypopituitarism resulting from hemochromatosis usually occurs at a much younger age and is more common in men. An elevated α-subunit level (Answer D) would only point more strongly to the need for an MRI, and if the α-subunit level were normal, it would not provide evidence for one to argue against performing an MRI.

EDUCATIONAL OBJECTIVE:
Evaluate hypopituitarism in older patients.

REFERENCE(S):
Higham CE, Johannsson G, Shalet SM. Hypopituitarism. *Lancet*. 2016;388(10058): 2403-2415.

23 **ANSWER: D) Start conivaptan**
Conivaptan (Answer D) is a vasopressin receptor antagonist that is given intravenously for 1 to 4 days, and it is very effective in the treatment of modest hyponatremia in the setting of congestive heart failure and cirrhosis. Alternatively, tolvaptan, an oral vasopressin receptor antagonist, could be given. If fluid restriction is to be successful, it should be to less than 1000 mL/24 h. A 1500-mL limit (Answer A) is too high. Hypertonic saline administration (Answer B) would most likely worsen his pulmonary edema.

Demeclocycline (Answer C) causes partial nephrogenic diabetes insipidus and may be useful for patients with chronic, symptomatic hyponatremia; it is generally not used when hyponatremia develops acutely and is contraindicated in patients with cirrhosis. Although furosemide (Answer E) causes an increase in urinary excretion of water in excess of sodium, correction of hyponatremia is minimal with its use. As with all acute management, the rate of correction is important to avoid demyelination, so the rate of correction should be less than or equal to 10 to 12 mEq/24 h.

EDUCATIONAL OBJECTIVE:
Manage modest hyponatremia in the setting of fluid overload.

REFERENCE(S):
Verbalis JG, Goldsmith SR, Greenberg A, et al. Diagnosis, evaluation, and treatment of hyponatremia: expert panel recommendations. *Am J Med*. 2013;126(10 Suppl 1):S1-S42.
Miller PD, Linas SL, Schrier RW. Plasma demeclocycline levels and nephrotoxicity. Correlation in hyponatremic cirrhotic patients. *JAMA*. 1980;243(24):2513-2515.

24 **ANSWER: A) Hypopituitarism**
Hyponatremia after head trauma can be due to a variety of causes. However, several months after trauma, the most likely cause is hypopituitarism (Answer A). Both glucocorticoids and thyroxine are necessary for free water clearance, and, in their absence, hyponatremia may ensue. Varying degrees of hypopituitarism occur in almost half of patients after severe head trauma and may occur at varying time points after the trauma. Although the syndrome of inappropriate antidiuretic hormone secretion (Answer B), excessive diuretic use (Answer C), cerebral salt wasting (Answer D), and iatrogenic water intoxication (Answer E) may all cause hyponatremia, they generally occur relatively soon after trauma and surgery, not many weeks later. With cerebral salt wasting, there is evidence of dehydration, and the patient's serum urea nitrogen and creatinine values argue against that. Furthermore, someone who is eating and drinking and has intact thirst mechanisms will generally compensate for developing hyponatremia by becoming nauseated and not drinking more water.

EDUCATIONAL OBJECTIVE:
Diagnose hypopituitarism after head trauma and review its manifestations.

REFERENCE(S):

Verbalis JG. Hyponatremia with intracranial disease: not often cerebral salt wasting. *J Clin Endocrinol Metab*. 2014;99(1):59-62.

Tritos NA, Yuen KC, Kelly DF; AACE Neuroendocrine and Pituitary Scientific Committee. American Association of Clinical Endocrinologists and American College of Endocrinology disease state clinical review: A neuroendocrine approach to patients with traumatic brain injury. *Endocr Pract*. 2015;21(7): 823-831.

25 ANSWER: C) Craniopharyngioma

The key feature in this vignette is that the patient has diabetes insipidus, which indicates a primarily hypothalamic origin of his tumor. One tends to think of craniopharyngiomas as occurring mainly in children, but there is a distinct second peak in older adults (age 50-74 years). Diabetes insipidus is very uncommon in patients with pituitary adenomas (Answers A, B, and D) and is common in patients with craniopharyngiomas (Answer C). Craniopharyngiomas are typically described on MRI as calcified, solid, and/or cystic lesions, usually with a lobular shape and diameter of 20 to 40 mm. The solid elements are often isointense or hypointense on T1-weighted images, exhibit inhomogeneous high intensity on T2-weighted images, and heterogeneously enhance after gadolinium administration. The cystic elements of adamantinomatous craniopharyngiomas typically display high intensity on T1-weighted images, high or mixed intensity on T2-weighted images, and contrast enhancement of the cyst wall. The squamous-papillary subtype is found in approximately one-third of adults with craniopharyngioma, and it rarely shows calcification. Overall, the mortality is much higher for patients with craniopharyngiomas than for those with pituitary adenomas. Studies suggest that activating mutations in the gene encoding β-catenin may be involved in the pathogenesis of the adamantinomatous variety of craniopharyngiomas.

The very mild prolactin elevation in this case is from hypothalamic damage rather than from a prolactinoma (Answer B) and could accompany any of these other tumors/lesions. Sarcoidosis (Answer E) usually presents as an infiltrative disease of the hypothalamus and stalk, with stalk thickening on MRI rather than as a mass lesion.

EDUCATIONAL OBJECTIVE:
Differentiate among hypothalamic and pituitary mass lesions.

REFERENCE(S):

Karavitaki N, Cudlip S, Adams CB, Wass JA. Craniopharyngiomas. *Endocr Rev*. 2006; 27(4):371-397.

Zada G, Lin N, Ojerholm E, Ramkissoon S, Laws ER. Craniopharyngioma and other cystic epithelial lesions of the sellar region: a review of clinical, imaging, and histopathological relationships. *Neurosurg Focus*. 2010;28(4):E4.

Martinez-Barbera JP. 60 years of neuroendocrinology: biology of human craniopharyngioma: lessons from mouse models. *J Endocrinol*. 2015;226(2):T161-T172.

Diabetes Mellitus, Section 2 Board Review

Michelle F. Magee, MD ● Georgetown University

31 **ANSWER: C) Ask her to show you how she self-administers insulin injections**

This patient is overweight and is taking 288 units of insulin daily, corresponding to 2.8 units/kg per day. This is a large dose for a woman of her size (BMI = 25 kg/m^2). When the patient was asked to demonstrate how she self-administers an injection of insulin aspart (Answer C), she dialed the dose into the pen correctly and administered the shot in her upper arm. The dose appeared to have been delivered (as the pen read "zero"); however, there was a stream of insulin dribbling down her arm from the injection site. Thus, it was not clear what insulin dose she had actually received. This patient clearly needs instruction in insulin self-administration technique, and this emergency department visit represents an opportunity to initiate basic diabetes self-management education.

Many patients with diabetes do not receive adequate diabetes self-management education to support optimal self-care outcomes. Despite evidence that diabetes self-management education reduces the number of emergency department visits and hospitalizations, lowers hemoglobin A$_{1c}$, and improves other outcomes, less than 55% of US patients with diabetes receive this type of education over the course of their illness and less than 7% receive it within the first year of diagnosis.

Her blood glucose has responded well to hydration and subcutaneous insulin. She is therefore clinically stable for discharge home. Thus, admitting her to the hospital (Answer A) is incorrect.

U500 regular insulin (Answer B) is used to treat patients with insulin resistance. If she had been taking all of the insulin prescribed and her blood glucose values were indeed persistently high, then this concentrated insulin would be a reasonable choice for her glycemic management. This patient was actually receiving an insulin dose that would be high for her if the entire dose were being delivered correctly. She does not require such a high total daily dose of insulin.

Increasing the insulin doses by 20% (Answer D) is the rule of thumb that her endocrinologist has been following when making insulin adjustments. However, in view of her size and the high number of units of insulin per kg body weight—and yet still no response in terms of blood glucose lowering—something else is going on.

EDUCATIONAL OBJECTIVE:
Evaluate the need for diabetes self-management and skills education in patients with poorly controlled diabetes.

REFERENCE(S):

Powers MA, Bardsley J, Cypress M, et al. Diabetes self-management education and support in type 2 diabetes: a joint position statement of the American Diabetes Association, the American Association of Diabetes Educators, and the Academy of Nutrition and Dietetics. *Diabetes Care*. 2015;38(7):1372-1382.

Magee MF, Nassar CN, Reyes-Castano J, McDonnell ME. In: Draznin B, ed. Emergency Department Management of Diabetes Patients with Non-crisis Hyperglycemia. *Managing Diabetes and Hyperglycemia in the Hospital Setting*. American Diabetes Association; 2016.

Lowery JB, Donihi AC , Korytkowski MT. U-500 insulin as a component of basal bolus insulin therapy in type 2 diabetes. *Diabetes Technol Ther*. 2012;14(6):505-507.

Rodriguez K, Meneghini L, Seley JJ, Magee MF. In: Draznin B, ed. Patient Education. *Managing Diabetes and Hyperglycemia in the Hospital Setting*. American Diabetes Association; 2016.

32 ANSWER: C) Change basal insulin to 20 units in the morning, stop the mealtime insulin, and start an oral agent

Many patients with inadequately controlled type 2 diabetes are treated with multiple daily insulin injections. This can impose a self-care burden, particularly among older patients, requiring them to measure blood glucose and inject insulin multiple times daily and, where appropriate, problem solve in order to adjust insulin doses and/or take correction doses. The use of rapid-acting or short-acting insulin also increases hypoglycemia risk, which is of particular concern in older patients, such as the one presented in this vignette.

Hypoglycemia in elderly patients with diabetes increases the risk of cardiovascular and cerebrovascular events, progression of dementia, injurious falls, emergency department visits, and hospitalization. Hypoglycemic episodes are difficult to diagnose in this population and are easily missed by intermittent fingerstick blood glucose measurements. Recent large studies have shown lack of benefit and sometimes higher risk of morbidity and mortality with tight glycemic control, especially in older adults. Therefore, the American Geriatric Society and the American Diabetes Association recommend relaxing glycemic control for vulnerable patients (hemoglobin A_{1c} <8.0% [<64 mmol/mol] instead of the usual <7.0% [<53 mmol/mol]).

Munshi et al used continuous glucose monitoring to evaluate hypoglycemia in older patients with type 2 diabetes who had a hemoglobin A_{1c} level greater than 8.0% (>64 mmol/mol). Community-living older patients seen at a diabetes center with a hemoglobin A_{1c} level greater than 8.0% were evaluated with blinded continuous glucose monitoring for a 3-day period while they continued their usual daily activities. Patients checked their blood glucose concentration 4 times daily while wearing the continuous glucose monitor and recorded symptoms suggestive of hypoglycemia. Forty adults aged 75 ± 5 years were evaluated. The mean hemoglobin A_{1c} level was 9.3% ± 1.3%. Most patients (58%) were taking insulin alone. Twenty-six of 40 patients (65%) had at least 1 episode of hypoglycemia (median glucose value of 63 mg/dL (3.5 mmol/L) (range, 42-69 mg/dL [2.3-3.8 mmol/L]) over the 3-day period. Among those with a hemoglobin A_{1c} value between 8.0% and 9.0% (64 to 75 mmol/mol)

and greater than 9.0% (>75 mmol/mol), the hypoglycemia rate was 54% and 46%, respectively.

This patient's basal insulin dose should clearly be reduced, as she becomes hypoglycemic when lunch is late. Her erratic morning blood glucose values suggest that she is also having nocturnal hypoglycemia. Her multiple daily insulin injection regimen requires problem solving, as she must determine when and how to take correction insulin doses. Her C-peptide level indicates that she is still making insulin. She is taking fewer than 10 units of rapid-acting analogue before meals, so it is reasonable to discontinue her mealtime insulin and to add an oral agent to her regimen per national guidelines (Answer C).

Referring her to a diabetes educator (Answer A) is a reasonable adjunctive measure, but it will not lower her risk for hypoglycemia without a concurrent adjustment in her antihyperglycemic medication regimen. Reducing her insulin doses and continuing the multiple daily injection regimen (Answer B) may reduce the frequency of hypoglycemia, but this would still require her to do problem solving, which seems to be challenging for her. Finally, if her risk for hypoglycemia is reduced via medication regimen simplification, her basal insulin dose is lowered sufficiently that it is appropriate for her, and an oral agent that does not increase risk for hypoglycemia is added to her regimen, she can continue to live independently (thus, Answer D is incorrect).

EDUCATIONAL OBJECTIVE:
Simplify the antihyperglycemic regimen in older adults with type 2 diabetes mellitus in order to prevent hypoglycemia.

REFERENCE(S):

Kirkman MS, Briscoe VJ, Clark N, et al. Diabetes in older adults. *Diabetes Care*. 2012;35(12): 2650-2664.

Munshi MN, Segal AR, Suhl E, et al. Frequent hypoglycemia among elderly with poor glycemic control. *Arch Intern Med*. 2011;171(4):362-364.

Munshi MN, Slyne C, Segal AR, Saul N, Lyons C, Weinger K. Simplification of insulin regimen in older adults and risk of hypoglycemia. *JAMA Intern Med*. 2016;176(7):1023-1025.

33

ANSWER: D) Lipohypertrophy

This patient clearly has lipohypertrophy (Answer D). In a study of 430 outpatients injecting insulin, nearly two-thirds had some degree of lipohypertrophy as determined by nurse examination and confirmed by use of ultrasonography, which allows for description of an "echo signature" for lipohypertrophy. Among those with lipohypertrophy, 39.1% had unexplained hypoglycemia and 49.1% had glycemic variability, compared with only 5.9% and 6.5%, respectively, in those without lipohypertrophy.

Several variables are associated with the presence of lipohypertrophy. This condition occurs in about 5% of patients who rotate insulin injection sites correctly; conversely, in those with lipohypertrophy, 98% either do not rotate sites or rotate sites incorrectly. Lipohypertrophy is also seen with needle reuse, with the risk increases significantly when needles are used more than 5 times. The duration of insulin use and education received also have a role. This particular patient had not rotated her insulin injection sites for many years and was reusing her insulin needles. With implementation of injection site rotation, which included her arms, opposite thigh, and abdomen, and stopping needle reuse, both her glycemic control and her hypoglycemic sensing improved.

Gastrointestinal autonomic neuropathy (Answer A) is a cause of erratic glycemic control due to variable absorption of nutrients depending on the rate at which the stomach empties following a meal. This patient does not have any classic symptoms suggestive of gastrointestinal autonomic neuropathy, which include early satiety, bloating sensation after meals, nausea, vomiting, and lower gastrointestinal motility disorders (constipation and/or diarrhea. She does not have symptoms that are otherwise suggestive of adrenal insufficiency (Answer B), which is most commonly detected when there is a trend for hypoglycemia and an otherwise unexplained reduction in insulin requirements in a patient with type 1 diabetes over time, rather than increased glycemic variability. Finally when a patient attempts tight glycemic control (Answer C), if hypoglycemia occurs frequently it can blunt insulin counterregulatory responses and cause blunted glycemic awareness. Frequent hypoglycemic episodes also increase glycemic variability due to the phenomenon of rebound hyperglycemia.

EDUCATIONAL OBJECTIVE:
List risk factors for erratic glycemic control, including lipohypertrophy.

REFERENCE(S):
Vardar B, Kizilci S. Incidence of lipohypertrophy in diabetic patients and a study of influencing factors. *Diabetes Res Clin Pract*. 2007;77(2): 231-236.

Blanco M, Hernandez MT, Strauss KW, Amaya M. Prevalence and risk factors of lipohypertrophy in insulin-injecting patients with diabetes. *Diabetes Metab*. 2013;39(5):445-453.

34

ANSWER: A) Rotate the pump insertion sites more widely

Localized involutional lipoatrophy of subcutaneous adipose tissue is a rare condition, characterized by reduction of fat cells in size, and, occasionally, in number. The fat tissue involution develops without symptomatic inflammation (as evidenced by the lack of erythema in this patient's lesion, although histopathology can show some inflammation). The cause of insulin-induced localized involutional lipoatrophy is hypothesized to be due to insulin delivered at the site. This phenomenon has been reported in cases where insulin is delivered via injection or pump and with a variety of insulin types, including currently available insulin analogues. Rotating away from the area where the lipoatrophy has developed (Answer A) usually allows the area to recover, and this should be the first intervention. Increasing the number of sites used in the rotation will reduce the risk that additional areas of lipoatrophy will develop.

If rotating the pump insertion sites more widely does not work, then switching to a different insulin preparation (Answer B) is the second-line strategy. Evidence that the injected hormonal agent itself has a role in the pathogenesis of localized lipoatrophy is indirectly supported by evidence from a small placebo-controlled study in which 13% of patients injecting pegylated GH developed lipoatrophy. None of the patients injecting a placebo (containing the same components as the vehicle in which the pegylated GH was delivered, namely water, sodium phosphate, mannitol, and glycine) developed lipoatrophy. The lipoatrophy in these patients resolved spontaneously within 2 to 3 months after the GH injections were stopped. Finally, several case reports in the literature describe use of oral glucocorticoids (Answer C) (prednisone, 10 mg daily for several months) in patients with large lesions with resolution.

Lipoatrophy is an autoimmune phenomenon associated with insulin use rather than the modality of delivery, so switching to a different insertion set (Answer D) is also incorrect.

EDUCATIONAL OBJECTIVE:
Recommend the steps for treating localized lipoatrophy.

REFERENCE(S):

Arranz A, Andia V, López-Guzmán A. A case of lipoatrophy with lispro insulin without insulin pump therapy. *Diabetes Care*. 2004;27(2):625-626.

Ernst A Chantelau EA, Prätor R, Prätor J. Insulin-induced localized lipoatrophy preceded by shingles (herpes zoster): a case report. *J Med Case Rep*. 2014;8:223.

35 ANSWER: B) Insulin degludec/liraglutide combination injectable

The basal insulin/glucagonlike peptide 1 analogue fixed-ratio coformulations have a lower risk of nausea than glucagonlike peptide 1 analogues given alone. The combined formulation makes it possible to titrate both the basal insulin and the glucagonlike peptide 1 analogue, starting at a low dose and titrating upwards at a slow and steady rate, which is hypothesized to be the reason that nausea rates are lower than when the glucagonlike peptide 1 analogues are given as single agents. Nausea rates for both fixed-ratio coformulations are relatively low. In the DUAL studies, the rate was reported to be in the 8% to 9% range for the combination insulin degludec/liraglutide injection, and in the pooled clinical trials for the combination insulin glargine/lixisenatide combination, the rate was 10% (thus, Answer B is correct and Answer D is incorrect).

When administered as single agents, nausea rates for liraglutide (Answer A) and lixisenatide (Answer C) are higher than for the fixed-ratio coformulations and are reported to be in the range of 25% to 35%.

Combination insulin degludec/liraglutide injection (Answer B) is a fixed-ratio combination of 100 units/mL of insulin degludec with 3.6 mg/mL of liraglutide. It is prescribed to improve glycemic control in adults with type 2 diabetes who have inadequate glycemic control on less than 50 units of basal insulin daily or less than or equal to 1.8 mg of liraglutide daily. It is administered as a once-daily injection from a prefilled pen and can be taken with or without food. Each 100/3.6 dosage unit contains 1 unit of insulin degludec and 0.036 mg of liraglutide. The starting dosage is 16 units (16 units of insulin degludec and 0.58 mg of liraglutide). The maximum dosage of 50 units corresponds to 50 units of insulin degludec and 1.8 mg of liraglutide. The most common adverse events seen during the DUAL clinical development program included nasopharyngitis, headache, nausea, diarrhea, increased lipase, and upper respiratory tract infection.

The fixed-ratio combination of 100 units of insulin glargine (U100) and 33 mcg/mL of lixisenatide is indicated as an adjunct to diet and exercise to improve glycemic control in adults with type 2 diabetes mellitus inadequately controlled on basal insulin (less than 60 units daily) or lixisenatide. In patients with inadequate glycemic control on less than 30 units of basal insulin or who are taking lixisenatide, the starting dosage is 15 units (15 units of insulin glargine and 5 mcg of lixisenatide) given subcutaneously once daily. In patients with inadequate glycemic control on 30 to 60 units of basal insulin, the starting dosage is 30 units (30 units of insulin glargine and 10 mcg of lixisenatide) given subcutaneously once daily, within the hour prior to the first meal of the day. The maximum daily dosage is 60 units (60 units of insulin glargine and 20 mcg of lixisenatide). Adverse reactions commonly associated with this combination injection include hypoglycemia, allergic reactions, nausea, nasopharyngitis, diarrhea, upper respiratory tract infection, and headache.

EDUCATIONAL OBJECTIVE:
Explain the relative potential for gastrointestinal adverse effects of glucagonlike peptide 1 analogues alone compared with new fixed-ratio combination basal plus glucagonlike peptide 1 analogue formulations.

REFERENCE(S):

Rosenstock J, Aronson R, Grunberger G, et al; LixiLan-O Trial Investigators. Benefits of LixiLan, a titratable fixed-ratio combination of insulin glargine plus lixisenatide, versus insulin glargine and lixisenatide monocomponents in type 2 diabetes inadequately controlled on oral agents: the LixiLan-O randomized trial. *Diabetes Care.* 2016;39(11):2026-2035.

Freemantle N, Mamdani M, Visboll T, Kongso JH, Kvist K, Bain SC. IDegLira versus alternative intensification strategies in patients with type 2 diabetes inadequately controlled on basal insulin therapy. *Diabetes Ther.* 2015;6(4):573-591.

Minze MG, Chastain LM. Combination therapies in the management of type 2 diabetes: the use of insulin degludec/liraglutide. *Ther Clin Risk Manag.* 2016;12:471-478.

36 **ANSWER: D) Reduced albuminuria**

With regard to nephropathy 5 to 10 years after successful pancreas transplant, mesangial volume and mesangial matrix volume are significantly decreased as compared with the same measurements at 0 and 5 years. In some patients, the width of the glomerular and tubular basement membranes and the mesangial volumes return to normal, and nodular glomerular lesions disappear. Tubular atrophy appears improved, possibly due to reabsorption of diseased nephrons. In all patients, urine albumin excretion improves significantly. Thus, reduced albuminuria (Answer D) can be expected within 5 years after a successful pancreas transplant.

In addition, after successful pancreas transplant, the velocity of motor and sensory nerve conduction, as well as clinical neuropathy, stabilizes but does not regress (Answer B). Abnormalities of gastric motility do not improve (Answer C). Quality-of-life studies consistently demonstrate benefits, such as return to work and successful pregnancies. Although initial reports indicated that established retinopathy does not improve, one study has shown that retinopathy was more likely to be arrested in patients who were successful pancreas recipients, when compared with those who lost the allograft. However, retinopathy does not regress (Answer A).

EDUCATIONAL OBJECTIVE:
Describe the potential benefits of pancreas transplant 5 to 10 years after successful transplant.

REFERENCE(S):

de Sá JR, Monteagudo PT, Rangel EB, et al. The evolution of diabetic chronic complications after pancreas transplantation. *Diabetol Metab Syndr.* 2009;1(1):11.

Boggi U, Rosati CM, Marchetti P. Follow-up of secondary diabetic complications after pancreas transplantation. *Curr Opin Organ Transplant.* 2013;18(1):102-110.

37 **ANSWER: D) Indeterminate**

Given the increased risk of type 2 diabetes mellitus in women with a history of gestational diabetes, the American Diabetes Association guidelines recommend screening for undiagnosed type 2 diabetes at the time that pregnancy is established in patients such as this one. Screening is done using the established criteria for the diagnosis of diabetes in adults.

Hemoglobin A_{1c}, fasting plasma glucose, and the 75-g oral glucose tolerance test may all be used as screening tests for type 2 diabetes. The oral glucose tolerance test is the most sensitive modality. However, in this case, her hemoglobin A_{1c} level is less than 6.5% (<48 mmol/mol)—the diagnostic threshold for diabetes—but her 2-hour plasma glucose value is greater than 200 mg/dL (>11.1 mmol/L) during the 75-g oral glucose tolerance test, which meets the criteria for type 2 diabetes. In the absence of unequivocal hyperglycemia, discordant results should be confirmed by repeated testing. Thus, the best assessment of this woman's current glycemic status is indeterminate (Answer D).

Establishing a diagnosis of type 2 diabetes that has not previously been recognized in the first trimester of pregnancy is important. If diabetes was preexisting, glycemic control before and during the pregnancy has implications for the health of both the mother and the baby. Management targeting glycemic control throughout the pregnancy is required for optimal outcomes.

If type 2 diabetes is not present, the oral glucose tolerance test should be repeated at 24 to 28 weeks' gestation to screen for gestational diabetes. This could consist of a 2-step process (50-g oral glucose tolerance test and then, depending on threshold criteria, the 100-g oral glucose tolerance test) or a 1-step process (75-g oral glucose tolerance test). The 1-step process has significantly increased the number of women identified with gestational diabetes because it requires only 1 abnormal value rather than 2. However, because this increased identification has not clearly translated into improved maternal or neonatal outcomes, the 2-step approach to diagnosing gestational diabetes is still supported by several organizations, including the American College of Obstetrics and Gynecology.

EDUCATIONAL OBJECTIVE:
Recommend a screening protocol for early pregnancy in a patient with a history of gestational diabetes.

REFERENCE(S):
American Diabetes Association. Standards of medical care in diabetes--2017. *Diabetes Care.* 2016;39(Suppl 1):S13-S22.
Committee on Practice Bulletins--Obstetrics. Practice Bulletin No. 137: gestational diabetes mellitus. *Obstet Gynecol.* 2013;122(2 Pt 1):406-416.

38 **ANSWER: B) Increase her basal insulin to 15 units in the morning**
"Pattern management" allows interpretation of fingerstick blood glucose results relative to the time of day and insulin doses taken in order to determine adjustments to the insulin regimen to help optimize glycemic control.

Her fasting blood glucose values are consistently higher than the recommended target of less than 90 to 95 mg/dL (5.0 to 5.3 mmol/L) for pregnant women with diabetes, so her basal insulin dose should be increased (Answer B). The 2-hour postmeal blood glucose goal is less than 120 mg/dL (<6.7 mmol/L). On Day 2, her lower 2-hour postbreakfast value is explained by her physical activity after the meal, so making an adjustment on the basis of this single reading (Answer A) is not warranted. If this postexercise pattern persists, it may later be appropriate to advise her to take a reduced dose of mealtime insulin on days she knows she will exercise after breakfast. On Day 2, the 2-hour postlunch value is consistent with rebound hyperglycemia in response to the hypoglycemia earlier on, so it also does not warrant an adjustment in the insulin acting at this time of day (ie, the lunch insulin dose). The value of 145 mg/dL (8.0 mmol/L) 2 hours after dinner on Day 1 is explained by the pizza meal; her other postdinner readings are under the recommended target of 120 mg/dL (<6.7 mmol/L). Therefore, the dinner dose of insulin aspart should not be increased (Answer C). Finally, basal insulin is not responsible for hypoglycemia on Day 2, as this is a postprandial value, so decreasing her basal insulin (Answer D) is also incorrect.

EDUCATIONAL OBJECTIVE:
Perform "pattern management" to enable targeted glycemic control for women with pregestational diabetes.

REFERENCE(S):
American Diabetes Association. Standards of medical care in diabetes--2016. *Diabetes Care.* 2016;39(Suppl 1):S94-S98.
ACOG Committee on Practice Bulletins. ACOG Practice Bulletin. Clinical management guidelines for obstetrician-gynecologists. Number 60, March 2005. Pregestational diabetes Mellitus. *Obstet Gynecol.* 2005;105(3):675-685.

39 **ANSWER: B) Reduction in hemoglobin A_{1c} of about 3% points**
Insulin patch pumps provide a method to offer basal-bolus insulin delivery to cover both fasting and postprandial glucose excursions for adults requiring insulin therapy. One application of the device is made every 24 hours. They are filled with U100 rapid-acting insulin, are applied to the skin, and deliver a preset basal rate of insulin via a subcutaneous needle for 24 hours. Mealtime boluses are delivered by simple button pushes.

When results for patients using one such device were stratified by baseline hemoglobin A_{1c}, the following reductions were observed:

Baseline Hemoglobin A_{1c}	Hemoglobin A_{1c} Reduction
7.2%-8.9%	0.8%
9.0%-10.4%	1.9%
10.5%-13.9%	3.2%

Therefore, this patient might be expected to have potential reduction in hemoglobin A_{1c} of about 3% points (Answer B).

Patients previously treated with a basal-bolus regimen consisting of a total daily dose of insulin of 120 + 58 units/day have been reported to have a 49% reduction in the total daily dose of insulin when switched to a patch pump (thus, Answer A is incorrect). This is postulated to be due to improved adherence to the prescribed regimen. The incidence of patient-reported hypoglycemia remains similar to baseline (thus, Answer C is incorrect). Finally, on the basis of direct pharmacy costs before and on patch pump therapy, there are significant reductions in costs with this therapy modality (based on actual prescription data and medication changes, including stopping noninsulin glucose-lowering medications documented in the electronic medical record) (thus, Answer D is incorrect).

EDUCATIONAL OBJECTIVE:
Explain the potential advantages of therapy using disposable insulin patch pumps.

REFERENCE(S):
Lajara R, Nikkel C, Abbott S. The clinical and economic impact of the V-Go disposable insulin delivery device for insulin delivery in patients with poorly controlled diabetes at high risk. *Drugs Real World Outcomes.* 2016;3(2):191-199.

40 ANSWER: E) More than 90%
Understanding the pathogenesis, natural history, and available treatment options for patients with diabetic retinopathy is critical because targeted glycemic control has clearly been shown to reduce both the incidence and progression of retinopathy.

For this reason, the American Diabetes Association recommends retinopathy screening by an eye specialist within 5 years of the diagnosis of type 1 diabetes in adults. Patients with type 2 diabetes should have an initial dilated and comprehensive eye examination by an ophthalmologist or optometrist at the time of the diabetes diagnosis, as microvascular changes can begin before diagnosis if prediabetes has been present. Female patients should be made aware that an eye exam should be done before conception or during the first trimester of pregnancy, and then every trimester and for 1 year post partum. If any level of diabetic retinopathy is present, subsequent dilated retinal examinations for patients with type 1 (or type 2) diabetes should be repeated at least annually by an ophthalmologist or optometrist. If retinopathy is progressive or sight-threatening, examinations are required more frequently.

Management recommendations call for optimizing glycemic control, blood pressure, and lipids to reduce the risk or slow progression of retinopathy. It is important to emphasize to the patient that attention to lifestyle and pharmacotherapeutic measures to optimize blood glucose, blood pressure, and lipids can be highly effective and would indeed reduce risk for progression of his eye changes by more than 90% (Answer E). Effective metabolic control will significantly reduce his risk for progression to proliferative retinopathy, macular edema, and the need for laser or alternative treatments, thus protecting sight.

If retinopathy does advance, current therapeutic options can be remarkably effective at preventing severe vision loss when administered in an appropriate and timely manner.

EDUCATIONAL OBJECTIVE:
Define the impact of appropriate medical care on the risk of vision loss in type 1 diabetes mellitus.

REFERENCE(S):
American Diabetes Association. Standards of Medical Care for Diabetes. Retinopathy. *Diabetes Care.* 2016(Suppl 1):S74-S76.
Bloomgarden ZT. Screening for and managing diabetic retinopathy: current approaches. *Am J Health Syst Pharm.* 2007;64(17 Suppl 12):S8-S14.

41 **ANSWER: C) Stereo views of the retina**
Diabetic retinopathy, one of the most common microvascular complications in both type 1 and type 2 diabetes, is classified as nonproliferative when it consists of retinal microhemorrhages and hard exudates, the latter representing lipid deposition. With progressive ischemia, more ominous signs such as ischemic infarcts (cotton wool spots) and neovascularization occur, and the changes are then classified as proliferative.

The image in the vignette shows extensive nonproliferative retinopathy, with retinal hemorrhages and hard exudates. In view of the extensive nature of the lesions and her recent change in vision, it would be important to determine whether she has coexisting macular edema, as this would warrant specific therapy. Stereo views of the retina (Answer C) are needed to determine whether thickening of the macula is present in order to make this diagnosis. Unless macular edema is diagnosed on the basis of further examination, intravitreal antivascular endothelial growth factor (anti-VEGF) injections such as ranibizumab (Answer A) are not indicated.

The Early Treatment of Diabetic Retinopathy Study examined the effect of treating eyes with mild nonproliferative diabetic retinopathy or early proliferative diabetic retinopathy to determine the best timing of photocoagulation. Rates of vision loss were low with either treatment applied early or delayed until development of high-risk characteristics, namely disc neovascularization or vitreous hemorrhage with any retinal neovascularization. Because of this low rate and the risk of complications, the report suggests that scatter photocoagulation be deferred in eyes with mild-to-moderate nonproliferative diabetic retinopathy. As this patient does not have high-risk characteristics, photocoagulation (Answers B and D) is not indicated now. In proliferative retinopathy with neovascularization, panretinal laser photocoagulation has been demonstrated to protect against vision loss. Focal laser photocoagulation is typically used for isolated areas of neovascularization.

EDUCATIONAL OBJECTIVE:
Recommend appropriate management of nonproliferative diabetic retinopathy.

REFERENCE(S):
Fong DS, Aiello L, Gardner TW, et al; American Diabetes Association. Diabetic retinopathy. *Diabetes Care.* 2003;26(Suppl 1):S99-S102.
Giuliari GP. Diabetic retinopathy: current and new treatment options. *Curr Diabetes Rev.* 2012;8(1):32-41.

42 **ANSWER: D) Intravitreal anti-VEGF agent injections once each month for the first year**
Diabetic macular edema, a manifestation of diabetic retinopathy that impairs central vision, affects approximately 750,000 people in the United States and is a leading cause of vision loss. Until recently, focal laser therapy (Answer B) had been the first-line therapy for this condition. Vascular endothelial growth factor (VEGF) is an important mediator of abnormal vascular permeability in diabetic macular edema and the emergence of multiple clinical trials have generated evidence that the addition of intravitreal anti-VEGF agents (Answer D) to the care of diabetic macular edema improves visual acuity better than focal laser alone. The evidence-based recommendation for frequency of anti-VEGF injections is once monthly for the first year. Multiple clinical trials have demonstrated that diabetic macular edema has high disease activity in the first year after diagnosis, but the need for treatment tapers in the second year. Patients in these trials received, on average, 9 to 10 anti-VEGF shots in the first year.

Relative to how these recommendations are being applied in real-world/nonclinical trial settings, a retrospective cohort study from a large, national US insurer that examined medical claims data from 2002 to 2012 representing 4743 patients with diabetes and diabetic macular edema recently reported its findings. Types and frequencies of treatment were analyzed and compared over time. Data for individual patients were examined for 1 or 2 years. Although the percentage of treated patients increased across the 2-year cohorts, no more than 41% of patients diagnosed with diabetic macular edema ever received treatment in any of the 1- or 2-year cohorts. The percentage of patients receiving therapy for diabetic macular edema and the number of treatments given increased for *both* focal laser and anti-VEGF (*P*<.001). The highest use of anti-VEGF agents in any of the cohorts was in 2012, the last year data were examined. This is not unexpected, as the Diabetic Retinopathy Clinical Research Network's Protocol I study, which was the first study to definitively show that anti-VEGF injections (with or without supplemental laser) dramatically improved the visual acuity results for patients with diabetic macular edema compared with laser alone, was not published until June 2010.

Regardless of the treatment modality (laser or injection), patients in real-world settings with diabetic macular edema received significantly fewer treatments than patients in randomized controlled trials. Despite the proven superior vision outcomes of anti-VEGF agents over focal laser in the setting of diabetic macular edema, focal laser is still used more frequently in patients with macular edema. The endocrinologist can therefore have a key role in explaining the importance of completing a 1-year series of shots, with or without focal laser when also indicated, in order to enhance adherence to this vision-saving treatment for patients with diabetic macular edema.

Observation may sometimes be appropriate within the accepted standards of care, but because the course of progression of diabetic macular edema is most rapid in the first year following diagnosis, waiting 6 months for follow-up observation (Answer A) is too long.

Panretinal photocoagulation (Answer C) is indicated for the treatment of proliferative diabetic retinopathy and venous occlusive diseases.

EDUCATIONAL OBJECTIVE:
Recommend the best treatment for patients with diabetic macular edema.

REFERENCE(S):
Diabetic Retinopathy Clinical Research Network, Elman MJ, Aiello LP, et al. Randomized trial evaluating ranibizumab plus prompt or deferred laser or triamcinolone plus prompt laser for diabetic macular edema. *Ophthalmology*. 2010;117(6):1064-1077.
Diabetic Retinopathy Clinical Research Network, Wells JA, Glassman AR, et al. Aflibercept, bevacizumab, or ranibizumab for diabetic macular edema. *N Engl J Med*. 2015;372(13):1193-1203.

VanderBeek BL, Shah N, Parikh PC, Ma L. Trends in the care of diabetic macular edema: analysis of a national cohort. *PLoS ONE*. 2016;11(2):e0149450.

43 ANSWER: B) Microalbuminuria represents a stage of diabetic nephropathy during which treatment is often successful in preventing progression to macroalbuminuria

The development of microalbuminuria in type 1 diabetes typically begins 5 to 15 years after disease onset (thus, Answer A is incorrect) and increases over time. Several studies have shown that ACE inhibitors and angiotensin-receptor blockers are not effective interventions for primary prevention of microalbuminuria (thus, Answer C is incorrect); however, this patient does not have microalbuminuria and he is normotensive, so treatment with one of these agents would not be appropriate now.

High total and LDL-cholesterol levels (not low HDL cholesterol [Answer D]) are also associated with increased risk for microalbuminuria. Risk of nephropathy is associated with risk of retinopathy and it is thought that they likely share many common etiologic pathways (thus, Answer E is incorrect).

Should microalbuminuria develop, several studies have shown that treating to recommended targets for glycemic control and blood pressure can prevent progression of diabetic nephropathy to more advanced stages of chronic kidney disease.

EDUCATIONAL OBJECTIVE:
List factors that affect microalbuminuria risk and progression and the rationale for its treatment.

REFERENCE(S):
Chaturvedi N, Bandinelli S, Mangili R, Penno G, Rottiers RE, Fuller JH. Microalbuminuria in type 1 diabetes: rates, risk factors and glycemic threshold. *Kidney Int*. 2001;60(1):219-227.
Rossing P, Hougaard P, Parving HH. Risk factors for development of incipient and overt diabetic nephropathy in type 1 diabetic patients: a 10-year prospective observational study. *Diabetes Care*. 2002;25(5):859-864.
Microalbuminuria Collaborative Study Group. Predictors of the development of microalbuminuria in patients with type 1 diabetes mellitus: a

seven-year prospective study. *Diabetic Med.* 1999;16(11):918-925.

Hovind P, Tarnow L, Rossing P, et al. Predictors for the development of microalbuminuria and macroalbuminuria in patients with type 1 diabetes: inception cohort study. *BMJ.* 2004;328(7448):1105.

Bilous R, Charturvedi N, Sjolie AK, et al. Effect of candesartan on microalbuminuria and albumin excretion rate in diabetes: three randomized trials. *Ann Intern Med.* 2009;151(1):11-20.

Randomised placebo-controlled trial of lisinopril in normotensive patients with insulin-dependent diabetes and normoalbuminuria or microalbuminuria. The EUCLID Study Group. *Lancet.* 1997;349(9068):1787-1792.

Mauer M, Zinman B, Gardiner R, et al. Renal and retinal effects of enalapril and losartan in type 1 diabetes. *N Engl J Med.* 2009;361(1):40-51.

44 ANSWER: D) Begin sildenafil

This patient has longstanding diabetes, macrovascular disease, retinopathy, and peripheral and autonomic neuropathy. It is not surprising that he has erectile dysfunction given the key role that endothelial function and autonomic innervation have in penile tumescence.

Use of phosphodiesterase 5 inhibitors such as sildenafil (Answer D) is the mainstay of therapy for erectile dysfunction, and although patients with diabetes do not respond as well as those without diabetes, response rates are still approximately 50%. This patient may have a reduced chance of responding because of his longstanding erectile dysfunction and other co-morbidities; nonetheless, neither the presence of endothelial dysfunction nor autonomic neuropathy predicts response to sildenafil. The simplicity and safety of phosphodiesterase 5 inhibitor treatment make this the best first step in this patient. Although use of nitrates is a contraindication for use of drugs such as sildenafil, the presence of cardiovascular disease is not.

Improvement of glycemic control (Answer B) has not been demonstrated to improve sexual function in cases of erectile dysfunction. Intracavernosal alprostadil (Answer C) and penile implants (Answer A) are effective treatments, but they are more invasive than sildenafil and are thus relegated to second- or third-line therapy.

It should also be noted that many medications, including antihypertensive agents (ie, metoprolol, which this patient is taking), antidepressants, anti-anxiety and anticonvulsant drugs, antihistamines, and some nonsteroidal anti-inflammatory agents (eg, naproxen and indomethacin) may also cause erectile dysfunction. If his neuropathy and/or cardiac disease were not so advanced, it would be worth asking his cardiologist to consider substituting another class of antihypertensive drug for the β-adrenergic blocker.

EDUCATIONAL OBJECTIVE:
Manage erectile dysfunction in the setting of diabetes mellitus.

REFERENCE(S):
Price D, Hackett G. Management of erectile dysfunction in diabetes: an update for 2008. *Curr Diab Rep.* 2008;8(6):437-443.

Pegge NC, Twomey AM, Vaughton K, Gravenor MB, Ramsey MW, Price DE. The role of endothelial dysfunction in the pathophysiology of erectile dysfunction in diabetes and in determining response to treatment. *Diabet Med.* 2006;23(8):873-878.

45 ANSWER: A) Diabetic radiculopathy

Diabetic neuropathy is generally more common in patients with long disease duration and poor glycemic control. Classification is subdivided into somatosensory, motor, and autonomic.

Diabetes-related radiculopathy manifests as acute sensory and/or motor neuropathy characterized by sudden pain and dysesthesias and/or muscle weakness in the distribution of 1 or more individual peripheral nerves or nerve roots. The patient in this vignette has right-sided facial pain and muscle weakness in the distribution of the facial (seventh cranial) nerve. This is an acute mononeuropathy or radiculitis (Answer A). There is no specific therapy for this complication. The patient can be reassured that it typically resolves after 2 to 3 months. Neuropathy pain relief medications such as tricyclic antidepressants or selective serotonin and norepinephrine reuptake inhibitors may be given in the interim. The most common presentation of neuropathy with diabetes involves damage to sensory nerve fibers and typically affects the distal extremities in a "stocking-glove" distribution as this patient has on exam. Patients describe numbness, paresthesias, and occasionally sharp pains.

Autonomic dysfunction (Answer B) may affect 1 or several organ systems including the vasculature (orthostatic hypotension), the heart (silent ischemia, abnormal cardiac rhythms), the gastrointestinal tract (gastroparesis, constipation, diarrhea from bacterial overgrowth), and the urinary bladder (atonic bladder, chronic urinary tract infections, overflow incontinence). It does not cause pain syndromes.

Herpes zoster (Answer C) can cause localized pain in a pattern similar to that described here, and pain can precede the typical rash but not usually for about 1 week after the onset of pain. Otitis media (Answer D) can spread to the facial nerve and inflame it, causing compression of the nerve in its canal; however, there is no evidence of otitis on her exam. Findings on her head CT do not suggest cerebrovascular accident (Answer E).

EDUCATIONAL OBJECTIVE:
Diagnose less common manifestations of diabetic neuropathy.

REFERENCE(S):

Tesfaye S, Boulton AJ, Dyck PJ, et al; Toronto Diabetic Neuropathy Expert Group. Diabetic neuropathies: update on definitions, diagnostic criteria, estimation of severity, and treatments. *Diabetes Care*. 2010;33(10):2285-2293.

Casellini CM, Vinik AI. Clinical manifestations and current treatment options for diabetic neuropathies. *Endocr Pract*. 2007;13(5):550-566.

46 ANSWER: A) Measure serum vitamin B_{12}

This patient has new neuropathic symptoms superimposed on a history and examination findings consistent with peripheral polyneuropathy. The symptoms and physical findings suggest posterior column and upper motor neuron disease, and in this setting, a positive Romberg sign and Babinski response would likely be present. Although this may represent progression of diabetic neuropathy, the latter findings are not typical for this alone. He has anemia, and the combination of neurologic and hematologic disturbance is compatible with vitamin B_{12} deficiency. Use of metformin has been associated with lowered plasma vitamin B_{12} levels in up to 30% of patients and it doubles the risk of clinically significant B_{12} deficiency. While the mechanism is not entirely clear, most evidence points to interference with food-derived B_{12} absorption, primarily in the ileum. Replacement with oral or parenteral vitamin B_{12} is usually successful and precludes discontinuation of metformin.

Numerous laboratory testing options are available to assess for the presence of B_{12} deficiency. Serum vitamin B_{12} measurement (Answer A) is most commonly used for initial assessment, while others, such as the tests that access levels of holotranscobalamin, methylmalonic acid, or homocysteine, are reserved for confirmatory testing.

Electromyelography and nerve conduction studies (Answer D) would most likely be abnormal in this man, but they are not specific for subacute combined degeneration (neuropathy due to vitamin B_{12} deficiency). Vitamin B_6 (Answer B), pyridoxine, has a role in serotonin and norepinephrine metabolism and in the formation of myelin. Clinical symptoms of B_6 deficiency are bilateral, distal limb numbness (appears early) and distal limb burning paresthesia (replaces numbness later in the course). Distal limb weakness is rare.

This patient's presentation is not consistent with spinal or nerve root irritation from C-spine disease, which can manifest as pain in the neck and pain and numbness or weakness radiating down to the shoulder, arm, and hand. Thus, MRI of the cervical spine (Answer C) is incorrect.

EDUCATIONAL OBJECTIVE:
Diagnose adverse effects of metformin.

REFERENCE(S):

Pierce SA, Chung AH, Black KK. Evaluation of vitamin B12 monitoring in a veteran population on long-term, high-dose metformin therapy. *Ann Pharmacother*. 2012;46(11):1470-1476.

Pflipsen MC, Oh RC, Saguil A, Seehusen DA, Seaquist D, Topolski R. The prevalence of vitamin B(12) deficiency in patients with type 2 diabetes: a cross-sectional study. *J Am Board Fam Med*. 2009;22(5):528-534.

Ting RZ, Szeto CC, Chan MH, Ma KK, Chow KM. Risk factors of vitamin B(12) deficiency in patients receiving metformin. *Arch Intern Med.* 2006;166(18):1975-1979.

Ward PC. Modern approaches to the investigation of vitamin B12 deficiency. *Clin Lab Med.* 2002;22(2): 435-445.

47 **ANSWER: C) Empagliflozin**
Cardiovascular disease and heart failure are major causes of morbidity and mortality in type 2 diabetes. Once congestive heart failure is present, mortality is increased 10-fold and 5-year survival is only 12.5%. Several diabetes drugs have been associated with an unexpected increase in heart failure risk during clinical trials and postmarketing surveillance, raising concerns about overall risks and benefits.

Recently completed cardiovascular outcome trials for type 2 diabetes drugs for patients with or at high risk of cardiovascular disease have provided new evidence that can be factored in when making choices about which antihyperglycemic agents to use. On the basis of proven cardiovascular and renal benefit, the antihyperglycemic drugs empagliflozin (Empa-Reg Outcomes study), liraglutide (LEADER study), and semaglutide (SUSTAIN study) may be preferentially used as second-line treatments in these patient populations, typically in addition to metformin (semaglutide is still under review by the US FDA).

Relevant specifically to heart failure risk, which is high in this patient, use of empagliflozin (Answer C) in the EMPA-Reg Outcomes study resulted in a hazard ratio for hospital admissions due to congestive heart failure of 0.64 (95% confidence interval, 0.50-0.85; *P* = .002). Empagliflozin is therefore the best choice.

The US FDA has added a warning to the drug labels for saxagliptin (Answer B) and alogliptin regarding increased risk of heart failure, particularly in those who have heart disease or kidney disease. In the SAVOR-TIMI 53 trial, saxagliptin was associated with an unexpected 27% increase in heart failure hospital admissions, representing 3.5% of patients who received the drug. In the EXAMINE trial, 3.9% of alogliptin-treated patients were hospitalized for heart failure vs 3.3% in the placebo group.

Thiazolidinediones such as pioglitazone (Answer A) have long been associated with increased risk for heart failure, and insulin glargine (Answer D) in the ORIGIN study had a neutral effect on cardiovascular outcomes, including risk for hospitalizations for heart failure.

EDUCATIONAL OBJECTIVE:
Select empagliflozin over other antihyperglycemic agents for patients at high risk for heart failure.

REFERENCE(S):
Standl E, Schnell O, McGuire DK, Ceriello A, Ryden L. Integration of recent evidence into management of patients with atherosclerotic cardiovascular disease and type 2 diabetes. *Lancet Diabetes Endocrinol.* 2017;5(5):391-402.

Zinman B, Wanner C, Lachin JM, et al; EMPA-REG OUTCOME Investigators. Empagliflozin, cardiovascular outcomes, and mortality in type 2 diabetes. *N Engl J Med.* 2015;373(22):2117-2128.

McGuire DK, Van de Werf F, Armstrong PW, et al; Trial Evaluating Cardiovascular Outcomes With Sitagliptin (TECOS) Study Group. Association between sitagliptin use and heart failure hospitalization and related outcomes in type 2 diabetes mellitus: secondary analysis of a randomized clinical trial. *JAMA Cardiol.* 2016;1(2):126-135.

Green JB, Bethel MA, Armstrong PW, et al; TECOS Study Group. Effect of sitagliptin on cardiovascular outcomes in type 2 diabetes. *N Engl J Med.* 2015;373(3):232-242.

ORIGIN Trial Investigators. Basal insulin and cardiovascular and other outcomes in dysglycemia. *N Engl J Med.* 2012;367(4):319-328.

48 **ANSWER: B) Vascular segmental pressures and pulse volume recordings**
This patient has multiple risk factors for atherosclerosis, including diabetes, retinopathy, chronic kidney disease, hypertension, and hyperlipidemia. His diabetes, blood pressure, and lipids are well controlled on his current regimen. Diagnosing peripheral vascular disease is clinically important for several reasons. The first is to identify whether the patent is at high risk for cardiovascular disease and stroke. The second is to reduce the risk for foot ulcers, functional disability, and limb amputations.

The third is so that revascularization may be considered in cases where the limb is threatened or a foot ulcer fails to heal.

You are concerned that he has peripheral arterial disease with intermittent claudication. It should be noted that dorsalis pedis pulses are reported to be absent in 8.1% of healthy individuals, and the posterior tibial pulse is absent in 2.0%. Nevertheless, the absence of both pedal pulses strongly suggests the presence of vascular disease.

His ankle brachial index is 1.4. The diagnostic criteria for peripheral arterial disease based on the ankle brachial index are as follows:

- 0.91-1.30 = normal
- 0.70-0.90 = mild obstruction
- 0.40-0.69 = moderate obstruction
- <0.40 = severe obstruction
- >1.30 = poorly compressible

An ankle brachial index greater than 1.3 suggests poorly compressible arteries at the ankle due to the presence of calcification, which is a common finding in patients with diabetes and atherosclerosis. Calcification makes the diagnosis of peripheral arterial disease by ankle brachial index alone less reliable, so the diagnosis should be confirmed by sending this patient to the vascular lab to have his vascular segmental pressures and pulse volumes checked (Answer B). In patients with confirmed peripheral arterial disease, these tests are used to localize disease and determine its severity. As in this patient's case, these tests are also helpful when poorly compressible vessels are present. Finally, these tests are also used when the ankle brachial index is normal and when there is high suspicion of peripheral arterial disease. Segmental pressures help with lesion localization. Pulse volume recordings provide segmental waveform analysis for a qualitative assessment of blood flow.

The other listed assessments are used in different case scenarios or at intermediate points in the workup of peripheral arterial disease. Treadmill functional testing (Answer D) is used if the patient has a normal ankle brachial index with typical symptoms of claudication. Further noninvasive studies are used to guide clinical decision-making regarding potential for revascularization to be done when a patient has a nonhealing foot ulcer or

rest ischemic pain. Transcutaneous oxygen pressure (Answer A) is used to predict capacity to heal a foot ulcer. A value less than 30 mm Hg is associated with poor wound healing or amputations. A systolic toe pressure (Answer C) less than 40 mm Hg or toe waveform less than 4 mm also predicts poor wound healing. Systolic toe pressure may be also be used as an adjunctive test to evaluate patients who have medial arterial calcification, for whom the ankle brachial index is less accurate.

EDUCATIONAL OBJECTIVE:
Order appropriate initial tests when a patient is suspected to have peripheral arterial disease.

REFERENCE(S):
American Diabetes Association. Peripheral arterial disease in people with diabetes. *Diabetes Care.* 2003;26(12):3333-3341.

49 **ANSWER: A) Clindamycin**
Patients with diabetes mellitus who present with a foot ulcer should be evaluated at 3 levels: the clinical presentation of the patient as a whole, the extent of involvement of the affected foot or limb, and the likelihood that the wound is infected. Presence of infection in a diabetic foot ulcer is defined by 2 or more classic findings of inflammation or purulence. This patient has erythema, some swelling, and increased skin temperature. His infection would be classified as mild (superficial and limited in size and depth), rather than moderate (deeper/more extensive), or severe (accompanied by systemic signs or metabolic perturbations).

Empiric antibiotic therapy can be narrowly targeted at gram-positive cocci in many acutely infected patients, but those at risk for infection with antibiotic-resistant organisms (recent antibiotic therapy) or with chronic, previously treated, or severe infections usually require broader-spectrum regimens.

This patient has a mild foot infection associated with a superficial ulcer. The probable pathogens are methicillin-sensitive *Staphylococcus aureus* and *Streptococcus* species. Empiric therapy with clindamycin (Answer A), dicloxacillin, cephalexin, levofloxacin, or amoxicillin-clavulanate would therefore be appropriate choices for oral therapy.

If the patient were at high risk for methicillin-resistant *Staphylococcus aureus* (eg, recent hospitalization), then a mild infection should be treated with doxycycline (Answer B) or trimethoprim-sulfamethoxazole (Answer C). He is, however, not at risk for methicillin-resistant *Staphylococcus aureus*.

When infection is chronic and severe and there has been previous antibiotic therapy, a broader-spectrum combination of agents, such as vancomycin plus ceftazidime (Answer D) would be required. Finally, definitive therapy should be based on the results of an appropriately obtained culture and sensitivity testing of a wound specimen, as well as the patient's clinical response to the empiric regimen.

EDUCATIONAL OBJECTIVE:
Select the appropriate antibiotic to treat a diabetes-related foot ulcer.

REFERENCE(S):

Lipsky BA, Berendt AR, Cornia PB, et al. 2012 Infectious Diseases Society of America clinical practice guideline for the diagnosis and treatment of diabetic foot infections. *Clin Infect Dis.* 2012; 54(12):e132-e173.

50 ANSWER: B) Temporarily relax tight glucose targets

Up to 30% of patients with type 1 or longstanding type 2 diabetes mellitus have impaired or absent awareness of hypoglycemia. As plasma glucose levels fall, compromised physiologic counterregulatory defenses include failure of an increase in glucagon secretion and attenuated epinephrine secretion. This, together with inability to reduce circulating insulin levels, results in the clinical syndrome of defective counterregulation, which markedly increases the risk of recurrent severe hypoglycemia. Hypoglycemia-attenuating defense against subsequent hypoglycemia is a concept referred to as hypoglycemia-associated autonomic failure. The mainstay of treatment for this condition is the scrupulous avoidance of hypoglycemia. Patients with hypoglycemia unawareness and/or severe hypoglycemia and tight control should be advised to relax their glucose targets (Answer B) for a period to allow awareness to potentially return with adrenergic symptoms.

This patient should continue his usual dietary regimen (consistent carbohydrate or matching insulin to carbohydrates). Frequent small meals (Answer A) would not get at the root of his problem. Switching to insulin pump therapy (Answer C) would not address the underlying cause of the hypoglycemia unawareness (repetitive hypoglycemic episodes) or guarantee its avoidance. A pump with a closed-loop suspend or auto-suspend for hypoglycemia function might be considered in his long-term management plan; however, he has had tight glycemic control on a multiple daily injection regimen as evidenced by his hemoglobin A_{1c} level and again, the urgent need here is to address the blunted glycemic awareness. There would also be a delay in initiating pump therapy and a learning curve regarding its use. While a number of educational programs focusing on hypoglycemia detection and avoidance (Dose Adjustment for Normal Eating [DAFNE], Blood Glucose Awareness Training [BGAT], Hypoglycemia Awareness and Avoidance [HAAT]) have demonstrated effectiveness in reducing the occurrence of hypoglycemia, such an education program (Answer D) is not the most immediate fix for this patient, nor would it address the cause.

EDUCATIONAL OBJECTIVE:
Recommend management for severe hypoglycemia and hypoglycemia unawareness in type 1 diabetes mellitus.

REFERENCE(S):

Alsahli M, Gerich JE. Hypoglycemia. *Endocrinol Metab Clin North Am.* 2013;42(4):657-676.

Little SA, Leelarathna L, Barendse SM, et al. Severe hypoglycaemia in type 1 diabetes mellitus: underlying drivers and potential strategies for successful prevention. *Diabetes Metab Res Rev.* 2014;30(3):175-190.

Choudhary P, Amiel SA. Hypoglycaemia: current management and controversies. *Postgrad Med.* 2011;87(1026):298-306.

Oyer DS. The science of hypoglycemia in patients with diabetes. *Curr Diabetes Rev.* 2013;9(3): 195-208.

Cryer PE. Mechanisms of hypoglycemia-associated autonomic failure in diabetes. *N Engl J Med.* 369(4):362-372.

Awoniyi O, Rehman R, Dagogo-Jack S. Hypoglycemia in patients with type 1 diabetes: epidemiology, pathogenesis, and prevention. *Curr Diab Rep.* 2013;13(5):669-678.

Morales J, Schneider D. Hypoglycemia. *Am J Med.* 2014;127(Suppl 10):S17-S24.

51 ANSWER: A) Intravenous U100 regular insulin infusion titrated to achieve blood glucose between 140 and 180 mg/dL (7.8-10.0 mmol/L)

This critically ill patient, who has no history of diabetes, has severe hyperglycemia precipitated by high-dosage glucocorticoid therapy compounded by insulin counterregulatory hormones due to illness-related stress. Evidence-based national guidelines from the American Association of Clinical Endocrinologists and the American Diabetes Association recommend that hyperglycemic patients in the intensive care unit should receive intravenous insulin to control their glucose and that the glucose levels should be maintained between 140 and 180 mg/dL (7.8-10.0 mmol/L) (Answer A). The NICE-SUGAR study (Normoglycemia in Intensive Care Evaluation and Surviving Using Glucose Algorithm Regulation) demonstrated no benefit from lowering blood glucose to less than 110 mg/dL (<6.1 mmol/L) and showed an increase in morbidity and mortality when more stringent control was attempted.

Regular insulin by intermittent subcutaneous injection (Answers B and D) has little role in the intensive care unit, since blood glucose control can be achieved more quickly and more reliably with intravenous administration. Achieving a lower target of 80 to 110 mg/dL (4.4-6.1 mmol/L) with intravenous insulin (Answer C) markedly increases the risk of severe hypoglycemia (more than 6-fold). A basal and prandial insulin regimen, such as insulin glargine and insulin aspart, is appropriate upon transfer out of the intensive care unit, but, as with regular insulin, it is not rapid enough in its action and is not as easily adaptable as is an intravenous infusion.

Given that his blood glucose before initiation of the insulin drip was 183 mg/dL (10.2 mmol/L) (may not be normal), his glucose tolerance status should be reassessed after discontinuation of the steroids and discharge from the hospital to ensure that it is normal. Measurement of hemoglobin A_{1c} in the hospital lab may also help to make this distinction.

EDUCATIONAL OBJECTIVE:
Manage blood glucose in acutely ill hospitalized patients.

REFERENCE(S):
American Diabetes Association. Standards of medical care in diabetes--2016. *Diabetes Care.* 2016;39(Suppl 1):S99-S104.

Moghissi ES, Korytkowski MT, DiNardo M, et al; American Association of Clinical Endocrinologists; American Diabetes Association. American Association of Clinical Endocrinologists and American Diabetes Association consensus statement on inpatient glycemic control. *Diabetes Care.* 2009;32(6): 1119-1131.

52 ANSWER: D) Insulin glargine, 58 units in the morning, and insulin lispro, 5 units before meals, and a correction dose if blood glucose is >180 mg/dL (>10.0 mmol/L)

Patients with type 1 diabetes mellitus being treated with continuous subcutaneous insulin infusion who are stabilized clinically and will be sent to a medical-surgical ward require transition to subcutaneous insulin, with determination of appropriate basal, nutritional, and correction (or supplemental) insulin dosing. It is extremely important to allow time for onset of action of the first dose(s) of subcutaneous insulin before stopping the drip in order to prevent rebound hyperglycemia. If rapid analogue insulin will be given, then the drip can be stopped when it is administered. If basal insulin is given alone (eg, if the patient is not going to eat), then the drip would need to be stopped 2 to 3 hours after administration of the first dose. Under-insulinization following transition from intravenous to subcutaneous insulin is also a common cause of hyperglycemia following the transition. If there is concern that allocation of 80% of the estimated daily basal insulin requirement at the time of transition is high, then a more conservative approach is appropriate. Another approach to support the transition is to co-treat the patient with a low dose of basal insulin (0.25 units/kg body weight) starting within 12 hours of initiating intravenous insulin, so that basal insulin will be on board at the time that transition to subcutaneous injections is made.

Basal Insulin Dose Calculation

While the patient is acutely ill and not eating, the insulin delivered by continuous subcutaneous insulin infusion is serving to meet basal insulin requirements.

- An extrapolated total daily basal insulin dose at the time the drip will be stopped can be made based on the amount of insulin delivered via the drip in the 4 to 6 hours before the infusion is stopped. This represents the patient's daily basal insulin requirement at the time the drip is stopped. In this patient, the rate was 3 units/h, which is multiplied by 6 to give a 6 hours' dose of 18 units. The estimated 24-hour basal dose is then calculated by multiplying by 4, which equals 72 units of insulin daily.
- Current guidelines and evidence in the literature suggest that it is acceptable to give 50% to 80% of the estimated total daily basal insulin dose to enable optimal glycemic control while avoiding risk for hypoglycemia (eg, in this case, 80% of 72 units equals 58 units). The percentage of estimated daily basal insulin dose chosen as the multiplier varies depending on the clinical circumstances (eg, higher requirements after major surgical procedures such as coronary bypass and institutional factors/experience). It should be noted that the basal dose is often underestimated due to concern for hypoglycemia, which in turn results in post-transition hyperglycemia.

Meal Subcutaneous Insulin Dose Determination

Dosing of prandial insulin, which will be given as a rapid-acting insulin analogue either at the start or the end of the meal, is commonly provided as follows:

- Using a weight-based calculation (eg, 0.1 units/kg before each meal, which in this patient would be 8 or 9 units with each meal).
- Using a small fixed dose of insulin, such as 5 units, that is given to cover carbohydrates

consumed as the patient begins to eat and can then be adjusted per the resulting blood glucose values. Nutritional coverage must be provided if enteral feeds or parenteral infusions are being given.

Finally, a correction or supplemental dose insulin scale, preferably using a rapid-acting analogue, is provided when blood glucose values are greater than 180 mg/dL (>10.0 mmol/L).

Insulin glargine, 58 units in the morning will meet this patient's basal needs. This is 80% of the estimated daily basal insulin requirement at the time of drip discontinuation. Insulin lispro, 5 units before meals, will meet his nutritional insulin needs as he begins to eat. Correction doses will be provided if blood glucose values are greater than 180 mg/dL (>10.0 mmol/L). Thus, Answer D is correct.

While the daily basal insulin requirement will be met using split doses in Answer A, this patient will be eating and will need rapid-acting analogue with each meal despite his premeal blood glucose level. While the basal insulin dose in Answer B is correct, he will be eating and regular insulin every 6 hours will not be matched to his meal times. The basal insulin dose of 29 units in Answer C will only meet 50% of his total daily requirement. The dose of 10 units of rapid-acting analogue with each meal may be high as he is just beginning to eat.

EDUCATIONAL OBJECTIVE:
Devise a rational plan for transitioning from intravenous insulin to a subcutaneous insulin regimen in hospitalized patients.

REFERENCE(S):

Lien LF, Low Wang CC, Kreider KE, Baldwin D Jr. Transitioning from IV to SC insulin. In: Draznin B, ed. *Managing Diabetes and Hyperglycemia in the Hospital Setting.* American Diabetes Association; 2016:115-128.

American Diabetes Association. Standards of medical care in diabetes--2017. *Diabetes Care.* 2014;37(Suppl 1).

Hsia E, Seggelke S, Gibbs J, et al. Subcutaneous administration of glargine to diabetic patients receiving insulin infusion prevents rebound hyperglycemia. *J Clin Endocrinol Metab.* 2012;97(9):3132-31327.

Moghissi ES, Korytkowski MT, DiNardo M, et al; American Association of Clinical Endocrinologists ; American Diabetes Association. American Association of Clinical Endocrinologists and American Diabetes Association consensus statement on inpatient glycemic control. *Endocr Pract.* 2009;15(4): 353-369.

Schmeltz LR, DeSantis AJ, Schmidt K, et al. Conversion of intravenous insulin infusions to subcutaneously administered insulin glargine in patients with hyperglycemia. *Endocr Pract.* 2006;12(6):641-650.

53 ANSWER: A) Once-daily basal insulin, plus correction insulin dose regimen every 4 to 6 hours

Subcutaneous insulin is the recommended treatment for glycemic management in postoperative patients with type 2 diabetes who are in a noncritical care unit. If the patient were in the critical care setting, continuous intravenous insulin infusion (Answer D) would be the recommended method of glycemic management. However, if the patient is in a noncritical care setting, as in this case, a regimen of scheduled subcutaneous insulin injections is the best method for achieving glycemic targets.

This patient's glycemic status warrants basal insulin in addition to correction dose insulin. As she is not eating, meal insulin will not be provided. The frequency of dosing of correction dose insulin depends on the type of insulin used. If a rapid-acting analogue is used, it may be given every 4 hours, and if regular insulin is used, it will be given every 6 hours (Answer A). These time intervals correspond with the known duration of action of each insulin and will help avoid stacking of insulin and resulting hypoglycemia. Injections should align with meals and bedtime or every 4 to 6 hours if the patient is not consuming meals (thus, Answer B is incorrect). Evidence clearly shows that sliding-scale insulin used alone (Answer C) is associated with increased rates of both hypoglycemia and hyperglycemia and its use is therefore not recommended. In addition, evidence from randomized controlled trials has demonstrated that a scheduled basal plus bolus treatment regimen results in better glycemic control and reduced hospital complications when compared with outcomes with sliding-scale insulin alone in general surgery patients with type 2 diabetes, further making the case for a basal plus bolus regimen. When this patient begins to eat, scheduled meal insulin will be added to her regimen.

EDUCATIONAL OBJECTIVE:
Manage inpatient insulin treatment in the noncritical care setting.

REFERENCE(S):
American Diabetes Association. Standards of medical care in diabetes--2016. *Diabetes Care.* 2016;39(Suppl 1):S99-S104.

Umpierrez GE, Smiley D, Jacobs S, et al. Randomized study of basal-bolus insulin therapy in the inpatient management of patients with type 2 diabetes undergoing general surgery (RABBIT 2 surgery). *Diabetes Care.* 2011;34(2):256-261.

54 ANSWER: B) Insulin glargine U100, 8 units twice daily plus regular insulin every 6 hours

When selecting a subcutaneous insulin regimen for patients with diabetes mellitus, an effort is made to prescribe a physiologic basal-bolus regimen that will meet both basal insulin requirements and nutritional insulin needs.

The underlying principles of subcutaneous insulin therapy for patients receiving enteral nutrition call for use of judicious basal insulin therapy, so that if the tube feedings are interrupted the patient will not become hypoglycemic. For the basal insulin dosing, a weight-based starting dose of 0.2 units/kg per day (16 units daily in this case) (Answer B) or 40% of the total daily dose of insulin administered via insulin infusion before the transition (22 units/day in this case) are the rules of thumb. This may be administered as insulins glargine or detemir once daily or in a split dose twice daily, or as short (regular U100 insulin) every 6 hours—the latter can also provide a steady 24-hour basal action profile. Use of NPH insulin (2 to 3 times daily) has also been reported in this clinical setting. However, NPH insulin once daily (Answer A) is incorrect because this would not provide continuous basal insulin coverage.

Regular insulin administered every 4 hours (Answer C) would lead to insulin stacking and hypoglycemia. Insulin glargine U300 (Answer D) has not been evaluated for use in the inpatient setting. Nutritional insulin needs will be met using regular insulin via a scaled dose of either regular U100 insulin every 6 hours or rapid-acting insulin analogue every 4 hours.

Only one published randomized controlled trial has examined specific subcutaneous insulin regimens in patients with diabetes receiving enteral nutrition. Fifty patients were randomly assigned to sliding-scale regular insulin alone or sliding-scale regular insulin plus glargine. By the end of the insulin titration period, 48% of the patients randomly assigned to sliding-scale regular insulin alone required the addition of NPH insulin to the regimen for persistent hyperglycemia (blood glucose >180 mg/dL [>10 mmol/L]).

The Endocrine Society Clinical Practice Guideline on management of hyperglycemia in the hospital outlines approaches depending on which type of enteral nutrition is being given (see table).

Enteral Nutrition Administration Method	Potential Approach to Subcutaneous Insulin Therapy
Continuous	Basal insulin once daily (glargine or detemir) or twice-daily detemir or NPH
	Short- or rapid-acting every 4 hours (rapid) or every 6 hours (regular)
Cycled	Basal insulin once daily (glargine, detemir, or NPH) with short- or rapid-acting at start of enteral nutrition
	Repeat the rapid-acting every 4 hours or the regular every 6 hours
Bolus	Short- or rapid-acting insulin before each bolus*

*With judicious dose of basal insulin as described above if indicated (eg, if on insulin therapy before hospital admission and/or there is persistent hyperglycemia across a 24-hour period).

EDUCATIONAL OBJECTIVE:
Order a physiologic basal-bolus insulin regimen for patients treated with enteral nutrition.

REFERENCE(S):
Korytkowski MT, Salata RJ, Koerbel GL, et al. Insulin therapy and glycemic control in hospitalized patients with diabetes during enteral nutrition therapy. *Diabetes Care.* 2009;32(4):594-596.

Umpierrez GE, Hellman R, Korytkowski MT, et al; Endocrine Society. Management of hyperglycemia in hospitalized patients in non-critical care setting: an Endocrine Society Clinical Practice Guideline. *J Clin Endocrinol Metab.* 2012; 97(1):16-38.

Low Wang CC, Hawkins M, Gianchandani R, Dungan K. Glycemic control in the setting or parenteral nutrition or enteral nutrition via tube-feeding. In: Draznin B, ed. *Managing Diabetes and Hyperglycemia in the Hospital Setting.* American Diabetes Association; 2016.

55 ANSWER: B) U200 basal insulin degludec once daily plus mealtime insulin

The new ultralong-acting basal insulins (U100 degludec, U200 degludec, and U300 glargine) have a longer duration of action than the long-acting insulins U100 detemir and U100 glargine. An ultralong-acting basal insulin, such as U200 degludec (Answer B) which has a duration of action of up to 42 hours, would offer this patient increased dosing flexibility and reduce the likelihood of developing diabetic ketoacidosis when he misses an insulin dose. Importantly, it would be necessary to obtain preauthorization from his Medicaid plan to provide him with this new insulin analogue.

While a recently released hybrid closed-loop continuous subcutaneous insulin infusion pump with a sensor system (Answer A) would be ideal for this patient in terms of autoregulation of his insulin dosing, there are several major hurdles to this possibility from a practical perspective. These obstacles include the fact that he is homeless (access to supplies issues), he has severe mental illness that would most likely interfere with his ability to use such a pump when an exacerbation occurs, and preauthorization for payment would likely be a challenge to obtain.

A 24-hour insulin patch pump system (Answer C) that delivers a low basal insulin rate continuously over a 24-hour period with ability to activate a bolus by pressing a button for meal coverage might also be considered as an option for this patient. However, these are relatively new on the market, expensive, and usually used for treatment of type 2 diabetes. This system would also require him to have access to a new pump system every 24 hours so that insulin delivery would not be interrupted. This, of course, could be a challenge for this patient, as would episodes of exacerbation of his serious mental illness.

U500 regular human insulin (Answer D) has delayed onset and a longer duration of action than U100 regular human insulin as it has both basal and prandial properties. It may be given 2 (or 3) times daily, which would be convenient for this patient; however, its niche is for patients with insulin resistance who require high total daily doses of insulin (typically in excess of 200 units daily), which is not the case in this young man with type 1 diabetes.

EDUCATIONAL OBJECTIVE:
Appropriately prescribe the new ultralong-acting insulin analogues.

REFERENCE(S):

American Diabetes Association. Standards of care for medical management of diabetes. *Diabetes Care*. 2017;40(Suppl 1):S1-S135.

Garber AJ, Abrahamson MJ, Barzilay JI, et al. Consensus statement by the American Association of Clinical Endocrinologists and American College of Endocrinology on the comprehensive type 2 diabetes managaement algorithm – 2017 executive summary. *Endocr Pract*. 2017;23(2):207-238.

Riddle MC, Bolli GB, Home PD, et al. Efficacy and safety of flexible versus fixed dosing intervals of insulin glargine 300 U/mL in people with type 2 diabetes. *Diabetes Technol Ther*. 2016;18(4): 252-257.

Meneghini L, Atkin SL, Gough SC, et al; NN1250-3668 (BEGIN FLEX) Trial Investigators. The efficacy and safety of insulin degludec given in variable one-daily dosing intervals compared with insulin glargine and insulin degludec dosed at the same time daily: a 26-week, randomized, open-label, parallel-group, treat-to-target trial in individuals with type 2 diabetes. *Diabetes Care*. 2013;36(4):858-864.

56 ANSWER: A) Adrenal insufficiency

This patient with type 1 diabetes, primary ovarian insufficiency, and possible hypothyroidism (as evidenced by her elevated TSH) has adrenal insufficiency (Answer A), part of an autoimmune polyendocrine syndrome. It may manifest as hypoglycemia despite progressive reduction in insulin doses and orthostatic hypotension, defined as a decrease in systolic blood pressure greater than 20 mm Hg and a reflex increase in heart rate with standing. Other suggestive features of adrenal insufficiency, such as hypoglycemia and mild hyperkalemia, may not be present.

Orthostatic hypotension may also result from cardiovascular autonomic neuropathy (Answer B), but one would not expect a reflex increase in heart rate if this were present. In the setting of cardiovascular autonomic neuropathy, signs of peripheral neuropathy (Answer D) are usually also present (they are not in this case). Although this patient with longstanding type 1 diabetes mellitus may also have hypothyroidism (Answer C), it should not cause orthostatic hypotension. Because the patient's serum sodium concentration is normal, there is no evidence to suspect a salt-wasting nephropathy (Answer E).

EDUCATIONAL OBJECTIVE:
Recognize the clinical signs and symptoms suggestive of adrenal insufficiency in the setting of type 1 diabetes mellitus.

REFERENCE(S):

Barker JM. Clinical review: type 1 diabetes-associated autoimmunity: natural history, genetic associations, and screening. *J Clin Endocrinol Metab*. 2006;91(4):1210-1217.

Cutolo M. Autoimmune polyendocrine syndromes. *Autoimmun Rev*. 2014;13(2):85-89.

Pop-Busui R. Cardiac autonomic neuropathy in diabetes: a clinical perspective. *Diabetes Care*. 2010;33(2):434-441.

Vinik AI, Ziegler D. Diabetic cardiovascular autonomic neuropathy. *Circulation*. 2007;115(3): 387-397.

57

ANSWER: C) Dumping syndrome

Bariatric surgery is a potentially useful treatment for patients with type 2 diabetes mellitus and morbid obesity. Observational studies and randomized controlled trials have shown that procedures including Roux-en-Y gastric bypass, sleeve gastrectomy, gastric banding, and biliopancreatic diversion significantly improve glycemic control and favorably affect cardiovascular risk factors.

Hypoglycemia following gastric bypass surgery procedures may be complicated by early or late hypoglycemia, and it may occur in patients with or without diabetes. Hyperinsulinemic (or reactive) hypoglycemia, which is seen within an hour of eating (early dumping), is attributed to concentrated nutrients and carbohydrates rapidly entering the small bowel. This disorder is seen early in the postoperative course. It is controlled by dietary intervention and most likely represents a different pathophysiology than late post–gastric bypass hypoglycemia. This patient had surgery several months ago, so her episode is consistent with early dumping syndrome (Answer C).

Hypoglycemia is also recognized as a late sequela of gastric bypass surgery. Patients present with hypoglycemia associated with neuroglycopenic symptoms (including confusion, syncope, and seizures). This disorder presents 2 to 4 years after surgery. The potential mechanisms are hypothesized to be nesidioblastosis (Answer A) that is most likely due to the trophic effects of gastric inhibitory polypeptide and glucagonlike peptide 1 on pancreatic islet cells, increased insulin sensitivity (Answer D), and/or increased islet functional activity (Answer B). Risk is not increased with vertical banded gastroplasty or gastric banding. The clinical syndrome is seen only in patients who have Roux-en-Y bypass procedures, and it occurs in 0.2% of patients. Treatment for late postbypass hypoglycemia involves a low-carbohydrate diet. Diazoxide, octreotide, or calcium-channel blockers may be required. If necessary, surgical treatment involves consideration of a restrictive bariatric procedure, with or without reconstitution of gastrointestinal continuity.

EDUCATIONAL OBJECTIVE:
Distinguish between early and late development of hypoglycemia after gastric bypass surgery.

REFERENCE(S):

Cui Y, Elahi D, Anderson DK. Advances in the etiology and management of hyperinsulinemic hypoglycemia after Roux-en-Y Gastric Bypass. *J Gastrointest Surg.* 2011;15(10):1879-1888.

Marsk R, Jonas E, Rasmussen F, Naslund E. Nationwide cohort study of post-gastric bypass hypoglycaemia including 5,040 patients undergoing surgery in for obesity in 1986-2006 in Sweden. *Diabetologia.* 2010;53(11):2307-2311.

Schauer PR, Bhatt DL, Kirwan JP, et al; STAMPEDE Investigators. Bariatric surgery versus intensive medical therapy for diabetes--3-year outcomes. *N Engl J Med.* 2014;370(21):2002-2013.

Schauer PR, Bhatt DL, Kirwan JP, et al; STAMPEDE Investigators. Bariatric surgery versus intensive medical therapy for diabetes - 5-year outcomes. *N Engl J Med.* 2017;376(7):641-651.

De León DD, Stanley CA. Determination of insulin for the diagnosis of hyperinsulinemic hypoglycemia. *Best Pract Res Clin Endocrinol Metab.* 2013;27(6):763-769.

58

ANSWER: B) Duration of diabetes less than 8 years

Duration of diabetes less than 8 years (Answer B) was the main predictor of achieving a favorable glycated hemoglobin level after surgery in the 2017 report of 5-year outcomes in the STAMPEDE study. This emphasizes the importance of considering early surgical intervention for maximal glycemic benefit in this population. Over the last 5 years, an increasing body of data has emerged on the benefits of bariatric surgery on glucose control in patients with type 2 diabetes.

The STAMPEDE trial (Surgical Therapy and Medications Potentially Eradicate Diabetes Efficiently) is one of the first prospective randomized controlled trials to compare traditional medical therapy for type 2 diabetes with either gastric bypass surgery or sleeve gastrectomy. These investigators defined remission as a hemoglobin A_{1c} level less than 6.0% (<42 mmol/mol) while on no glucose-lowering medications.

At the 3-year time point, 38% of patients in the surgical group still met the criteria for the primary endpoint, while only 5% of the medically treated patients had a hemoglobin A_{1c} level less than 6.0% (<42 mmol/mol) and all of these individuals were being treated with glucose-lowering medications. The number of patients who enter and remain in remission after gastric bypass surgery is higher if one uses a higher cutoff for defining remission (ie, 58% of patients having a hemoglobin A_{1c} level less than 7.0% (<53 mmol/mol) while on no medications 3 years after gastric bypass surgery). These results suggest that, indeed, bariatric surgery appears to be the best treatment we currently have for type 2 diabetes.

After 5 years, when compared with intensive medical therapy alone, the proportion of patients who achieved the primary outcome was greater among patients undergoing gastric bypass surgery (5% vs 29%; $P = .01$, unadjusted; $P = .03$, adjusted; $P = .08$, intent-to-treat) and among patients undergoing sleeve gastrectomy (5% vs 23%; $P = .03$, unadjusted; $P = .07$, adjusted; $P = .17$, intent-to-treat). Duration of diabetes (<8 years), randomization to gastric bypass, and weight loss at 1 year (not 2 years [Answer D]) were associated with achieving a glycated hemoglobin less than 6.0%.

In the STAMPEDE 5-year follow-up, beneficial effects of bariatric surgery on glycemic control were durable, even among patients with mild obesity (BMI of 27-34 kg/m^2), and led to a sustained reduction in the use of diabetes and cardiovascular medications (thus, Answer A is incorrect). While changes in quality of life after surgery are superior to the changes observed after medical therapy alone, the duration of diabetes is, as mentioned earlier, the best predictor of outcomes following bariatric surgery (thus, Answer C is incorrect).

EDUCATIONAL OBJECTIVE:
Explain predictors based on data from randomized controlled trials that predict remission of diabetes after gastric bypass surgery.

REFERENCE(S):
Schauer PR, Bhatt DL, Kirwan JP, et al; STAMPEDE Investigators. Bariatric surgery versus intensive medical therapy for diabetes - 5-year outcomes. *N Engl J Med.* 2017;376(7):641-651.
Schauer PR, Bhatt DL, Kirwan JP, et al; STAMPEDE Investigators. Bariatric surgery versus intensive medical therapy for diabetes--3-year outcomes. *N Engl J Med.* 2014;370(21):2002-2013.

Schauer PR, Kashyap SR, Wolski K, et al. Bariatric surgery versus intensive medical therapy in obese patients with diabetes. *N Engl J Med.* 2012; 366(17):1567-1576.

59 ANSWER: C) Glucagonoma syndrome
The development of type 2 diabetes mellitus, particularly in a relatively abrupt fashion, is unusual and should prompt consideration of a secondary cause. The presence of new-onset diabetes and necrotizing migratory erythema accompanied by weight loss suggests glucagonoma syndrome (Answer C), which has a mean age of presentation of 55 years. Other clinical features can include anemia, stomatitis, thromboembolism (as seen in this patient), and gastrointestinal and neuropsychiatric disturbances.

Necrolytic migratory erythema is the typical rash associated with glucagonoma syndrome, as observed in this patient. It is present in 80% of cases. It can be itchy and painful and it often affects the genital and anal region, groin, buttocks, and lower legs but any site may be involved. It is nontender with irregular borders, sometimes associated with scaling or crusting, and it progresses through an initial ring-shaped red area that blisters, erodes, then crusts over and leaves behind a brown mark.

Glucagonomas are rare neuroendocrine tumors of the pancreas (others include insulinomas, somatostatinomas, carcinoid, and nonsecreting neuroendocrine tumors). In this setting, hyperglycemia, which is typically quite severe, results predominantly through the counterregulatory effects of glucagon. In larger tumors, destruction of nearby islet cells and pancreatic insulin secretion may also have an etiologic role.

Glucagonomas are often malignant and frequently present already metastatic to the liver. If localized, surgical resection is necessary. Unless large portions of the pancreas are sacrificed, hyperglycemia typically resolves relatively rapidly postoperatively. If metastatic or residual tumor is demonstrated after surgery, somatostatin receptor agonist therapy (eg, octreotide, lanreotide) should be considered.

Other etiologies of secondary diabetes include medication-induced (eg, corticosteroids), other endocrinopathies (eg, acromegaly [Answer A]), Cushing disease [Answer D]), pancreatic diseases (eg, pancreatitis), infections (eg, cytomegalovirus), and genetic conditions (eg, Rabson-Mendenhall syndrome [Answer B]).

EDUCATIONAL OBJECTIVE:
Diagnose glucagonoma as a secondary cause of diabetes mellitus.

REFERENCE(S):

Jabbour SA. Skin manifestations of hormone-secreting tumors. *Dermatol Ther*. 2010;23(6):643-650.

Warner RR. Enteroendocrine tumors other than carcinoid: a review of clinically significant advances. *Gastroenterology*. 2005;128(6):1668-1684.

Chastain MA. The glucagonoma syndrome: a review of its features and discussion of new perspectives. *Am J Med Sci*. 2001;321(5):306-320.

Female Reproduction Board Review

Margaret E. Wierman, MD • University of Colorado

1 **ANSWER: D)** *FGFR1*

In the last 10 years, our understanding of the genetic causes of GnRH deficiency, including both anosmic and normosmic idiopathic hypogonadotropic hypogonadism, has greatly expanded. In this patient with absent sexual maturation and no sense of smell, the associated abnormalities point to a defect in the gene encoding the fibroblast growth factor receptor 1 (*FGFR1*) (Answer D) or its ligand, fibroblast growth factor 8 (*FGF8*). This patient's syndrome is inherited in autosomal dominant manner. Mutations in *FGFR1* are much more common than mutations in *KAL1* (Answer B), which also presents with anosmia. Also, because *KAL1* is located on the X chromosome, women with *KAL1* mutations are not usually symptomatic. The fibroblast growth factor system cross-talks with anosmin (product of *KAL1*) during GnRH neuron migration to target the GnRH neurons to the hypothalamus. Patients with *KAL1* or *FGFR1* mutations often have midline defects, such as cleft palate.

KISS1R (previously known as *GPR54*) (Answer A) is a G-protein–coupled receptor known as the kisspeptin receptor. Together with its ligand kisspeptin, it has been identified as an up-stream activator of GnRH secretion at the time of puberty. Very few cases of *KISS1R* mutations have been identified and affected persons do not have anosmia. However, a constitutively active *KISSR1* mutation was identified as a putative cause of precocity in a young girl, which is further evidence of the importance of this ligand/G-protein–coupled receptor system. Mutations in *NR0B1* (previously known as *DAX1*) (Answer C) result in hypogonadism and adrenal insufficiency because the protein is expressed in the pituitary and the adrenal. It is extremely rare and usually presents at birth with adrenal crisis. However, a few cases have been reported with adrenal failure occurring later in childhood, which suggests the involvement of

modifying genes. Mutations in the gene encoding leptin (*LEP*) or its receptor (*LEPR*) (Answer E) result in morbid obesity and failure to undergo puberty. Although leptin signals fat stores to the brain, it is necessary but not sufficient for pubertal development.

Despite an explosion of new research in the genetics of pubertal development, fewer than 40% of all patients with idiopathic hypogonadotropic hypogonadism have a known genetic mutation. New approaches such as exome sequencing of families and large cohorts of probands will increase the discovery of new players in the control of the reproductive axis.

EDUCATIONAL OBJECTIVE:
Differentiate among the genetic causes of hypogonadotropic hypogonadism.

REFERENCE(S):

Wierman ME, Kiseljak-Vassiliades K, Tobet S. Gonadotropin-releasing hormone (GnRH) neuronal migration: initiation, maintenance and cessation as critical steps to ensure normal reproductive function. *Front Neuroendocrinol.* 2011;32(1):43-52.

Sykiotis GP, Pitteloud N, Seminara SB, Kaiser UB, Crowley WF Jr. Deciphering genetic disease in the genomic era: the model of GnRH deficiency. *Sci Transl Med.* 2010;19(2):32rv2.

Bianco SD, Kaiser UB. The genetic and molecular basis of idiopathic hypogonadotropic hypogonadism. *Nat Rev Endocrinol.* 2009;5(10):569-576.

2 **ANSWER: C) Androgen insensitivity**

This patient is phenotypically female, with excellent breast development but an absent uterus and high LH >> FSH levels. This is the presentation of a patient with complete androgen insensitivity syndrome (testicular feminization) (Answer C).

In androgen insensitivity syndrome, an individual with a 46,XY karyotype presents with a female phenotype because testosterone is unable to activate its receptor. This is confirmed by the absence of a cervix and uterus, as the mullerian ducts are needed for development of the upper one-third of the vagina, cervix, uterus, and fallopian tubes. A testosterone level distinguishes androgen insensitivity syndrome from the even more rare congenital absence of the uterus and vagina, which would present with absent menarche but normal pubertal development because of normal ovarian function. In androgen insensitivity syndrome, pubic and axillary hair is sparse because of lack of androgen in combination with estrogen action.

Aromatization of testosterone in peripheral tissues results in high estrogen as well. Individuals with complete androgen insensitivity syndrome can usually function as phenotypic females, although they are unable to bear children. The testes are often located in the groin and should be removed after puberty because of the potential for tumor formation (2%-5%). At that time, physiologic hormone therapy or oral contraceptives can be used as estrogen replacement modalities. With more subtle defects in the androgen receptor, patients can present with genital ambiguity or even as phenotypic males with hypospadias, oligospermia, undervirilization, and infertility.

In females, Fragile X syndrome (Answer A) presents with premature menopause, with earlier loss of ovarian function in each successive generation. Gonadal dysgenesis (Answer B) (or Turner syndrome) is associated with high FSH and LH, low estradiol, and failure of pubertal development. 5α-Reductase deficiency (Answer D) is an autosomal recessive disorder in which XY males present with ambiguous genitalia and virilize to a more male phenotype at puberty.

EDUCATIONAL OBJECTIVE:
Outline the manifestations and diagnosis of patients with androgen insensitivity syndrome.

REFERENCE(S):

Souhail R, Amine S, Nadia A, et al. Complete androgen insensitivity syndrome or testicular feminization: review of literature based on a case report. *Pan Afr Med J.* 2016;25:199.

Lucas-Herald A, Bertelloni S, Juul A, et al. The long-term outcome of boys with partial androgen insensitivity syndrome and a mutation in the androgen receptor gene. *J Clin Endocrinol Metab.* 2016;101(11):3959-3967.

Hughes IA, Davies JD, Bunch TI, Pasterski V, Mastroyannopoulou K, MacDougall J. Androgen insensitivity syndrome. *Lancet.* 2012;380(9851): 1419-1428.

Tadokoro-Cuccaro R, Hughes IA. Androgen insensitivity syndrome. *Curr Opin Endocrinol Diabetes Obes.* 2014;21(6):499-503.

3 ANSWER: D) Nonclassic congenital adrenal hyperplasia

Congenital adrenal hyperplasia (CAH) (Answer D) is a rare cause of hyperandrogenic anovulation in adolescence (hirsutism with irregular menses). The incidence varies from 1 to 10 per 20,000 live births. Nonclassic CAH is more common in those of Italian, Hispanic, Ashkenazi Jewish, and Eskimo descent. In women with nonclassic CAH, basal morning serum 17-hydroxyprogesterone concentrations (during the follicular phase of the menstrual cycle) are usually greater than 200 ng/dL (>6.1 nmol/L) (high-normal or high). The diagnosis of 21α-hydroxylase deficiency is confirmed by documenting stimulated levels of 17-hydroxyprogesterone greater than 1000 to 1500 ng/dL (30.3 to 45.5 nmol/L) 30 minutes after ACTH stimulation. Treatment of nonclassic CAH consists of a combination oral contraceptive with a less androgenic progestin and an androgen-receptor blocker (spironolactone) to treat the hirsutism until pregnancy is desired. Glucocorticoids are sometimes needed for induction of ovulation to suppress circulating progesterone to allow optimal folliculogenesis and LH surge.

A patient with polycystic ovary syndrome (Answer A) could present with a scenario similar to that of this patient, but not with an elevated 17-hydroxyprogesterone value. Thus, the presented scenario is more consistent with nonclassic CAH. A virilizing adrenal tumor (Answer B) would present with a very high DHEA-S level (>800 µg/dL [>21.7 µmol/L]) or rarely a very high testosterone level. A patient with adrenal Cushing syndrome (Answer C) would present with low levels of DHEA-S and ACTH. One would perform a dexamethasone suppression test to confirm the diagnosis. Ovarian tumors (Answer E) may make a combination of ovarian androgens, but affected patients usually have a testosterone level in the male range and would not have just an elevated 17-hydroxyprogesterone level.

EDUCATIONAL OBJECTIVE:
Diagnose nonclassic congenital adrenal hyperplasia and evaluate a patient with hyperandrogenic anovulation.

REFERENCE(S):

Bachelot A, Grouthier V, Courtillot C, Dulon J, Touraine P. Management of endocrine disease: congenital adrenal hyperplasia due to 21-hyroxlase deficiency: update on the management of adult patients and prenatal treatment. *Eur J Endocrinol*. 2017;176(4):R167-R181.

Falhammar H, Nordenstrom A. Nonclassic congenital adrenal hyperplasia due to 21-hydroxylase deficiency: clinical presentation, diagnosis, treatment, and outcome. *Endocrine*. 2015;50(1): 32-50.

Krone N, Rose IT, Willis DS, et al; United Kingdom Congenital Adrenal Hyperplasia Adult Study Executive (CaHASE). Genotype-phenotype correlation in 153 adult patients with congenital adrenal hyperplasia due to 21-hydroxylase deficiency: analysis of the United Kingdom Congenital Adrenal Hyperplasia Adult Study Executive (CaHASE) cohort. *J Clin Endocrinol Metab*. 2013;98(2):E346-E354.

Speiser PW, Azziz R, Baskin LS, et al; Endocrine Society. Congenital adrenal hyperplasia due to steroid 21-hydroxylase deficiency: an Endocrine Society clinical practice guideline [published correction appears in *J Clin Endocrinol Metab*. 2010;95(11):5137]. *J Clin Endocrinol Metab*. 2010;95(9):4133-4160.

4 ANSWER: C) Cardiac MRI

Recent guidelines have reviewed the treatment options for and complications of pregnancy in women with Turner syndrome (or gonadal dysgenesis). The most common risk related to body size, metabolic issues, and hypertension is an increased risk of preeclampsia. However, rare but life-threatening risks include stroke and, very rarely, a ruptured aorta. Thus, all women with gonadal dysgenesis considering ovulation induction and in vitro fertilization with a donor embryo must have had a recent cardiac MRI (Answer C) to exclude a dilated aorta or other congenital heart disease.

There are no abnormal brain findings in patients with gonadal dysgenesis, so brain MRI (Answer A) is incorrect. Duplication of the renal collecting system assessed by renal ultrasonography (Answer B) is useful to know, but it is not the most important screening test. Patients with Turner syndrome have been reported to have coronary disease later in life, but an exercise stress test (Answer D) in a young woman with gonadal dysgenesis is not indicated.

Turner syndrome occurs in 1 in 2500 live births and is associated with growth failure, pubertal delay, and cardiac abnormalities. Current recommendations include cardiac MRI or echocardiography for all girls with Turner syndrome to assess for congenital cardiovascular abnormalities (present in 50%), and this is the most important test to perform next in this patient. Congenital cardiac abnormalities associated with Turner syndrome include coarctation of the aorta, bicuspid aortic valve, and partial anomalous pulmonary venous return. MRI follow-up is recommended every 5 to 10 years in adulthood to assess for aortic dissection (0.65% to 1.4%), which is predicted by aortic dilation. Women with Turner syndrome have an increased standardized mortality ratio of 3.5 for coronary disease (presumably due to lack of estrogen therapy in the past, metabolic phenotype, obesity, hypertension.

Patients with Turner syndrome are at increased risk for several other morbidities. Diabetes risk is increased in women with Turner syndrome (related to their short stature and obesity), and hemoglobin A_{1c} measurement or glucose tolerance testing can be used for screening. Mosaicism is present in 10% of patients with Turner syndrome, and 5% may have Y chromosomal material. In these cases, ultrasonography is needed to assess for the risk of gonadoblastoma (5% to 30%). Women with Turner syndrome have an increased risk of autoimmune thyroid disease and appropriate screening would be TSH and thyroid antibody assessment.

In most cases, Turner syndrome is diagnosed when girls present with short stature and/or pubertal delay. Although girls with Turner syndrome are not strictly GH deficient, GH can be used before sex steroids to improve predicted adult stature. In this syndrome, short stature is due to the loss of the short stature homeobox gene (*SHOX*), which also contributes to the cubitus valgus and short fourth metacarpals. Induction of puberty should be accomplished with low-dosage estradiol that is subsequently increased to mimic normal puberty to induce breast development. Progestin is added last to differentiate the ductules of the breast. Oral contraceptives or continuous estrogen and progestin are not used initially because the progestin may inhibit breast development. Some suggest that low-dosage hormone therapy similar to that used in menopause may be preferable to oral contraceptives long term because of the cardiovascular and metabolic risks in these patients.

EDUCATIONAL OBJECTIVE:
Recommend prescreening tests before considering pregnancy in women with gonadal dysgenesis.

REFERENCE(S):

Pinsker JE. Clinical review: Turner syndrome: updating the paradigm of clinical care. *J Clin Endocrinol Metab.* 2012;97(6):994-1003.

Conway GS, Band M, Doyle J, Davies MC. How do you monitor the patient with Turner's syndrome in adulthood? *Clin Endocrinol (Oxf).* 2010;73(6): 696-699.

Davenport ML. Approach to the patient with Turner syndrome. *J Clin Endocrinol Metab.* 2010;95(4): 1487-1495.

Ross JL, Quigley CA, Cao D, et al. Growth hormone plus childhood low-dose estrogen in Turner's syndrome. *N Engl J Med.* 2011;364(13):1230-1242.

5 ANSWER: A) Oral contraceptive containing norethindrone

Contraception in women with polycystic ovary syndrome should be targeted not only to protect from unplanned pregnancy, but also to control the metabolic and hyperandrogenic phenotype. An oral contraceptive with a less androgenic progestin such as norethindrone (Answer A) is preferred to suppress ovarian and adrenal androgens and to ensure shedding of the endometrial lining. An intrauterine device is a consideration, but the levonorgestrel-releasing intrauterine device (Answer B) has an androgenic progestin and will not help,

and may worsen, the hyperandrogenism. In addition, the third-generation progestins (desogestrel and norgestimate) and drospirenone (Answer C), a spironolactone-like progestin that gained popularity for treatment of hirsutism, have recently lost favor because of increased risk of deep venous thrombosis. Depo-medroxyprogesterone (Answer D) is an effective contraceptive, but it often causes weight gain and would not be indicated in a patient with polycystic ovary syndrome. The vaginal ring contains ethinyl estradiol (15 mcg) and etonogestrel (120 mcg) (Answer E), while the contraceptive hormonal patch contains ethinyl estradiol (20 mcg) and norelgestromin (150 mcg). Neither has been well studied in the treatment of hirsutism and both are associated with an increased risk of deep venous thrombosis compared with oral contraceptives.

EDUCATIONAL OBJECTIVE:
Differentiate among contraceptive options for women with polycystic ovary syndrome.

REFERENCE(S):

Gialeraki A, Valsami S, Pittaras T, Panayiotakopoulos G, Politou M. Oral contraceptives and HRT risk of thrombosis. *Clin Appl Thormb Hemost.* 2016 [Epub ahead of print]

Legro RS, Pauli JG, Kunselman AR, et al. Effects of continuous versus cyclical oral contraception: a randomized controlled trial. *J Clin Endocrinol Metab.* 2008;93(2):420-429.

Legro RS, Arslanian SA, Ehrmann DA, et al; Endocrine Society. Diagnosis and treatment of polycystic ovary syndrome: an Endocrine Society Clinical Practice Guideline. *J Clin Endocriol Metab.* 2013;98(12):4565-4592.

6 ANSWER: D) Sertoli-Leydig–cell tumor of the ovary

Premenopausal hirsutism or virilization is most commonly associated with obesity or hyperthecosis. However, the rapid onset and severity of the symptoms and signs in this patient raise the concern of an ovarian tumor (usually Sertoli-Leydig–cell tumor [Answer D], arrhenoblastoma, or hilus-cell tumor) that is secreting testosterone and causing virilization. A granulosa-cell tumor of the ovary (Answer A) would present with high estrogens and endometrial hyperplasia but without virilization. An adrenal virilizing tumor (Answer C) would usually present with high DHEA-S, but rarely can secrete testosterone. However, they are very rare. Exposure to exogenous androgens (Answer B) might also be in the differential diagnosis because many men now use testosterone gel. Testosterone therapy for women is not approved for hypoactive sexual desire disorder in the United States. If it were administered, a physiologic—not pharmacologic—level would be the goal. In addition, exposure to exogenous supraphysiologic testosterone administration would result in suppressed, usually undetectable FSH and LH levels.

EDUCATIONAL OBJECTIVE:
Evaluate premenopausal hyperandrogenism.

REFERENCE(S):

Sherf S, Martinez D. Leydig cell tumor in the post-menopausal woman: case report and literature review. *Acta Biomed*. 2017;87(3): 310-313.

Alpañés M, González-Casbas JM, Sánchez J, Pián H, Escobar-Morreale HF. Management of postmenopausal virilization. *J Clin Endocrinol Metab*. 2012;97(8):2584-2588.

Vollaard ES1, van Beek AP, Verburg FA, Roos A, Land JA. Gonadotropin-releasing hormone agonist treatment in postmenopausal women with hyperandrogenism of ovarian origin. *J Clin Endocrinol Metab*. 2011;96(5):1197-1201.

Rothman MS, Wierman ME. How should postmenopausal androgen excess be evaluated? *Clin Endocrinol (Oxf)*. 2011;75(2):160-164.

7 ANSWER: A) Spironolactone and ethinyl estradiol, 30 mcg, with norethindrone, 0.5 mg
Hirsutism in women is defined as excessive terminal hair growth in a male pattern. With the Ferriman-Gallwey scoring method, a score of 8 or higher is indicative of hirsutism in white women. The Endocrine Society Clinical Practice Guidelines on the Evaluation and Treatment of Hirsutism in Premenopausal Women recommend screening androgen levels in women with moderate or severe hirsutism or any hirsutism associated with irregular menses or infertility, central obesity, acanthosis nigricans, rapid onset or progression, or clitoromegaly. Testosterone levels do not always correlate with the severity of the hirsutism. About 50% of patients with hirsutism have no other issues, and in these cases the hirsutism is deemed familial, ethnic, or idiopathic. When associated with other symptoms and signs, evaluation for polycystic ovary syndrome, Cushing syndrome, congenital adrenal hyperplasia, hyperprolactinemia, and, rarely, ovarian or adrenal tumors is appropriate.

Treatment of excessive hair growth can be accomplished with local measures such as shaving, waxing, depilatories, photoepilation, etc. The antiandrogen spironolactone is useful as a treatment in dosages of 50 to 100 mg daily, often as an adjunct to an oral contraceptive with a less androgenic progestin such as ethinyl estradiol with norethindrone (thus, Answer A is correct). Spironolactone alone is not recommended in premenopausal women because it can cause irregular menses and has the theoretical risk of inducing ambiguous genitalia in a male fetus if taken during early pregnancy. The Endocrine Society Clinical Practice Guidelines on the Evaluation and Treatment of Hirsutism in Premenopausal Women recommend that the first-line pharmacologic therapy be an oral contraceptive with a less androgenic progestin (ie, norethindrone or drospirenone, not norgestrel or levonorgestrel). Use of the oral contraceptive pill of ethinyl estradiol, 20 mcg, with levonorgestrel, 1 mg, (Answer C) is incorrect because it consists of a low ethinyl estradiol dose with an androgenic progestin that is more often used in perimenopausal women. Oral contraceptives reduce hirsutism via several mechanisms, including suppression of gonadotropins (the stimulus to ovarian androgen production); increase in sex hormone–binding globulin, which decreases free testosterone levels; and some suppression of adrenal androgens. In addition, they optimize menstrual cycle regularity and flow and provide contraception. Flutamide is a pure antiandrogen with effectiveness similar to that of spironolactone but it is more costly than spironolactone and has a risk of hepatic toxicity. Combination with a more androgenic oral contraceptive (Answer B) would not be recommended. Topical antiandrogen and ethinyl estradiol, 30 mcg, with norethindrone, 0.5 mg, (Answer D) would have some effect, but the topical antiandrogens have very limited effectiveness in this setting and thus are not recommended.

EDUCATIONAL OBJECTIVE:
Recommend therapy for hirsutism.

REFERENCE(S):

Van Zuuren EJ, Fedorowicz Z. Interventions for hirsutism excluding laser and photoepilation therapy alone: abridged Cochrane systematic review including GRADE assessments. *Br J Dermatol.* 2016;175(1):45-61.

Martin KA, Chang RJ, Ehrmann DA, et al. Evaluation and treatment of hirsutism in pre-menopausal women: an Endocrine Society clinical practice guideline. *J Clin Endocrinol Metab.* 2008;93(4):1105-1120.

Hagag P, Steinschneider M, Weiss M. Role of the combination spironolactone-norgestimate- estrogen in hirsute women with polycystic ovary syndrome. *J Reprod Med.* 2014;59(9-10):455- 463.

8   ANSWER: B) Letrozole

Women with polycystic ovary syndrome can have intermittent ovulation or anovulation, hyper-androgenism, and insulin resistance. Before planning for fertility, lifestyle should be optimized with diet and exercise. Weight loss can decrease androgen levels, but lifestyle intervention is difficult to use alone to control all the manifestations of polycystic ovary syndrome. Oral contraceptives with a less androgenic progestin, rather than an intrauterine device with a more androgenic progestin, are preferred to suppress androgens effectively (both testosterone and DHEA-S), improve hirsutism and acne, regulate menstrual cycles, and prevent endometrial hyperplasia before planned pregnancies. Addition of metformin as an insulin sensitizer can also help regulate cycles and suppress androgens, and it may make lifestyle intervention more effective. In an effort to prevent gestational diabetes in those at risk and to improve insulin sensitivity, the initial use of lifestyle intervention and metformin before attempting pregnancy is a rational option. An exercise program is important, but weight loss, suppression of androgens, and improvement of insulin sensitivity by other means are usually necessary.

Historically, if fertility was desired, clomiphene citrate (Answer A) (50-150 mg on cycle days 5 through 9) was prescribed to induce ovulation. Clomiphene citrate is more effective than metformin therapy (Answer D) to achieve live births. In addition, results from recent meta- analyses suggest that combination therapy with clomiphene and metformin may be more useful to increase live births. Although clomiphene citrate is a potential approach to induce ovulation, the recent Reproductive Network trial comparing the second-generation aromatase inhibitor letrozole with clomiphene citrate demonstrated a convincingly higher rate of ovulation induction and live births with letrozole, especially in obese women with polycystic ovary syndrome (thus, Answer B is correct). On the basis of this landmark study and multiple other smaller studies with the more potent second-generation aromatase inhibitor, this approach is being rapidly adopted in most centers. An initial concern about an increase in congenital abnormalities (4 vs 1 NS) in this large study has not been detected in follow-up studies.

Spironolactone (Answer C) is an androgen receptor blocker used to treat hirsutism in polycystic ovary syndrome. It should be stopped 3 months before planning conception because of the theoretical risk of ambiguous genitalia in a male fetus due to blocking of dihydrotestosterone action in early gestation. Progesterone suppositories (Answer E) are sometimes prescribed for women with hypothalamic amenorrhea and inadequate luteal phase—not for women with polycystic ovary syndrome. They improve menstrual cyclicity, but they have not been shown to increase rates of ovulation induction.

EDUCATIONAL OBJECTIVE:
Compare treatment effectiveness of clomiphene citrate with that of aromatase inhibitors for ovulation induction in women with polycystic ovary syndrome who would like to become pregnant.

REFERENCE(S):

Palomba S. Aromatase inhibitors for ovulation induction. *J Clin Endocrinol Metab.* 2015;100(5): 1742-1747.

Legro RS, Brzyski RG, Diamond MP, et al; NICHD Reproductive Medicine Network. Letrozole versus clomiphene for infertility in the polycystic ovary syndrome [published correction appears in *N Engl J Med.* 2014;317(15):1465]. *N Engl J Med.* 2014;371(2):119-129.

Franik S, Kremer JA, Nelen WL, Farquhar C, Marjoribanks J. Aromatase inhibitors for subfertile women with polycystic ovary syndrome: summary of a Cochrane review. *Fertil Steril.* 2015;103(2):353-355.

Fauser BC, Tarlatzis BC, Rebar RW, et al. Consensus on women's health aspects of polycystic ovary syndrome (PCOS): the Amsterdam ESHRE/ASRM-Sponsored 3rd PCOS Consensus Workshop Group. *Fertil Steril.* 2012;97(1):28-38.

Azziz R, Carmina E, Dewailly D, et al; Androgen Excess Society. Positions statement: criteria for defining polycystic ovary syndrome as a predominantly hyperandrogenic syndrome: an Androgen Excess Society guideline. *J Clin Endocrinol Metab.* 2006;91(11):4237-4245.

Legro RS, Arslanian SA, Ehrmann DA, et al; Endocrine Society. Diagnosis and treatment of polycystic ovary syndrome: An Endocrine Society Clinical Practice Guideline. *J Clin Endocriol Metab.* 2013;98(12):4565-4592.

9 ANSWER: A) Obstructive sleep apnea

Polycystic ovary syndrome is a common disorder that occurs in 6% to 8% of women. Affected patients usually present with hirsutism, acne, and irregular menses. Sixty percent of affected women become obese. Occasionally, girls with polycystic ovary syndrome can exercise and implement lifestyle interventions to mask the symptoms of the disorder and actually induce a picture of hypothalamic amenorrhea. Their polycystic ovary syndrome phenotype then manifests when their diet, lifestyle, or exercise regimen is modified or they stop therapy with oral contraceptives.

Two major definitions have been used to define polycystic ovary syndrome:

1. National Institutes of Health criteria, which include oligoovulation and clinical and/or biochemical hyperandrogenism after excluding congenital adrenal hyperplasia, hyperprolactinemia, Cushing syndrome, and other disorders.

2. Revised Rotterdam criteria, which suggest that a woman must have 2 of the following 3 findings: hyperandrogenism, oligo-ovulation or anovulation, and ultrasonography findings of polycystic ovary syndrome morphology (ie, at least 12 small cysts around the periphery of the ovary or enlarged ovarian volume).

This patient has not had ultrasonography, but she fits the criteria with hirsutism and anovulation. At least 20% of women have polycystic ovary syndrome morphology on ultrasonography, so it should not be a major criterion for making the diagnosis.

Recently, investigators have emphasized the increased risk of obstructive sleep apnea (Answer A) in women with polycystic ovary syndrome. The risk is worse with concomitant obesity, but it is also increased when compared with BMI-matched control women. Treatment of obstructive sleep apnea may improve some of the symptoms and metabolic components of the disorder as women age.

Women with polycystic ovary syndrome are at risk for impaired glucose tolerance and type 2 diabetes mellitus with a risk 5 to 10 times that of age-matched control women. In women with polycystic ovary syndrome, the prevalence of impaired glucose tolerance is 30% to 35% and the prevalence of type 2 diabetes mellitus is 3% to 10%. The risk of prediabetes and diabetes is higher in those women who are obese. For example, in normal-weight women with polycystic ovary syndrome, the risk is 10% to 15% for impaired glucose tolerance and 1% to 2% for diabetes. But, taken together, all women with polycystic ovary syndrome have an increased risk compared with that of age-matched and weight-matched control women. Metabolic complications are more common when there is a family history of type 2 diabetes mellitus. The recent Endocrine Society guidelines recommend use of a 75-g oral glucose tolerance test to screen for impaired glucose intolerance in women with polycystic ovary syndrome because of increased sensitivity, but state that hemoglobin A_{1c} measurement may be more practical and cost effective.

Despite an increase in metabolic syndrome and cardiac risk factors, studies have not yet shown an increased risk of cardiovascular disease (ie, myocardial infarction [Answer C] or stroke [Answer B]) in women with polycystic ovary syndrome. Studies have suggested that women with polycystic ovary syndrome are at risk for endometrial hyperplasia and endometrial cancer at an earlier age. In addition, women with polycystic ovary syndrome have a higher risk of nonalcoholic fatty liver disease, but it is unclear whether any treatment strategies alter this risk. Autoimmune thyroid disease (Answer D) is not increased in polycystic ovary syndrome. If a patient undergoes ovulation induction with anti-estrogens (clomiphene or letrozole) or gonadotropins, she will have an increased risk of multiple gestations. Pregnancy complications in women with polycystic ovary syndrome include gestational diabetes mellitus, preterm delivery, and preeclampsia.

EDUCATIONAL OBJECTIVE:
Identify increased risks associated with polycystic ovary syndrome.

REFERENCE(S):

McCartney CR, Marshall JC. Clinical Practice. Polycystic ovary syndrome. *N Engl J Med*. 2016; 375(1):54-64.

Legro RS, Arslanian SA, Ehrmann DA, et al; Endocrine Society. Diagnosis and treatment of polycystic ovary syndrome: an Endocrine Society Clinical Practice Guideline. *J Clin Endocrinol Metab*. 2013;98(12):4565-4592.

Ehrmann DA. Metabolic dysfunction in pcos: relationship to obstructive sleep apnea. *Steroids*. 2012;77(4):290-294.

Tasali E, Chapotot F, Leproult R, Whitmore H, Ehrmann DA. Treatment of obstructive sleep apnea improves cardiometabolic function in young obese women with polycystic ovary syndrome. *J Clin Endocrinol Metab*. 2011;96(2): 365-374.

Ramezani-Binabaj M, Motalebi M, Karimi-Sari H, Rezaee-Zavareh MS, Alavian SM. Are women with polycystic ovarian syndrome at a high risk of non-alcoholic fatty liver disease; a meta-analysis. *Hepat Mon*. 2014;14(11):e23235.

10 **ANSWER: A) Oral contraceptive containing progestin only**

An oral contraceptive containing progestin only (Answer A) is often used in the postpartum period to avoid any negative effects on the ability to continue breastfeeding. An oral contraceptive containing ethinyl estradiol, 20 mcg, and levonorgestrel, 1 mg, (Answer C) is a low-dose oral contraceptive, but the estrogen component may inhibit breast milk production. A levonorgestrel-containing intrauterine device (Answer B) would be effective contraception, but it can worsen acne and hirsutism and would therefore not be the first choice. The postpartum period is one of increased risk for deep venous thrombosis and pulmonary embolism. Transdermal patch contraceptives (Answer D) have been associated with an increased risk of clotting and thus would not be the best contraceptive option in this patient now.

EDUCATIONAL OBJECTIVE:
Recommend the optimal birth control method in the postpartum period depending on the individual issues in each patient.

REFERENCE(S):

Pieh Holder KL. Contraception and breastfeeding. *Clin Obstet Gynecol*. 2015;58(4):928-935.

Roach RE, Helmerhorst FM, Lijfering WM, Stijnen T, Algra A, Dekkers OM. Combined oral contraceptives: the risk of myocardial infarction and ischemic stroke. *Cochrane Database Syst Rev*. 2015;8:CD011054.

Evans G, Sutton EL. Oral contraception. *Med Clin North Am*. 2015;99(3):479-503.

11 **ANSWER: A) Levonorgestrel, 3.0 mg**

Emergency contraception is used to prevent unintended pregnancy after unprotected intercourse and is endorsed by the World Health Organization and the American Congress of Obstetricians and Gynecologists. Most physicians have limited knowledge or understanding of the options and efficacy of currently available alternatives. Insertion of a copper intrauterine device is the most effective method with a pregnancy rate of less than 0.1%. However, because of cost and availability, this is not an option for many women. Levonorgestrel is usually prescribed at a dose of 1.5 mg. However, this would not be enough post LH surge (she is on day 17 in her cycle) or in an obese woman, so 3.0 mg would be recommended (Answer A). Oral emergency contraception is less effective in obese women, especially levonorgestrel-based methods, with increased failure rates 1.5 times higher than in women with a BMI less than 25 kg/m^2. Some advocate a double dose of levonorgestrel for obese women.

Ulipristal acetate (Answer B) is a progesterone receptor modulator dosed at 30 mg, and it is the most effective oral emergency contraceptive pill, which acts by delaying ovulation. However, she is postovulatory. The Yuzpe regimen, which consists of 2 doses of 100 mcg of ethinyl estradiol and 1.0 mg of levonorgestrel, is the least effective method with nausea as an adverse effect. Low-dose mifepristone (10-25 mg) would be effective, but it is only available in China, Russia, and Vietnam.

EDUCATIONAL OBJECTIVE:
Explain the options and effectiveness of emergency contraception medications.

REFERENCE(S):
Fok WK, Blumenthal PD. An update on emergency contraception. *Curr Opin Obstet Gynecol.* 2016;28(6):522-529.

Chau VM, Stamm CA, Borgelt L, et al. Barriers to single-dose levonorgestrel-only emergency contraception access in retail pharmacies. *Womens Health Issues.* 2017;pii: S1049-3867(16)30304-8.

12 ANSWER: C) Normal FSH, normal LH, normal estradiol, and no response to progestin withdrawal

In the evaluation of amenorrhea, one considers whether the problem is due to a hormonal or mechanical problem, then assesses the locus of the defect. This young woman had normal menarche and was able to conceive. She has no signs of hyperandrogenism. The most likely cause of her amenorrhea is Asherman syndrome, which would be associated with normal levels of FSH, LH, and estradiol but no withdrawal menses in response to progestin (Answer C). This is a mechanical form of amenorrhea related to vigorous curettage of the endometrial lining after a miscarriage or with endometrial ablation. Premature ovarian insufficiency (Answer B) would be associated with high FSH and LH and low estradiol, but in that scenario, she should have hot flashes and signs of estrogen deficiency.

Hyperprolactinemia due to mild thyroid dysfunction, medications, or tumors can turn off the GnRH pulse generator and present as amenorrhea. In these situations, FSH, LH, and estradiol would be low and there would be no response to progestin withdrawal (Answer A), but the vignette has no history to suggest these issues. A normal hypothalamic-pituitary axis would demonstrate normal laboratory values and response to progestin (Answer D), but this history was not observed in this amenorrheic woman. Women with polycystic ovary syndrome would have higher LH and FSH, normal estradiol, and normal response to progestin withdrawal (Answer E). They usually have oligoanovulation and irregular menses and would have signs of hyperandrogenism.

EDUCATIONAL OBJECTIVE:
Determine the most likely set of hormone patterns in a woman with Asherman syndrome.

REFERENCE(S):
Zupi E, Centini G, Lazzeri L. Asherman syndrome: an unsolved clinical definition and management. *Fertil Steril.* 2015;104(6):1380-1381.

Lemmers M, Verschoor MA, Hooker AB, et al. Dilatation and curettage increases the risk of subsequent preterm birth: a systematic review and meta-analysis. *Hum Reprod.* 2016;31(1): 34-45.

13 ANSWER: D) Premature ovarian insufficiency

Antimullerian hormone (AMH) is a marker of ovarian reserve and follicular number. Infertility specialists have used it extensively in clinical practice to evaluate older women with borderline elevated FSH levels to predict response to in vitro fertilization and to diagnose premature ovarian insufficiency. A woman with polycystic ovary syndrome (Answer A) would have a high AMH level and a lower FSH level. AMH levels are lower in women with impending premature ovarian insufficiency (with higher FSH levels) (Answer D). Importantly, women with hypothalamic amenorrhea (Answer C) also have a low AMH level but a low-normal FSH level. Autoimmune adrenal insufficiency (Answer B) would not be directly associated with a high FSH level or a low AMH level. AMH assays to date are not optimally standardized, and although levels correlate with ultimate time to menopause in population studies, some obstetricians use AMH as an index of follicle number to predict response to in vitro fertilization. However, it is important to remember that women with hypothalamic amenorrhea have low AMH and low FSH levels, while women with polycystic ovary syndrome have low FSH and high AMH levels. To date, it is unclear whether AMH measurement offers more discriminatory data in an individual patient relative to menopause than FSH and estradiol with other clinical features. The literature is mixed on the usefulness of its measurement in routine practice.

EDUCATIONAL OBJECTIVE:
Describe the utility of measuring antimullerian hormone in women with amenorrhea.

REFERENCE(S):

Silva CA, Yamakami LY, Aikawa NE, Araujo DB, Carvalho JF, Bonfá E. Autoimmune primary ovarian insufficiency. *Autoimmun Rev.* 2014;13(4-5):427-430.

Welt CK. Primary ovarian insufficiency: a more accurate term for premature ovarian failure. *Clin Endocrinol (Oxf).* 2008;68(4):499-509.

Meczekalski B, Czyzyk A, Kunicki M, et al. Fertility in women of late reproductive age: the role of serum anti-Müllerian hormone (AMH) levels in its assessment. *J Endocrinol Invest.* 2016;39(11):1259-1265.

La Marca A, Ferraretti AP, Palermo R, Ubaldi FM. The use of ovarian reserve markers in IVF clinical practice: a national consensus. *Gynecol Endocrinol.* 2016;32(1):1-5.

Iliodromiti S, Anderson RA, Nelson SM. Technical and performance characteristics of anti-müllerian hormone and antral follicle count as biomarkers of ovarian response. *Hum Reprod Update.* 2015;21(6):698-710.

14   ANSWER: B) Prescribe a serotonin reuptake inhibitor

Women with premenstrual syndrome experience a wide variety of cyclic and recurrent physical, emotional, behavioral, and cognitive symptoms that start in the luteal phase and diminish and stop after the onset of menses. Major symptoms include affective symptoms, such as depression, angry outbursts, irritability, and anxiety, and somatic symptoms, such as breast pain, bloating and swelling, and headache. Referral to a therapist (Answer A) may be helpful, but this has not been shown to be beneficial for this symptom complex. An antidepressant such as amitriptyline (Answer D) has been supplanted by newer targeted drugs and thus is not the best option. Controlled studies confirm that abrogation of ovulation with continuous oral contraceptives (Answer E) may help, but initiation of a selective serotonin reuptake inhibitor (Answer B) that targets mood directly is the treatment of choice. Some patients may benefit from taking the serotonin reuptake inhibitor only the week before their menses, but Answer C indicates prescription for the entire luteal phase (2 weeks each month). In addition, most women with premenstrual syndrome need medications throughout the cycle. Nonhormonal or levonorgestrel intrauterine devices have not been shown to help premenstrual syndrome. Multiple studies of supplements, including zinc and calcium, to treat premenstrual syndrome have had negative or modestly positive effects. Addition of progesterone-only medications is not effective. Some have advised low-dosage estrogens, but the long-term safety is unclear.

EDUCATIONAL OBJECTIVE:
Recommend treatment options for women with premenstrual dysphoria.

REFERENCE(S):

Schmidt PJ, Martinez PE, Nieman LK, et al. Premenstrual dysphoric disorder symptoms following ovarian suppression: triggered by change in ovarian steroid levels but not continuous stable levels. *Am J Psychiatry.* 2017 [Epub ahead of print]

Shobeiri F, Araste FE, Ebrahimi R, Jenabi E, Nazari M. Effect of calcium on premenstrual syndrome: a double-blind randomized clinical trial. *Obstet Gynecol Sci.* 2017;60(1):100-105.

Management of premenstrual syndrome: Green-top Guideline No. 48. *BJOG.* 2017;124(3):e73-e105.

Brown J, O'Brien PM, Marjoribanks J, Wyatt K. Selective serotonin reuptake inhibitors for premenstrual syndrome. *Cochrane Database Syst Rev.* 2009:CD001396.

Jarvis CI, Lynch AM, Morin AK. Management strategies for premenstrual syndrome/premenstrual dysphoric disorder. *Ann Pharmacother.* 2008;42(7):967-978.

15 **ANSWER: E) Weight gain**
New guidelines are available for hormone treatment of male transgender patients. Because hormone therapies induce physical changes that are not reversible, most experts suggest evaluation by a mental health professional to ensure there is no unstable mood disorder before hormone therapy is initiated, as well as cross-dressing full time for 6 months to deal with the psychosocial aspects of transition.

Weight gain (Answer E) is an expected adverse effect of pharmacologic androgen administration to genetic women. Myocardial infarction (Answer A) has been reported in genetic men given high-dosage anabolic steroids, but this has not been reported in female-to-male transgender patients. The risk for diabetes mellitus (Answer B) may be increased as a side effect of weight gain, but this has not been reported as an independent risk. Instead, androgen administration at pharmacologic levels in women causes increased hematocrit and risk of polycythemia, as well as increased risk of metabolic syndrome with increased BMI. No reports of increased risk of colon and breast cancer (Answers C and D) have been documented in male transgender patients to date. However, high-dosage physiologic testosterone gel was not approved for women by the US FDA because of concerns of breast cancer in the clinical trial. Thus, further research is needed in this population of patients.

Types of hormone therapy include GnRH analogue therapy that may be administered monthly or every 3 months (depending on the formulation) to induce and maintain medical castration, followed by low-dosage hormone therapy. Although this is the safest and most physiologic approach, this regimen is quite costly and not available in many centers. An alternative approach is to use injectable depotestosterone to achieve testosterone levels in the low male reference range to prevent menses and to allow transition to a male sex assignment. However, a dosage of 200 mg every 2 weeks may not be necessary achieve goals of virilization and prevent menses. Often 100 to 150 mg intramuscularly every 3 weeks is sufficient. Risks of pharmacologic testosterone therapy include polycythemia, abnormal lipid profile, and metabolic syndrome. Long-term risks are not known because most investigations thus far have been observational studies in young persons. Often testosterone gel options do not suppress the LH surge, and amenorrhea is not achieved.

EDUCATIONAL OBJECTIVE:
Counsel male transgender patients about the potential adverse effects of hormone treatment for masculinization.

REFERENCE(S):
Gorton RN, Erickson-Schroth L. Hormonal and surgical treatment options for transgender men (female-to-male). *Psychiatr Clin North Am.* 2017;40(1):79-97.
Hembree WC, Cohen-Kettenis P, Delemarre-van de Waal HA, et al; Endocrine Society. Endocrine treatment of treatment of transsexual persons: an Endocrine Society clinical practice guideline. *J Clin Endocrinol Metab.* 2009;94(9):3132-3154.
Spack NP. Management of transgenderism. *JAMA.* 2013;309(5):478-484.
Deutsch MB, Feldman JL. Updated recommendations from the world professional association for transgender health standards of care. *Am Fam Physician.* 2013;87(2):89-93.
Fernandez J, Tannock LR. Metabolic effects of hormone therapy in transgender patients. *Endocr Pract.* 2016;22(4):383-388.

16 **ANSWER: E) Levonorgestrel-releasing intrauterine device**
Options for contraception in women after their childbearing years are evolving. Cyclic progestin (Answer A) can help regularize menses in women who are anovulatory, but it is not an optimal contraceptive choice. In women who do not smoke cigarettes and do not have risks for clotting or cardiovascular events, low-dosage oral contraceptives can be used until menopause (ethinyl estradiol, decreasing from 30-35 mcg to 20 mcg). High-dosage oral contraceptives (50 mcg ethinyl estradiol) (Answer B) would not be recommended. A nonhormonal intrauterine device (Answer C) would be an effective contraceptive, but it is associated with increased menstrual bleeding, so it is not an optimal choice in this patient who is anemic. Barrier contraception (Answer D) has a higher failure rate than the other options and would not improve the heavy menstrual flow. The levonorgestrel-releasing intrauterine

device (Answer E) is being used more frequently in women who have heavy periods because it decreases menstrual flow. Few studies have addressed the systemic effects of the androgenic progestin in the intrauterine device on lipids or blood pressure, which may be issues in some women.

EDUCATIONAL OBJECTIVE:
Explain the treatment options for contraception in women with anemia.

REFERENCE(S):
Long ME, Faubion SS, MacLaughlin KL, Pruthi S, Casey PM. Contraception and hormonal management in the perimenopause. *J Womens Health (Larchmt)*. 2015;24(1):3-10.

Kaunitz AM. Clinical practice. Hormonal contraception in women of older reproductive age. *N Engl J Med*. 2008;358(12):1262-1270.

17 **ANSWER: B)** *FMR1* **genetic testing**
Fragile X premutation screening should be performed in women with premature ovarian insufficiency, especially in women who have a family history of premature ovarian insufficiency, male relatives with learning disorders, autism, or mental retardation, or family members with ataxia and/or dementia (suggestive of Fragile X–related ataxia). The screening is accomplished by *FMR1* genetic testing (Answer B). In Fragile X carriers, CGG repeats are in the premutation range.

Karyotype analysis (Answer A) would be indicated to rule out mosaic Turner syndrome in a younger patient, but such patients usually have few cycles in adolescence and subsequent ovarian insufficiency. Antibody testing unfortunately does not predict an autoimmune cause of premature ovarian insufficiency. 21-Hydroxylase antibodies (Answer C) predict future risk of adrenal insufficiency. Ovarian antibodies as currently developed are not clinically useful and have no predictive value. Thyroid antibodies (Answer D) may be positive in patients with autoimmune thyroid disease and concomitant autoimmune premature ovarian insufficiency, but an autoimmune etiology would not explain the family history of learning disability and early menopause in relatives. There is no indication for measurement of antimullerian hormone (Answer E), which is an indicator of follicle number

and is often low in premature ovarian insufficiency and high in polycystic ovary syndrome.

EDUCATIONAL OBJECTIVE:
Explain the differential diagnosis of premature ovarian insufficiency and appropriately recommend Fragile X carrier testing.

REFERENCE(S):
Welt CK. Primary ovarian insufficiency: a more accurate term for premature ovarian failure. *Clin Endocrinol (Oxf)*. 2008;68(4):499-509.

Wang T, Bray SM, Warren ST. New perspectives on the biology of fragile X syndrome. *Curr Opin Genet Dev*. 2012;22(3):256-263.

Hoyos LR, Thakur M. Fragile X premutation in women: recognizing the health challenges beyond primary ovarian insufficiency. *J Assist Reprod Genet*. 2017;34(3):315-332.

Hipp HS, Charen KH, Spencer JB, Allen EG, Sherman SL. Reproductive and gynecologic care of women with fragile X primary ovarian insufficiency (FXPOI). *Menopause*. 2016;23(9):993-999.

18 **ANSWER: B) Gallbladder disease**
The risk of gallbladder disease (Answer B) is increased in women and was increased in both arms of the Women's Health Initiative study (WHI). In the estrogen + progestin and estrogen-only arms of the WHI, an increased the risk of stroke (Answer C) was observed but only in a small subset of patients (8 cases/10,000 women per year). Whether this is related to underlying hypercoagulable risk or to another modifier is unclear. The incidence of deep venous thrombosis (not included as a choice) was the most frequent vascular risk in both the estrogen + progestin and estrogen-only arms of the WHI and in many other studies. It is unclear whether there is a genetic risk profile that could be identified to predict this risk. Of interest, when investigators were told to advise patients hospitalized with immobility to discontinue hormone therapy, the risk of deep venous thrombosis and pulmonary embolism decreased.

Risk for colon cancer (Answer A) was decreased, not increased, in the WHI estrogen + progestin arm and neutral in the estrogen-only arm. Risk for breast cancer (Answer D) was increased in the estrogen + progestin arm, at a much lower frequency than gallstones, but not in the estrogen-only arm (*see table*).

Substudies that have examined "dementia" (Answer E) indicate that estrogen + progestin in the WHI increased the risk of cognitive impairment. Although investigators initially suggested this was Alzheimer disease, adjudication indicated that the picture was more consistent with microvascular disease progression in older women studied 4 years after intervention.

Overall, the WHI study of women aged 50 to 79 years showed that estrogen + progestin hormone therapy was associated with an increased risk of deep venous thrombosis, stroke, and cardiovascular events, but had a protective effect against colon cancer and bone fractures. A reanalysis of the data suggests that in women aged 50 to 59 years, hormone therapy has a cardioprotective effect, whereas it increases adverse events in older women. These data support the role of primary prevention, but not secondary prevention,

of cardiac risk with estrogen + progestin. Because of risk-benefit modeling, most authorities do not recommend hormone therapy for asymptomatic women. Symptomatic woman (who often have low endogenous estrogens) may benefit the most from short-term hormone therapy.

The absolute risks in the WHI were different for estrogen + progestin continuously than for estrogen therapy alone, suggesting that daily medroxyprogesterone may have contributed to some of the increased risks of cardiac disease and breast cancer in the estrogen + progestin arm. Thus, many suggest cyclic estrogen and progestin therapy for postmenopausal women who have a uterus. The WHI used conjugated estrogen (Premarin, 625 mcg) with daily medroxyprogesterone (Provera, 5 mg). Many practitioners now use lower dosages of estrogens, often in the form of an estradiol patch or gel to bypass the liver and avoid alterations in clotting proteins, although no controlled studies have investigated the risk vs benefit in a head-to-head trial. Bioidentical hormones have not been tested

---

Benefits and risks (absolute risks per 10,000 women per year, rate differences, and relative risks) of menopausal hormone therapy on chronic disease outcomes in the overall study population of women aged 50–79 years in the Women's Health Initiative (WHI) estrogen-progestin (E+P) and estrogen-alone (EA) trials.[a]

| | Estrogen-progestin trial (n = 16,608) | | | | Estrogen alone trial (n = 10,739) | | | |
| | No. of cases per 10,000 women per year | | | | No. of cases per 10,000 women per year | | | |
Outcome	E+P	Placebo	Difference (b)	RR (95% CI)[b]	EA	Placebo	Difference (b)	RR (95% CI)[b]
Benefits (in addition to menopausal symptom management)								
Hip fracture	11	17	−6	0.67 (0.47–0.95)	13	19	−6	0.67 (0.46–0.96)
Type 2 diabetes	72	88	−16	0.81 (0.70–0.94)	134	155	−21	0.86 (0.76–0.98)
Risks								
Stroke	33	24	+8	1.37 (1.07–1.76)	45	34	+11	1.35 (1.07–1.70)
Pulmonary embolism	18	9	+9	1.98 (1.36–2.87)	14	10	+4	1.35 (0.89–2.05)
Deep vein thrombosis	25	14	+11	1.87 (1.37–2.54)	23	15	+8	1.48 (1.06–2.07)
Breast cancer[c]	43	35	+8	1.24 (1.01–1.53)	28	35	−7	0.79 (0.61–1.02)
Gallbladder disease	131	84	+47	1.57 (1.36–1.80)	164	106	+58	1.55 (1.34–1.79)
Neutral or uncertain risks and benefits[d]								
Coronary heart disease[e]	41	35	+6	1.18 (0.95–1.45)	55	58	−3	0.94 (0.78–1.14)
Myocardial infarction	35	29	+6	1.24 (0.98–1.56)	44	45	−1	0.97 (0.79–1.21)
Ovarian cancer	5	4	+1	1.41 (0.75–2.66)	–	–	–	Not available
Colorectal cancer	10	17	−7	0.62 (0.43–0.89)	17	15	+2	1.15 (0.81–1.64)
Dementia (age ≥65 y)	46	23	+23	2.01 (1.19–3.42)	44	29	+15	1.47 (0.85–2.52)
Total mortality	52	53	−1	0.97 (0.81–1.16)	80	77	+3	1.03 (0.88–1.21)
Global index[d,f]	189	168	+21	1.12 (1.02–1.24)	208	204	+4	1.03 (0.93–1.13)

[a] The estrogen-progestin arm of the WHI assessed a median of 5.6 years of conjugated equine estrogens (0.625 mg/d) plus medroxyprogesterone acetate (2.5 mg/d) versus placebo. The estrogen-alone arm of the WHI assessed a median of 7.2 years of conjugated equine estrogens (0.625 mg/d) versus placebo.
[b] RR = relative risk; CI = confidence interval. Rate difference is rate in the hormone arm minus rate in the placebo arm.
[c] Divergent results for the two interventions.
[d] Also includes outcomes with divergent results for the two interventions.
[e] Coronary heart disease is defined as nonfatal myocardial infarction or coronary death.
[f] The global index is a composite outcome representing the first event for each participant from among the following: coronary heart disease, stroke, pulmonary embolism, breast cancer, colorectal cancer, endometrial cancer (E+P trial only), hip fracture, and death. Because participants can experience more than one type of event, the global index can not be derived by a simple summing of the component events.
Source of data: Manson JE, Chlebowski RT, Stefanick ML, et al.; JAMA 2013; 310:1353–68.

Manson. *Clinical recommendations. Fertil Steril* 2014.

Reprinted from Manson JE. Current recommendations: what is the clinician to do? *Fertil Steril.* 2014;101(4):916-921. Reproduced with permission of Elsevier, Inc, in the format reuse in CME Materials via Copyright Clearance Center.

in any prospective randomized controlled studies and have not undergone testing by the US FDA for bioavailability. Thus, they cannot be recommended.

EDUCATIONAL OBJECTIVE:
Identify common increased risks associated with postmenopausal hormone therapy.

REFERENCE(S):
Henderson VW, Lobo RA. Hormone therapy and the risk of stroke: perspectives 10 years after the Women's Health Initiative trials. *Climacteric*. 2012;15(3):229-234.
Gompel A, Santen RJ. Hormone therapy and breast cancer risk 10 years after the WHI. *Climacteric*. 2012;15(3):241-249.
Kreatsoulas C, Anand SS. Menopausal hormone therapy for the primary prevention of chronic conditions. U.S. Preventive Services Task Force Recommendation Statement. *Pol Arch Med Wewn*. 2013;123(3):112-117.
Marjoribanks J, Farquhar C, Roberts H, Lethaby A. Long term hormone therapy for perimenopausal and postmenopausal women. *Cochrane Database Syst Rev*. 2012;7:CD004143.

19 **ANSWER: C) The timing of her first menses, pregnancies, and last menses**
Although estrogen therapy or combined estrogen and progestin hormone therapy was once offered to many menopausal women, results of studies such as the Women's Health Initiative (WHI) have suggested that the risks outweigh the benefits in many women, especially those without symptoms. Clinical considerations include age, time since menopause, current vascular health, risk for breast cancer, and genetic and family risk profile.

In this vignette, the timing of first menses, number and timing of pregnancies, and timing of menopause (Answer C) modulate the risk for breast cancer in response to hormone therapy, with early menarche, late menopause, and nulliparity all associated with increased risk. A family history of Alzheimer disease—not Parkinson disease—would be relevant (thus, Answer A is incorrect). A family history of premenopausal—not postmenopausal—breast cancer would be important to elicit (thus, Answer B is incorrect). Neither a history of autoimmune thyroid disease (Answer D) nor

kidney stones (Answer E) is considered in the risk vs benefit assessment of hormone therapy in symptomatic postmenopausal women.

EDUCATIONAL OBJECTIVE:
Evaluate the risks and benefits of postmenopausal hormone therapy.

REFERENCE(S):
Rosano G, Vitale C, Spoletini I, Fini M. Cardiovascular health in the menopausal woman: impact of the timing of hormone replacement therapy. *Climacteric*. 2012;15(4):299-305.
Gompel A, Santen RJ. Hormone therapy and breast cancer risk 10 years after the WHI. *Climacteric*. 2012;15(3):241-249.
Kreatsoulas C, Anand SS. Menopausal hormone therapy for the primary prevention of chronic conditions. U.S. Preventive Services Task Force Recommendation Statement. *Pol Arch Med Wewn*. 2013;123(3):112-117.
Marjoribanks J, Farquhar C, Roberts H, Lethaby A, Lee J. Long-term hormone therapy for perimenopausal and postmenopausal women. *Cochrane Database Syst Rev*. 2012;7:CD004143.
Mauvais-Jarvis F, Manson JE, Stevenson JC, Fonseca VA. Menopausal hormone therapy and type 2 diabetes prevention: evidence, mechanisms and clinical implications. *Endocr Rev*. 2017;38(3): 173-188.

20 **ANSWER: B) Hyperthecosis ovarii**
Postmenopausal hirsutism to frank virilization is most commonly associated with obesity or hyperthecosis. Hyperthecosis (Answer B) occurs when high gonadotropin levels drive androgen production from the theca cells, often in menopausal women. Whether women with hyperthecosis have polycystic ovary syndrome before menopause has not been clarified.

An adrenal virilizing tumor (Answer A) would present with a rapid onset, severe symptoms and signs, and usually high DHEA-S levels. A granulosa tumor of the ovary (Answer C) would present with high estrogen levels and endometrial hyperplasia and would not cause virilization. Obesity (Answer D) can cause hirsutism—adipose tissue can have increased 5α-reductase activity, as well as local aromatase activity, which can cause androgenic and estrogenic effects. However, it does not usually result in such high testosterone levels or virilization. Weight loss and suppression of androgens are the goals with obesity-induced hyperandrogenism. Ovarian tumors that cause hyperandrogenism include Sertoli-Leydig–cell tumors (Answer E), arrhenoblastomas, or hilus-cell tumors that secrete testosterone in the male normal range (>240 ng/dL [>8.3 nmol/L]) and cause virilization. Because these tumors are rare, more common causes of postmenopausal hirsutism and virilization should be considered.

EDUCATIONAL OBJECTIVE:
Outline the differential diagnosis of hyperandrogenism in a postmenopausal woman.

REFERENCE(S):
Rothman MS, Wierman ME. How should post-menopausal androgen excess be evaluated? *Clin Endocrinol (Oxf)*. 2011;75(2):160-164.

Pugeat M, Déchaud H, Raverot V, Denuzière A, Cohen R, Boudou P; French Endocrine Society. Recommendations for investigation of hyperandrogenism. *Ann Endocrinol (Paris)*. 2010; 71(1):2-7.

21 **ANSWER: C) Deep venous thrombosis**
In the estrogen-only arm of the Women's Health Initiative (WHI) study, the incidence of deep venous thrombosis (Answer C) was increased, suggesting effects through hypercoagulation pathways in susceptible individuals. The incidence of deep venous thrombosis was increased in both arms of the study, but the incidence was decreased when providers were instructed to stop hormone therapy when patients were hospitalized or immobilized. Risks for hypercoagulability and vascular risk include age, time since menopause, levels of LDL cholesterol and other lipids, metabolic syndrome, and factor V Leiden genotype. Women given 6.8 years of estrogen therapy had a neutral risk for coronary heart disease (Answer D), a relative risk of 1.4 for stroke, and a nonsignificant increase in pulmonary emboli compared with risks observed in women given placebo. Coronary heart disease risk was dependent of age: 0.76 (confidence interval, 0.50-1.16), 1.10 (confidence interval, 0.84-1.45), and 1.28 (confidence interval,

1.03-1.58) among women who were less than 10, between 10 and 19, and greater than 20 years after menopause, respectively, which supports the timing hypothesis. Risk of ovarian cancer (Answer A) was not increased. The incidence of breast cancer (Answer B) was not significantly increased. Risk of colon cancer (Answer E) was not significantly decreased with estrogen alone, but the incidence was not increased.

| Outcome | Intervention Phase | | | |
	Estrogen-Progestin, RR (95% CI)	P value	Estrogen Alone, RR (95% CI)	P value
Coronary heart disease	1.18 (0.95-1.45)	.13	0.94 (0.78-1.14)	.53
Myocardial infarction	1.24 (0.98-1.56)	.07	0.97 (0.79-1.21)	.81
Stroke	1.37 (1.07-1.76)	.01	1.35 (1.07-1.70)	.01
Pulmonary embolism	1.98 (1.36-2.87)	<.001	1.35 (0.89-2.05)	.15
Deep vein thrombosis	1.87 (1.37-2.54)	<.001	1.48 (1.06-2.07)	.02

Adapted with permission from the American Association for Clinical Chemistry, from Bassuk SS, Manson JE. Menopausal hormone therapy and cardiovascular disease risk: utility of biomarkers and clinical factors for risk stratification. *Clin Chem*. 2014;60(1):68-77; permission conveyed through Copyright Clearance Center, Inc.

EDUCATIONAL OBJECTIVE:
Identify the benefits and risks associated with estrogen-only hormone therapy at menopause.

REFERENCE(S):
Anderson GL, Limacher M, Assaf AR, et al; Women's Health Initiative Steering Committee. Effects of conjugated equine estrogen in postmenopausal women with hysterectomy: the Women's Health Initiative randomized controlled trial. *JAMA*. 2004;291(14):1701-1712.

Rossouw JE, Anderson GL, Prentice RL, et al; Writing Group for the Women's Health Initiative Investigators. Risks and benefits of estrogen plus progestin in healthy postmenopausal women: principal results from the Women's Health Initiative randomized controlled trial. *JAMA*. 2002;288(3):321-333.

Mauvais-Jarvis F, Manson JE, Stevenson JC, Fonseca VA. Menopausal hormone therapy and type 2 diabetes prevention: evidence, mechanisms and clinical implications. *Endocr Rev*. 2017;38(3): 173-188.

Male Reproduction Board Review

Frances J. Hayes, MD • Massachusetts General Hospital

1 **ANSWER: B) hCG injections**

The 3 key elements of this case are: (1) the patient has secondary as opposed to primary hypogonadism; (2) the cause of his central defect is a pituitary rather than a hypothalamic lesion, and (3) his hypogonadism is acquired as opposed to congenital. In men with primary hypogonadism, fertility options are typically limited to assisted reproductive techniques such as intracytoplasmic sperm injection, use of donor sperm, or adoption. In contrast, men whose infertility is due to secondary hypogonadism can have spermatogenesis induced with hormonal therapy in the form of either exogenous gonadotropins (hCG +/- FSH) or GnRH. Therefore, this patient who has hypogonadotropic hypogonadism is an appropriate candidate for medical therapy, so intracytoplasmic sperm injection (Answer A) is not the best initial treatment option.

All patients with hypogonadotropic hypogonadism who are interested in fertility should first have a semen analysis. The site of the defect in the hypothalamic-pituitary gonadal axis dictates which form of medical therapy is most appropriate to stimulate spermatogenesis in a given patient. GnRH (Answer C) is administered subcutaneously through a portable infusion pump every 120 minutes and stimulates the gonadotrope cells in the anterior pituitary to stimulate LH and FSH, which in turn stimulate the testes to make testosterone and sperm. Thus, an intact pituitary gland is a prerequisite for GnRH to effectively induce spermatogenesis, so this treatment is not appropriate for a patient who has had a hypophysectomy. In contrast, gonadotropin therapy is effective in patients with both pituitary and hypothalamic disease as gonadotropins act directly on the testes.

Gonadotropin therapy to induce spermatogenesis consists of subcutaneous administration of hCG alone or in combination with FSH. hCG bears strong structural homology to LH, and acting through the LH receptor on Leydig cells it causes an increase in both intratesticular and systemic testosterone production. In men who become hypogonadal after normal puberty has been completed and thus have normal testicular size, treatment with hCG alone is adequate to stimulate spermatogenesis. In contrast, patients who have congenital hypogonadotropic hypogonadism and prepubertal testes (<4 mL) need combination therapy with both hCG and FSH to stimulate growth of the seminiferous tubules. Thus, in this patient with acquired hypogonadism and testes of 20 mL, monotherapy with hCG (Answer B) is the correct answer and combination therapy with both hCG and FSH (Answer D) is incorrect.

EDUCATIONAL OBJECTIVE:
Recommend appropriate treatment to restore fertility in a man with acquired hypogonadotropic hypogonadism.

REFERENCE(S):

Burris AS, Rodbard HW, Winters SJ, Sherins RJ. Gonadotropin therapy in men with isolated hypogonadotropic hypogonadism: the response to human chorionic gonadotropin is predicted by initial testicular size. *J Clin Endocrinal Metab.* 1988;66(6):1144-1151.

Hayes FJ, Seminara SB, Crowley WF Jr. Hypogonadotropic hypogonadism. *Endocrinol Metab Clin North Am.* 1998;27(4):739-763.

King TF, Hayes FJ. Long-term outcome of idiopathic hypogonadotropic hypogonadism. *Curr Opin Endocrinol Diabetes Obes.* 2012;19(3):204-210.

2 ANSWER: C) Change the current regimen to 200 mg every 2 weeks

Testosterone esters including enanthate and cypionate have been used for the treatment of male hypogonadism for more than 7 decades. They have the advantage of being the least expensive of the testosterone replacement modalities and of predictably restoring testosterone levels to the normal range. However, they have unfavorable pharmacokinetics characterized by significant fluctuation in serum testosterone between peak and trough values. When administered by a deep intramuscular injection, testosterone is slowly released from this oily suspension into the circulation over a period of weeks. The esters are typically injected at 2-week intervals with levels reaching peak concentrations 24 to 48 hours after the injection followed by a gradual decline to the low-normal range before the next injection is due. When the interval between injections is extended to every 3 weeks, peak concentrations tend to be supraphysiologic and testosterone levels may fall to the hypogonadal range by the time the next injection is administered. Such wide excursions in serum testosterone concentrations can, in turn, cause undesirable swings in mood, libido, and energy levels.

In the case described, the serum testosterone level midway between injections is towards the upper end of the normal range. However, the fact that the patient becomes symptomatic in the days before his injection suggests that his trough levels are low. Therefore, reducing the dose while increasing the frequency of injections from every 3 to every 2 weeks (Answer C) will help to alleviate the patient's symptoms by reducing the fluctuation in his testosterone levels. In contrast, increasing the dose and further extending the interval to every 4 weeks (Answer D) would result in even greater peaks and troughs and would likely exacerbate his symptoms further. The fact that his tiredness and moodiness are limited to the period before his injections indicates they are related to his testosterone regimen rather than endogenous depression, so prescribing an antidepressant (Answer A) is incorrect. The pharmacokinetics of testosterone cypionate are similar to those of testosterone enanthate. Hence, switching esters (Answer B) would not address his problem.

EDUCATIONAL OBJECTIVE:
Describe the pharmacokinetics of injectable testosterone esters and manage adverse effects by altering the dose and frequency of administration.

REFERENCE(S):

Bhasin S, Cunningham GR, Hayes FJ, et al; Task Force, Endocrine Society. Testosterone therapy in men with androgen deficiency syndromes: an Endocrine Society clinical practice guideline. *J Clin Endocrinol Metab*. 2010;95(6):2536-2559.

Basaria S. Male hypogonadism. *Lancet*. 2014; 383(9924):1250-1263.

Snyder PJ, Lawrence DA. Treatment of male hypogonadism with testosterone enanthate. *J Clin Endocrinol Metab*. 1980;51(6):1335-1339.

3 ANSWER: A) Low gonadotropins and low sex hormone–binding globulin

This patient has glucocorticoid-induced hypogonadism. Glucocorticoid therapy in men can decrease serum testosterone levels because of combined effects on reduced GnRH secretion, as well as a direct effect on testosterone production from the testes. There is an inverse relationship between the dosage of glucocorticoids and serum testosterone levels, but in general prednisone dosages of 7.5 mg daily or higher result in testosterone suppression. Glucocorticoid-induced suppression of gonadal hormones can occur as early as 3 days after initiating therapy. Although both primary and secondary forms of hypogonadism have been described, most studies report low or inappropriately normal gonadotropin levels in association with low serum testosterone, indicating a predominantly central process. Prednisone also lowers sex hormone–binding globulin levels, so Answer A (low gonadotropins and low sex hormone–binding globulin) is correct. Answer B is incorrect because of the high sex hormone–binding globulin level, and Answers C and D are incorrect because they depict a predominantly gonadal defect.

EDUCATIONAL OBJECTIVE:
Explain the suppressive effects of glucocorticoids on the hypothalamic-pituitary gonadal axis in men.

REFERENCE(S):

Reid IR, Ibbertson HK, France JT, Pybus J. Plasma testosterone concentrations in asthmatic men treated with glucocorticoids. *Br Med J (Clin Res Ed)*. 1985;291(6495):574.

MacAdams MR, White RH, Chipps BE. Reduction of serum testosterone levels during chronic glucocorticoid therapy. *Ann Intern Med*. 1986;104(5):648-651.

4 ANSWER: B) Klinefelter syndrome

On a statistical basis, the most common cause of congenital primary gonadal failure is Klinefelter syndrome (Answer B), which has an incidence of approximately 1 in 600. There is wide variability in the phenotypic spectrum depending largely on the degree of mosaicism. However, gynecomastia and small testes, as described in this vignette, are common presenting features. Gonadotropin concentrations are invariably elevated (FSH > LH) in men with Klinefelter syndrome (and other causes of primary hypogonadism) because of impaired negative feedback by both sex steroids and inhibin B. Most patients have testosterone values in the low normal range or just below the lower end of normal. Sex hormone–binding globulin concentrations tend to be elevated in affected men because of increased estrogen production rates. Given that 98% or more of circulating testosterone is protein bound, the free testosterone fraction tends to be disproportionately lower than the total testosterone concentration in men with Klinefelter syndrome. The diagnosis is confirmed by karyotype analysis, which shows a 47,XXY pattern in more than 80% of cases. In the case described, the karyotype showed mosaicism (47,XXY and 46,XY), which explains why his testes are larger than those of many patients with Klinefelter syndrome.

Inactivating mutations in the gene encoding the FSH receptor (Answer A) are a rare cause of primary gonadal failure. Men harboring such mutations present with small testes and elevated FSH levels such as in the case described. However, unlike the patient in this vignette, they have normal testosterone and LH levels and do not develop gynecomastia.

17α-Hydroxylase deficiency (Answer C) is a rare form of congenital adrenal hyperplasia that causes decreased production of glucocorticoids and sex steroids and increased synthesis of mineralocorticoid precursors due to loss-of-function mutations involving the *CYP17A1* gene. Males with this disorder are undervirilized. The appearance of the external genitalia ranges from normal female to ambiguous to mildly underdeveloped male genitalia. The most commonly described phenotype is a small phallus, perineal hypospadias, and intra-abdominal or inguinal testes. Most patients with this disorder are hypertensive. The fact that the patient described in this vignette has scrotal testes with a normal phallus, no hypospadias, and normal blood pressure rules out this condition.

The incidence of mumps orchitis (Answer D) has declined dramatically since the introduction of the childhood vaccination program. However, in situations where parents decide not to have their children vaccinated, outbreaks of mumps can still occur. Orchitis is the most common complication of mumps in postpubertal men, affecting about 20% to 30% of cases. Thirty to fifty percent of affected testicles show some degree of atrophy. Mumps-associated orchitis results in severe pain, swelling, and tenderness at the affected site and is often associated with high fever, nausea, vomiting, and abdominal pain. In the case described, the absence of such a history makes mumps orchitis an unlikely diagnosis.

EDUCATIONAL OBJECTIVE:
Outline the differential diagnosis of primary hypogonadism.

REFERENCE(S):

Groth KA, Skakkebæk A, Høst C, Gravholt CH, Bojesen A. Clinical review: Klinefelter syndrome--a clinical update. *J Clin Endocrinol Metab*. 2013;98(1):20-30.

Tapanainen JS, Aittomäki K, Min J, Vaskivuo T, Huhtaniemi IT. Men homozygous for an inactivating mutation of the follicle-stimulating hormone (FSH) receptor gene present variable suppression of spermatogenesis and fertility. *Nat Genet*. 1997;15(2):205-206.

Braunstein GD. Clinical practice. Gynecomastia. *N Engl J Med*. 2007;357(12):1229-1237.

5 ANSWER: D) Sperm cryopreservation before chemotherapy

After 1 year of follow-up, azoospermia is seen in 90% of men with Hodgkin lymphoma who are treated with more than 3 courses of chemotherapy that includes an alkylating agent. The most reliable option for the preservation of male fertility is cryopreservation of sperm before treatment (Answer D). Cryopreservation of human sperm does not decrease its capability for fertilization, and studies have demonstrated successful pregnancies with cryopreserved sperm. Optimal semen collection procedures for cryopreservation include obtaining at least 3 samples after abstinence for a minimum of 48 hours. However, in men with Hodgkin lymphoma, semen analysis is frequently abnormal even before treatment and only 20% to 30% of patients meet traditional criteria for sperm cryopreservation for intrauterine insemination.

Infertility related to chemotherapy is due to loss of spermatogonial stem cells, and the recovery of spermatogenesis occurs via recolonization of the seminiferous tubules by these stem cells. Currently, cryopreservation and subsequent transplant of spermatogonial stem cells (Answer C) is considered experimental. It has been hypothesized that hormonal suppression and the resulting disruption of gametogenesis (Answer B) renders the gonad less sensitive to damage by the cytotoxic drugs. However, in clinical trials, hormonal suppression with GnRH agonists has not been shown to reliably afford gonadal protection and its use has led to recovery of spermatogenesis in only 20% of patients. The combination of exogenous testosterone and a progestin (Answer A) has been used in male contraceptive trials but has not been evaluated in the setting of cytotoxic chemotherapy.

EDUCATIONAL OBJECTIVE:
Counsel men planning to undergo cytotoxic chemotherapy on the options for fertility preservation.

REFERENCE(S):
Howell SJ, Shalet SM. Spermatogenesis after cancer treatment: damage and recovery. *J Natl Cancer Inst Monogr.* 2005;34:12-17.

Jahnukainen K, Ehmcke J, Hou M, Schlatt S. Testicular function and fertility preservation in male cancer patients. *Best Pract Res Clin Endocrinol Metab.* 2011;25(2):287-302.

Levine J, Canada A, Stern CJ. Fertility preservation in adolescents and young adults with cancer. *J Clin Oncol.* 2010;28(32):4831-4841.

Redman JR, Bajorunas DR, Goldstein MC, et al. Semen cryopreservation and artificial insemination for Hodgkin's disease. *J Clin Oncol.* 1987;5(2):233-238.

6 ANSWER: C) Referral for surgical consultation

The pathophysiology of gynecomastia involves an imbalance between free estrogen and free androgen actions in the breast tissue. During mid-to-late puberty, relatively more estrogen may be produced by the testes and peripheral tissues before testosterone secretion reaches adult levels, resulting in the gynecomastia that commonly occurs during this period. Most adolescents presenting with isolated gynecomastia have physiologic pubertal gynecomastia, which generally appears at 13 or 14 years of age, lasts for 6 months or less, and then regresses. Although the diagnosis is evident in most cases, a thorough history that includes review of medications, environmental exposures, and illicit drug use and physical examination are necessary. The case described fits the diagnosis of pubertal gynecomastia, but unlike most cases, it has failed to regress and is causing significant psychological distress. Thus, while reassurance and observation (Answer B) constitute the best approach for younger patients with gynecomastia present for less than 1 year, it is not appropriate for this patient. Surgical resection (Answer C) should be considered for adolescents with physiologic gynecomastia that is greater than 4 cm in diameter, has not responded to medical therapy, persists for more than 1 year or after the patient is age 17 years, or is associated with embarrassment that interferes with normal daily activities.

This patient's examination findings do not suggest any features of malignancy such as nipple retraction, discoloration, or serosanguinous discharge. There is also no risk of malignant transformation of the breast tissue in pubertal gynecomastia. Therefore, mammography (Answer A) is not indicated. There is no medication approved by the US FDA for the treatment of pubertal gynecomastia. In general, pharmacologic approaches to gynecomastia are most effective during the phase of active proliferation and thus would not be expected to be beneficial in this patient in whom it has been present for 3 years. Even in adolescents with a short history of gynecomastia, aromatase inhibitors (Answer D) such as anastrozole have not been shown to be beneficial.

EDUCATIONAL OBJECTIVE:
Diagnose and manage pubertal gynecomastia.

REFERENCE(S):
Braunstein GD. Clinical practice. Gynecomastia. *N Engl J Med*. 2007;357(12):1229-1237.

Nordt CA, DiVasta AD. Gynecomastia in adolescents. *Curr Opin Pediatr*. 2008;20(4):375-382.

Plourde PV, Reiter EO, Jou HC, et al. Safety and efficacy of anastrozole for the treatment of pubertal gynecomastia: a randomized, double-blind, placebo-controlled trial. *J Clin Endocrinol Metab*. 2004;89(9):4428-4433.

7 **ANSWER: D) Refer him to a urologist**
The diagnosis of hypogonadism made by the patient's primary care physician is correct based on the presence of symptoms of hypogonadism in association with 2 low morning testosterone levels. The issue at hand is whether the patient is an appropriate candidate for testosterone replacement. While the patient is eager to initiate testosterone therapy in the hope of improving his symptoms, it is the physician's responsibility to ensure that he is an appropriate candidate and that the risk-to-benefit ratio favors treatment. Endocrine Society clinical practice guidelines recommend that clinicians assess prostate cancer risk in men being considered for testosterone therapy. As a general rule, it is recommended that patients who have a palpable prostate nodule or induration or prostate-specific antigen level greater than 4.0 ng/mL (>4.0 µg/L) need further urologic evaluation before testosterone therapy is initiated. However, in subgroups of men considered to be at increased risk for prostate cancer, such as African American patients or men with first-degree relatives with prostate cancer, the baseline prostate-specific antigen level at which referral to a urologist is recommended is greater than 3.0 ng/mL (>3.0 µg/L). Thus, in the case described of an African American man with 2 baseline prostate-specific antigen measurements greater than 3.0 ng/mL (>3.0 µg/L), referral to a urologist (Answer D) is the best next step in his management. Should findings from this urological workup be reassuring, one could then proceed with testosterone replacement (Answer B).

While phosphodiesterase inhibitors (Answer A) would most likely help the patient's erectile dysfunction, they would not be an appropriate choice in this case as their use is contraindicated in patients taking nitrates given the risk of severe hypotension with this drug combination.

Testosterone therapy is not recommended in patients with untreated severe obstructive sleep apnea. However, this patient's sleep apnea is being treated with continuous positive airway pressure and appears well controlled based on the absence of daytime somnolence and the fact that his hematocrit is not elevated. Therefore, arranging a sleep study (Answer C) in a patient with an established diagnosis of obstructive sleep apnea and no symptoms would not yield any additional information.

EDUCATIONAL OBJECTIVE:
List indications for urologic evaluation before initiating testosterone therapy.

REFERENCE(S):
Bhasin S, Cunningham GR, Hayes FJ, et al; Task Force, Endocrine Society. Testosterone therapy in men with androgen deficiency syndromes: an Endocrine Society clinical practice guideline. *J Clin Endocrinol Metab*. 2010;95(6):2536-2559.

Wittert G. The relationship between sleep disorders and testosterone. *Curr Opin Endocrinol Diabetes Obes*. 2014;21(3):239-243.

8 **ANSWER: A) Measure free testosterone**
This patient's clinical presentation with decreased libido, erectile dysfunction, and fatigue is highly suggestive of hypogonadism. His physical examination also reveals gynecomastia. Despite this, 2 total testosterone values, both measured by liquid chromatography tandem mass spectrometry, are in the high-normal range. In such clinical scenarios, where the clinical phenotype is incongruent

with biochemical results, clinicians should consider alterations in serum sex hormone–binding globulin (SHBG) levels as a potential explanation. Certain clinical conditions are associated with elevated serum SHBG levels. These include aging, liver disease, hyperthyroidism, medications (anticonvulsant drugs, estrogen), and HIV infection. Although the exact mechanism behind SHBG elevation in HIV remains unclear, increased inflammatory milieu in these patients has been posited as one of the mechanisms (SHBG is an acute-phase reactant). As longevity is increasing in persons with HIV, quality-of-life issues in this patient population are gaining considerable attention. Furthermore, the prevalence of hypogonadism in men with HIV is higher than in the general population; therefore, an accurate diagnosis is important.

Thus, in cases such as this where the history is suggestive of hypogonadism and a disorder known to impact SHBG levels is present, measurement of free testosterone (Answer A) is required to diagnose androgen deficiency. Reliable methods of free testosterone measurement include (1) measurement by equilibrium dialysis (considered the gold standard, but is not routinely available in commercial laboratories); and (2) calculated free testosterone (derived from total testosterone and SHBG measurements using law of mass action equations). This patient's free testosterone level (measured by equilibrium dialysis) was low at 48 pg/mL (1.7 nmol/L) because of a markedly elevated SHBG level of 20.0 µg/mL (178 nmol/L), allowing a diagnosis of hypogonadism to be confirmed.

Referring this patient for psychiatric evaluation (Answer D) without taking further diagnostic steps would be inappropriate. Men with partial androgen insensitivity syndrome resulting from mutations in the gene encoding the androgen receptor (Answer C) may also present with symptoms and signs of hypogonadism in association with an elevated serum testosterone level. However, patients with partial androgen insensitivity syndrome tend to have additional clinical manifestations, including perineoscrotal hypospadias and infertility. Importantly, gonadotropin levels in such patients are elevated due to impaired testosterone negative feedback, unlike the gonadotropin profile of patients with HIV infection who typically have secondary hypogonadism. Epitestosterone is a biologically inactive 17-epimer of testosterone that is cosecreted by the Leydig cells of the testes. The urinary testosterone-to-epitestosterone ratio (Answer B) is measured in the evaluation of men suspected of androgen abuse. However, exogenous use of testosterone by this patient would be associated with suppressed gonadotropin levels.

EDUCATIONAL OBJECTIVE:
Identify the biochemical profile of men with HIV who experience alterations in the concentration of serum sex hormone–binding globulin.

REFERENCE(S):
Shea JL, Wong PY, Chen Y. Free testosterone: clinical utility and important analytical aspects of measurement. *Adv Clin Chem*. 2014;63:59-84.

Bhasin S, Cunningham GR, Hayes FJ, et al; Task Force, Endocrine Society. Testosterone therapy in men with androgen deficiency syndromes: an Endocrine Society clinical practice guideline. *J Clin Endocrinol Metab*. 2010;95(6):2536-2559.

Moreno-Pérez O, Escoín C, Serna-Candel C, et al. The determination of total testosterone and free testosterone (RIA) are not applicable to the evaluation of gonadal function in HIV-infected males. *J Sex Med*. 2010;7(8):2873-2883.

9 ANSWER: A) Y-Chromosome microdeletion

This patient has nonobstructive azoospermia based on a normal semen volume and presence of fructose in the ejaculate. He has normal LH and testosterone levels indicating normal Leydig-cell function but has an elevated FSH level due to lack of negative feedback from undetectable inhibin B indicating a selective defect in the seminiferous tubule compartment of the testis. This presentation is most likely due to a microdeletion in the Y-chromosome (Answer A), the second most common genetic cause of male infertility after Klinefelter syndrome. The male-specific region on the long arm of the Y chromosome has a locus known as the azoospermia factor (AZF) that contains genes needed for spermatogenesis. This AZF locus contains 3 regions: AZFa, AZFb, and AZFc. Deletions of the entire AZFa region result in complete atrophy of the tubular compartment, with only Sertoli cells seen on testicular biopsy, making retrieval of sperm for intracytoplasmic sperm injection virtually impossible. Large deletions in the AZFb region also result in Sertoli-cell–only syndrome. Mutations in the AZFc region are the most common and account for 80% of Y-chromosome microdeletions. AZFc deletions are compatible with residual spermatogenesis, with oligospermia being a common presentation. These men may be candidates for intracytoplasmic sperm injection. Infertile men who do not have obstructive azoospermia, hypogonadotropic hypogonadism, or a karyotype abnormality should be tested for Y-chromosome microdeletions.

This patient does not have Klinefelter syndrome (Answer: B) given his normal karyotype. Mutations in the *KISS1R* gene (Answer: C) result in Kallmann syndrome, a condition characterized by isolated hypogonadotropic hypogonadism in association with anosmia or hyposmia. This patient's history of normal puberty, normal testes size, and elevated FSH levels are not consistent with this condition. Mutations in the cystic fibrosis transmembrane conductance regulator gene (*CFTR*) are a relatively frequent cause of infertility in men with obstructive azoospermia and are associated with congenital bilateral absence of the vas deferens. However, given that his vas deferens is palpable and that he has normal semen volume and fructose in the ejaculate, a *CFTR* mutation (Answer: D) would not explain his presentation.

EDUCATIONAL OBJECTIVE:
Recognize the presentation of Y-chromosome microdeletions and outline the differential diagnosis of nonobstructive azoospermia.

REFERENCE(S):
Vogt PH, Edelmann A, Kirsch S, et al. Human Y chromosome azoospermia factors (AZF) mapped to different subregions in Yq11. *Hum Mol Genet*. 1996;5(7):933-943.

Pryor JL, Kent-First M, Muallem A, et al. Microdeletions in the Y chromosome of infertile men. *N Engl J Med*. 1997;336(8):534-539.

Stahl PJ, Schlegel PN. Genetic evaluation of the azoospermic or severely oligozoospermic male. *Curr Opin Obstet Gynecol*. 2012;24(4):221-228.

10 ANSWER: C) Adrenal hypoplasia congenita

The development of primary adrenal insufficiency in a patient with idiopathic hypogonadotropic hypogonadism should raise suspicion for adrenal hypoplasia congenita (Answer C), an X-linked recessive disease due to mutations in the *NR0B1* gene (also known as *DAX1*). The age at presentation and the severity of adrenal insufficiency are variable. Although adrenal insufficiency is most often diagnosed in childhood (some cases even presenting in the neonatal period), some patients present during adulthood, as in this vignette. Mutations in the *NR0B1* gene affect function of all levels of the hypothalamic-pituitary-gonadal axis, as well as the adrenal glands. There is a broad phenotypic spectrum for males with adrenal hypoplasia congenita. Unlike most patients with idiopathic hypogonadotropic hypogonadism, those with adrenal hypoplasia congenita fail to initiate spermatogenesis when treated with gonadotropin therapy due to the concomitant testicular defect.

Patients with partial hypopituitarism (Answer A) could present with hypogonadotropic hypogonadism and adrenal insufficiency but the latter would be secondary as opposed to primary. Autoimmune polyglandular endocrine deficiency syndromes (Answer B) could cause primary adrenal insufficiency but associated hypogonadism would be primary rather than secondary. Kallmann syndrome (Answer D) is the association of hypogonadotropic hypogonadism with anosmia. It is not the correct diagnosis for this patient as he has a normal sense of smell and it does not cause primary adrenal insufficiency.

EDUCATIONAL OBJECTIVE:
Describe the clinical and biochemical presentation of adrenal hypoplasia congenita.

REFERENCE(S):
Jadhav U, Harris RM, Jameson JL. Hypogonadotropic hypogonadism in subjects with DAX1 mutations. *Mol Cell Endocrinol*. 2011;346(1-2):65-73.

Lin L, Achermann JC. Inherited adrenal hypoplasia: not just for kids! *Clin Endocrinol (Oxf)*. 2004; 60(5):529-537.

Reutens AT, Achermann JC, Ito M, et al. Clinical and functional effects of mutations in the DAX-1 gene in patients with adrenal hypoplasia congenita. *J Clin Endocrinol Metab.* 1999;84(2):504-511.

11 ANSWER: D) Serum prolactin measurement

This patient has secondary hypogonadism (low serum testosterone and inappropriately normal gonadotropin levels). Given that his testes are adult sized and he is normally virilized, he has acquired secondary hypogonadism after the onset of puberty. The differential diagnosis of postpubertal secondary hypogonadism includes a pituitary macroadenoma, Cushing syndrome, hyperprolactinemia, opioid use, and iron-overload syndromes (including hemochromatosis). Given the frequency with which hyperprolactinemia can cause hypogonadotropic hypogonadism, prolactin should be measured in all men with secondary hypogonadism (thus, Answer D is correct).

In this patient, measurement of 24-hour urinary free cortisol (Answer A) is not indicated because of the absence of any features to suggest glucocorticoid excess (normal weight and blood pressure, no striae or evidence of proximal myopathy). The major indication for karyotype analysis in men with hypogonadism is to confirm a diagnosis of Klinefelter syndrome, the most common genetic cause of primary hypogonadism. Given that this patient does not have primary hypogonadism, screening for Klinefelter syndrome by karyotyping (Answer B) is not indicated.

Urine epitestosterone measurement (Answer C) is a test for exogenous testosterone abuse. Epitestosterone is produced by the testes, and the testosterone-to-epitestosterone ratio is elevated in patients who are taking exogenous testosterone. This patient is not abusing anabolic steroids as is evident from his physical examination and the fact that his gonadotropins are normal, not suppressed.

EDUCATIONAL OBJECTIVE:
Measure prolactin in the evaluation of men with secondary hypogonadism.

REFERENCE(S):
Bhasin S, Cunningham GR, Hayes FJ, et al; Task Force, Endocrine Society. Testosterone therapy in men with androgen deficiency syndromes: an Endocrine Society clinical practice guideline. *J Clin Endocrinol Metab.* 2010;95(6):2536-2559.

12 ANSWER: A) Refer him to a urologist

Although this patient's prostate-specific antigen (PSA) level remains within the reference range and he has no lower urinary tract symptoms, he should be referred for urologic evaluation (Answer A) on the basis of the magnitude of its change. PSA levels are known to fluctuate in an individual and also have considerable test-retest variability. However, an increase of greater than 1.4 ng/mL (1.4 µg/L) (confirmed by a repeated test) over the course of a year in a man on testosterone therapy cannot be attributed to random variation alone. A systematic review of prostate risk during testosterone therapy found that the average increase in PSA after initiation of testosterone therapy is 0.3 ng/mL and 0.44 ng/mL in young and old men, respectively. A cutoff of 1.4 ng/mL has been adopted on the basis of the findings of a clinical trial that evaluated the effectiveness of finasteride vs placebo on lower urinary tract symptoms and prostate volume in men with benign prostatic hyperplasia. In that study, the upper limit of the 90% confidence interval for the change in PSA level in the placebo arm was 1.4 ng/mL (1.4 µg/L). Hence, on the basis of the findings of the finasteride study and the fact that the average increase in PSA levels on testosterone therapy is less than 0.5 ng/mL (0.5 µg/L) (regardless of patient age), the Endocrine Society's clinical practice guidelines recommend that patients with a PSA increase of greater than 1.4 ng/mL during testosterone therapy should be referred for urologic consultation. It is important to understand that this increase of 1.4 ng/mL in PSA concentration does not indicate prostate cancer, but only serves as a trigger for further evaluation. Simply providing reassurance and scheduling a follow-up visit without any action is inappropriate (Answer B).

This patient has experienced symptomatic improvement on his current testosterone dosage, and his on-treatment testosterone concentration is normal. Therefore, a decrease in dosage (Answer

C) is not indicated. Although this patient has an enlarged prostate on rectal examination, he does not have lower urinary tract symptoms. Therefore, treatment with a 5α-reductase inhibitor (Answer D) is not indicated.

EDUCATIONAL OBJECTIVE:
Outline the appropriate prostate monitoring for middle-aged and older patients receiving testosterone replacement.

REFERENCE(S):

Bhasin S, Cunningham GR, Hayes FJ, et al; Task Force, Endocrine Society. Testosterone therapy in men with androgen deficiency syndromes: an Endocrine Society clinical practice guideline. *J Clin Endocrinol Metab*. 2010;95(6):2536-2559.

Bhasin S, Singh AB, Mac RP, Carter B, Lee MI, Cunningham GR. Managing the risks of prostate disease during testosterone replacement therapy in older men: recommendations for a standardized monitoring plan. *J Androl*. 2003;24(3): 299-311.

Gormley GJ, Stoner E, Bruskewitz RC, et al. The effect of finasteride in men with benign prostatic hyperplasia. The Finasteride Study Group. *N Engl J Med*. 1992;327(17):1185-1191.

13 **ANSWER: C) MRI of the sella**
This patient has prepubertal hypogonadism as evidenced by his failure to develop secondary sexual characteristics or an increase in testicular size. Laboratory tests show profound secondary hypogonadism with otherwise normal pituitary function and prolactin levels. His presentation is thus consistent with idiopathic hypogonadotropic hypogonadism. However, before a definitive diagnosis of idiopathic hypogonadotropic hypogonadism can be made, structural abnormalities in the hypothalamus or pituitary must be excluded. Therefore, MRI of the sella (Answer C) should be the next step in his evaluation.

Once a diagnosis of congenital hypogonadotropic hypogonadism has been made, targeted genetic testing can be considered. In the last decade, considerable advances have been made in unraveling the genetic basis of congenital hypogonadotropic hypogonadism and to date, mutations have been identified in approximately 40% of cases. While in familial cases the mode of inheritance can be used to guide genetic testing, most cases of congenital hypogonadotropic hypogonadism are actually sporadic, as in the patient described in this vignette. However, a careful clinical evaluation can be helpful in prioritizing genetic testing. In an analysis of 219 patients with Kallmann syndrome, the following clinical features were highly associated with specific gene defects: synkinesia (*KAL1*), dental agenesis (*FGF8/FGFR1*), digital bony abnormalities (*FGF8/FGFR1*), and hearing loss (*CHD7*). In this case, genetic testing for a *KAL1* mutation (Answer A) would not be the appropriate next step as the diagnosis of idiopathic hypogonadotropic hypogonadism has not yet been confirmed. In any case, this patient would not be expected to harbor a *KAL1* mutation given his normal sense of smell, absence of cleft lip or palate, and absent mirror movements.

A GnRH stimulation test (Answer B) would not be helpful as it does not reliably differentiate among various etiologies of secondary hypogonadism, and even patients with a hypothalamic defect, as in this case, may not mount a gonadotropin response on initial exposure to stimulation with GnRH. Measurement of free testosterone (Answer D) would not provide any further insight in a patient who has eunuchoidism and prepubertal total testosterone levels.

EDUCATIONAL OBJECTIVE:
Guide the appropriate workup in a patient with secondary hypogonadism.

REFERENCE(S):

Palmert MR, Dunkel L. Clinical practice. Delayed puberty. *N Engl J Med*. 2012;366(5):443-453.

Hayes FJ, Seminara SB, Crowley WF Jr. Hypogonadotropic hypogonadism. *Endocrinol Metab Clin North Am*. 1998;27(4):739-763.

Costa-Barbosa FA, Balasubramanian R, Keefe KW, et al. Prioritizing genetic testing in patients with Kallmann syndrome using clinical phenotypes. *J Clin Endocrinol Metab*. 2013;98(5):E943-E953.

14

ANSWER: A) Measurement of transferrin saturation

This patient has secondary hypogonadism (symptoms and/or signs of hypogonadism, low serum testosterone, and low or inappropriately normal gonadotropin levels). Considering that his testes are adult size and he is normally virilized, one can conclude he has acquired secondary hypogonadism after the onset of puberty. The differential diagnosis of postpubertal, acquired secondary hypogonadism includes pituitary macroadenomas, Cushing syndrome, hyperprolactinemia, opioid use, and iron overload syndromes such as hemochromatosis. Hand arthralgias, chondrocalcinosis, hyperpigmentation, and secondary hypogonadism are the earliest manifestations of iron overload syndromes. In men, hereditary hemochromatosis often causes these sequelae in the third and fourth decades. Later in the disease course, patients may experience heart failure, cirrhosis, and diabetes mellitus. Acquired forms of iron overload syndromes (eg, due to multiple transfusions) also may cause disease earlier. Hemochromatosis is inherited in an autosomal recessive manner and has a prevalence of about 0.4% in populations of northern European descent, but it has much lower clinical penetrance, and disease severity is highly variable. Mutations in the *HFE* gene are responsible, and the most common genotype is homozygosity for the Cys282Tyr (C282Y) mutation. Assessment of transferrin saturation (Answer A) is the most useful initial test for hemochromatosis; a transferrin saturation less than 45% is enough to exclude the diagnosis. In the appropriate clinical setting, C282Y homozygosity suffices to diagnose hemochromatosis, but liver biopsy with iron staining remains the criterion standard for diagnosis.

Opioid abuse (Answer B) is a possibility in this man given his occupation and resultant access to opioids. However, opioids do not cause chondrocalcinosis and arthralgias. Cushing syndrome can be excluded as the etiology of secondary hypogonadism in this patient on the basis of his history and physical examination. Therefore, screening for Cushing syndrome with a dexamethasone suppression test (Answer C) is not indicated. Serial dilution of serum (Answer E) is done to assess for the "hook" effect when measuring prolactin in patients with marked hyperprolactinemia. This is unlikely in this man who has normal sellar imaging.

EDUCATIONAL OBJECTIVE:
Diagnose hemochromatosis as a cause of secondary hypogonadism.

REFERENCE(S):

Bhasin S, Cunningham GR, Hayes FJ, et al; Task Force, Endocrine Society. Testosterone therapy in adult men with androgen deficiency syndromes: an Endocrine Society clinical practice guideline. *J Clin Endocrinol Metab*. 2010;95(6):2536-2559.

Moyer TP, Highsmith WE, Smyrk TC, Gross JB Jr. Hereditary hemochromatosis: laboratory evaluation. *Clin Chim Acta*. 2011;412(17-18):1485-1492.

van Bokhoven MA, van Deursen CT, Swinkels DW. Diagnosis and management of hereditary haemochromatosis. *BMJ*. 2011;342:c7251.

15

ANSWER: C) Reevaluate his hypothalamic-pituitary-gonadal axis in 6 to 12 months

Although the incidence of pituitary dysfunction after traumatic brain injury varies widely in published studies, it appears that pituitary dysfunction occurs commonly in men who experience moderate to severe traumatic brain injury. Low GH and testosterone concentrations are the most common abnormalities. However, it is unclear whether treatment with GH and/or testosterone is beneficial. Furthermore, longitudinal follow-up has demonstrated that many men recover function of these axes 3 to 12 months after the traumatic brain injury. In this man who appears to be recovering well from his brain injury, the best option is to reassess his gonadal axis 6 to 12 months after the initial injury (Answer C).

Treatment with hCG (Answer A) would raise his testosterone concentrations and stimulate spermatogenesis; however, he does not wish to start a family for at least 1 year so there is no urgency in starting treatment until it is clear that his hypothalamic-pituitary-gonadal axis has not recovered. Given that his libido is already beginning to improve and he has no problem with erections, there is no indication to start testosterone (Answer B). A phosphodiesterase inhibitor (Answer D) would not be appropriate for a patient with low libido but normal erectile function.

EDUCATIONAL OBJECTIVE:
Counsel a patient regarding the time course of secondary hypogonadism following traumatic brain injury.

REFERENCE(S):
Schneider HJ, Schneider M, Saller B, et al. Prevalence of anterior pituitary insufficiency 3 and 12 months after traumatic brain injury. *Eur J Endocrinol.* 2006;154(2):259-265.

Tanriverdi F, Senyurek H, Unluhizarci K, Selcuklu A, Casanueva FF, Kelestimur F. High risk of hypopituitarism after traumatic brain injury: a prospective investigation of anterior pituitary function in the acute phase and 12 months after trauma. *J Clin Endocrinol Metab.* 2006;91(6): 2105-2111.

16 **ANSWER: A) Serum total testosterone measurement in 3 months**
Severe systemic illness suppresses the hypothalamic-pituitary-gonadal axis and results in a hormonal profile of secondary hypogonadism. Testing for hypogonadism should ideally be done at a time representative of an individual's baseline health status. Measurement of serum testosterone and gonadotropins should generally not be done in men with acute illness or an acute flare of chronic illness. For this man who was recently hospitalized for pneumonia, the best course of action would be to repeat the assessment of his gonadal access when he has fully recovered from the acute flare and he has returned to his baseline health (Answer A).

Answers B, C, and D are not indicated until hypogonadism has been confirmed. Assessment for hyperprolactinemia (Answer C) should be performed in all men with secondary hypogonadism. Younger men with secondary hypogonadism should be tested for iron overload. The diagnostic value of assessing iron saturation (Answer B) in older men with secondary hypogonadism is much lower because most older men with hemochromatosis tend to present with cirrhosis or heart failure, not isolated hypogonadotropic hypogonadism. Free testosterone (Answer D) is helpful in diagnosing hypogonadism in situations where an altered sex hormone–binding globulin level is suspected; however, this patient does not have any conditions that one would expect to alter sex hormone–binding globulin concentrations.

EDUCATIONAL OBJECTIVE:
Identify severe systemic illness as a cause of reversible suppression of the gonadal axis.

REFERENCE(S):
Bhasin S, Cunningham GR, Hayes FJ, et al; Task Force, Endocrine Society. Testosterone therapy in men with androgen deficiency syndromes: an Endocrine Society clinical practice guideline. *J Clin Endocrinol Metab.* 2010;95(6):2536-2559.

17 **ANSWER: D) Testosterone abuse**
This patient has tender gynecomastia. Breast tenderness suggests benign breast growth of recent onset (<6 months). He also has a high-normal testosterone concentration, and his high-normal calculated free testosterone concentration confirms that this is not strictly due to high sex hormone–binding globulin concentrations, which can be seen in hepatitis and would decrease the free testosterone concentration. He also has high estradiol and low gonadotropin concentrations. This combination can be due to exogenous testosterone use or abuse (Answer D), endogenous or exogenous testosterone precursors (eg, dehydroepiandrosterone from an adrenal tumor), and endogenous or exogenous hCG (eg, hCG from a germ-cell tumor).

Although chronic hepatitis (Answer A) is commonly associated with elevated sex hormone–binding globulin concentrations, the calculated free testosterone concentration remains normal unless the patient has underlying hypogonadism, so it would not explain this patient's hormone profile. An estrogen-secreting testicular tumor (Answer B) would cause elevated estradiol concentrations and suppressed gonadotropins but testosterone levels would not be high. Finasteride (Answer C) modestly raises serum testosterone concentrations by blocking the conversion of testosterone to dihydrotestosterone, but it would not cause suppressed gonadotropin concentrations.

EDUCATIONAL OBJECTIVE:
Identify the clinical and biochemical features of exogenous testosterone abuse.

REFERENCE(S):
Amory JK, Wang C, Swerdloff RS, et al. The effect of 5alpha-reductase inhibition with dutasteride and finasteride on semen parameters and serum hormones in healthy men [published correction appears in *J Clin Endocrinol Metab.* 2007; 92(11):4379]. *J Clin Endocrinol Metab.* 2007;92(5):1659-1665.

Anawalt BD. Gynecomastia. In: Jameson JL, De Groot LJ, eds. *Endocrinology: Adult and Pediatric.* 7th ed. Philadelphia, PA: Saunders Elsevier; 2015.

Bhasin S, Cunningham GR, Hayes FJ, et al; Task Force, Endocrine Society. Testosterone therapy in men with androgen deficiency syndromes: an Endocrine Society clinical practice guideline. *J Clin Endocrinol Metab.* 2010;95(6):2536-2559.

18 ANSWER: D) Erythrocytosis

When considering testosterone replacement therapy, particularly in older men, the risks and benefits should be discussed before initiating therapy. Erythrocytosis (Answer D) is the most common adverse effect of testosterone therapy in older men. Meta-analyses of randomized controlled trials have shown that older men on testosterone are 4 to 5 times more likely to experience erythrocytosis than those on placebo. Testosterone-related erythrocytosis is dose-dependent and is more frequently encountered in older men and in patients on injectable testosterone preparations. Androgens stimulate erythropoiesis via various mechanisms: (1) direct stimulation of erythroid cell line in the bone marrow, (2) stimulation of erythropoietin synthesis and release from the kidneys, and (3) increasing iron availability for erythropoiesis. Although the mechanism(s) explaining why older men are predisposed to erythrocytosis remains unclear, reduced metabolic clearance rate of testosterone has been posited as a cause. Anecdotal reports also suggest that men with underlying hypoxic conditions may also be more predisposed to erythrocytosis during testosterone therapy.

Before initiating testosterone therapy, baseline hematocrit should be measured. The Endocrine Society clinical practice guidelines recommend against initiating testosterone therapy in patients with a baseline hematocrit level above 50% and suggest that the underlying cause of erythrocytosis be investigated before androgen therapy is prescribed. Once testosterone therapy is initiated, it is suggested that hematocrit be assessed in 3 to 6 months and then annually. If the hematocrit level is above 54%, testosterone therapy should be discontinued until hematocrit normalizes (and testosterone therapy can then be initiated at a reduced dosage). Such patients should be evaluated for hypoxia and sleep apnea.

Prostate-specific antigen elevation to greater than 4 ng/mL (>4 µg/L) (Answer C) is seen more frequently in older men on testosterone compared with rates observed in men taking placebo, but meta-analyses of randomized controlled trials show that this risk is much less common than erythrocytosis (odds ratio, 1.22). Similarly, randomized controlled trials have not shown a higher frequency of urinary retention (Answer B) in older men. There are no data to suggest that physiologic testosterone replacement causes aggressive behavior (Answer A) in men.

EDUCATIONAL OBJECTIVE:
Identify the most likely adverse effect of testosterone therapy in older men.

REFERENCE(S):
Snyder PJ, Bhasin S, Cunningham GR, et al; Testosterone Trials Investigators. Effects of testosterone treatment in older men. *N Engl J Med.* 2016;374(7):611-624.

Roy CN, Snyder PJ, Stephens-Shields AJ, et al. Association of testosterone levels with anemia in older men: a controlled clinical trial. *JAMA Intern Med.* 2017;177(4):480-490.

Bhasin S, Cunningham GR, Hayes FJ, et al; Task Force, Endocrine Society. Testosterone therapy in men with androgen deficiency syndromes: an Endocrine Society clinical practice guideline. *J Clin Endocrinol Metab.* 2010;95(6):2536-2559.

Calof OM, Singh AB, Lee ML, et al. Adverse events associated with testosterone replacement in middle-aged and older men: a meta-analysis of randomized, placebo-controlled trials. *J Gerontol A Biol Sci Med Sci.* 2005;60(11):1451-1457.

Shahani S, Braga-Basaria M, Maggio M, Basaria S. Androgens and erythropoiesis: past and present. *J Endocrinol Invest*. 2009;32(8):704-716.

19 ANSWER: B) Start a GnRH agonist with a 0.05-mg estradiol patch

This patient has several risk factors for hypertriglyceridemia-induced pancreatitis, including familial hypertriglyceridemia, poorly controlled diabetes, and oral estrogen therapy. In male-to-female transgender patients, estrogen therapy is needed to develop female sexual characteristics. In patients with an intact hypothalamic-pituitary-gonadal axis, the estrogen dosage needed is supraphysiologic given the need to suppress testosterone secretion. However, combined use of a GnRH agonist with estrogen allows physiologic doses of estrogen to be used as testosterone secretion is already suppressed. Estrogen therapy can result in marked hypertriglyceridemia. However, the lipid effects of estrogen depend on the route of administration, with the transdermal route having less effect on HDL cholesterol and triglycerides than the oral route. Given this patient's history, the most appropriate hormone regimen would be a GnRH agonist and an initial low-dosage estrogen patch (Answer B), which can be titrated based on clinical response and triglyceride levels. Options that include oral estrogen such as conjugated equine estrogen (Answer A) and ethinyl estradiol (Answer D) are incorrect. Ethinyl estradiol has also been shown to increase the risk of venous thromboembolism significantly more than 17β-estradiol.

Given that the patient has been living as a woman for more than 2 decades, as well as the increased risk of depression and suicide in the transgender population, withholding further hormone therapy (Answer C) is likely to significantly affect her mental health. In addition, estrogen therapy was not her only risk factor for hypertriglyceridemia.

EDUCATIONAL OBJECTIVE:
Guide the hormonal care of a transgender patient with hypertriglyceridemia.

REFERENCE(S):
Aljenedil S, Hegele RA, Genest J, Awan Z. Estrogen-associated severe hypertriglyceridemia with pancreatitis. *J Clin Lipidol*. 2017;11(1):297-300.

Lufkin EG, Ory SJ. Relative value of transdermal and oral estrogen therapy in various clinical situations. *Mayo Clin Proc*. 1994;69(2):131-135.

Rosenthal SM. Approach to the patient: transgender youth: endocrine considerations. *J Clin Endocrinol Metab*. 2014;99(12):4379-4389.

Gooren LJ. Clinical practice. Care of transsexual persons. *N Engl J Med*. 2011;364(13):1251-1257.

Hembree WC, Cohen-Kettenis P, Delemarre-van de Waal HA, et al; Endocrine Society. Endocrine treatment of transsexual persons: an Endocrine Society clinical practice guideline. *J Clin Endocrinol Metab*. 2009;94(9):3132-3154.

20 ANSWER: B) Arrange for transrectal ultrasonography

The vas deferens is normally palpable as a thin ropelike structure within the spermatic cord. In this case, imaging using transrectal ultrasonography (Answer B) confirmed the clinical suspicion of bilateral absence of the vas deferens. This patient turned out to have mutations in the *CFTR* gene, which is associated with cystic fibrosis. Congenital absence of the vas deferens, without the typical pulmonary and pancreatic manifestations of cystic fibrosis, is associated with compound heterozygosity for a classic (severe) *CFTR* mutation and a mild *CFTR* mutation. Given the autosomal recessive mode of inheritance of cystic fibrosis, screening of the female partner and genetic counseling are key components of this patient's management to determine the risk of having a child with cystic fibrosis. When the records of his semen analyses were retrieved, they were consistent with an obstructive cause of azoospermia as evidenced by an ejaculate volume of 1 mL, absent fructose, and low pH (normal >7.2). The patient's initial low testosterone could be explained by his obesity and was not low enough to cause azoospermia.

In men with obstructive azoospermia, sperm can be retrieved by a technique called microsurgical epididymal sperm aspiration, which can then be used to fertilize their partners' eggs through assisted reproductive technology such as intracytoplasmic sperm injection.

Adding FSH injections (Answer A) would not be appropriate given his normal testicular size and endogenous FSH levels. Increasing his hCG dosage (Answer C) would not be appropriate given that his testosterone level is already near the upper end of the normal range. Clomiphene citrate (Answer D) would not be effective in a patient with obstructive azoospermia. Even in men with hypogonadotropic hypogonadism, clomiphene is not an approved medication to stimulate spermatogenesis and can have negative effects on bone health, libido, and body fat.

EDUCATIONAL OBJECTIVE:
Explain the association between congenital bilateral absence of the vas deferens and infertility.

REFERENCE(S):

Anawalt BD. Approach to male infertility and induction of spermatogenesis. *J Clin Endocrinol Metab.* 2013;98(9):3532-3542.

Kolettis PN. The evaluation and management of the azoospermic patient. *J Androl.* 2002;23(3): 293-305.

Finkelstein JS, Lee H, Burnett-Bowie SA, et al. Gonadal steroids and body composition, strength, and sexual function in men. *N Engl J Med.* 2013;369(11):1011-1022.

Thyroid Board Review

Elizabeth N. Pearce, MD, MSc ● Boston University

1 ANSWER: B) Repeated blood tests after stopping biotin

The recommended daily intake for biotin is 300 mcg daily, but dosages that are orders of magnitude higher than requirements are available in many nutritional supplements. The use of biotin supplements can cause artifactual interference with commonly used biotin-streptavidin immunoassays for TSH, thyroid hormone, and anti–thyrotropin receptor antibodies. High circulating biotin levels cause falsely low measurements in immunometric sandwich assays (such as that for TSH), but falsely high measurements for competitive immunoassays (such as those for free T_4, T_3, and thyroid-stimulating immunoglobulin). Thus, patients taking biotin may have laboratory results identical to those found in Graves hyperthyroidism. Artifactual thyroid function results have been reported in patients taking at least 1500 mcg of biotin daily. Test results normalize 2 to 7 days after stopping the biotin.

Radioactive iodine uptake and scan (Answer A) would be diagnostic if this patient truly had Graves disease, but would not be warranted if her blood tests normalize after ceasing biotin. Similarly, thyroid ultrasonography with color Doppler (Answer C) might provide clues about the presence or absence of Graves disease, but it is not the best next step. Finally, serum TPO antibody assays (Answer D) are also subject to biotin interference, and TPO antibody assessment is neither a sensitive nor a specific test for Graves disease.

EDUCATIONAL OBJECTIVE:
Describe the potential for biotin interference with thyroid function assays.

REFERENCE(S):
Kummer S, Hermsen D, Distelmaier F. Biotin treatment mimicking Graves' disease. *N Engl J Med.* 2016;375(7):704-706.

Elston MS, Sehgal S, Du Toit S, Yarndley T, Conaglen JV. Factitious Graves' disease due to biotin immunoassay interference-a case and review of the literature. *J Clin Endocrinol Metab.* 2016;101(9):3251-3255.

2 ANSWER: B) Figure B

The sample presented in Figure B (Answer B) shows typical features of papillary thyroid cancer, including nuclear overlap and inclusions. Figure A shows a colloid nodule, Figure C shows adenomatous hyperplasia, and Figure D shows cystic fluid with macrophages. Cytopathology of papillary cancers typically demonstrates large, nonuniform cells with sparse or absent colloid. Nuclei are large and may contain clefts or holes ("Orphan Annie eyes") due to intranuclear cytoplasmic inclusions. The cytoplasm has a "ground-glass" appearance. Psammoma bodies, small laminated calcifications, may be present. Benign nodules (Answer A) typically include abundant colloid, which stains blue on a Papanicolaou stain. Cells in benign nodules generally have a uniform appearance and are not crowded; microfollicles and macrofollicles may be present. Cyst fluid (Answer D) typically contains relatively few cells, but cellular debris and hemosiderin-laden macrophages may be seen. Adenomatous hyperplasia (Answer C) is characterized by the presence of abundant colloid and a variable number of follicular cells; the follicular cells are predominately arranged in flat sheets with a honeycomb configuration. Nuclei have a uniform appearance and there is minimal nuclear overlapping and crowding.

EDUCATIONAL OBJECTIVE:
Explain classic features of papillary carcinoma on thyroid cytopathology.

REFERENCE(S):
Papanicolaou Society of Cytopathology. Online Image Atlas. Available at: http://www.papsociety.com/atlas.html.

3 ANSWER: A) Increase the levothyroxine dosage to 500 mcg daily

Absorption of levothyroxine occurs in the distal small intestine. Patients with short bowels due to surgery or extensive small bowel disease may malabsorb levothyroxine. One study of 5 patients with surgically shortened small bowels (undergone removal of portions of jejunum and ileum) documented diminished levothyroxine absorption in each patient, despite the presence of an intact duodenum. Another study demonstrated an increased levothyroxine dosage requirement to as high as 600 mcg daily in a patient after a jejunoileal bypass procedure, with a diminished requirement following surgical reversal. Therefore, the distal small bowel is probably the most important site for absorption of levothyroxine. Variable effects on levothyroxine dosing have been reported following Roux-en-Y gastric bypass surgery, with most patients actually requiring lower dosages postoperatively than preoperatively, most likely due to reduced body weight. A subset of patients requires very high levothyroxine dosages postoperatively, however, due to malabsorption. The patient in this vignette needs a higher levothyroxine dosage. Changing to once-weekly levothyroxine (Answer B), changing to liothyronine (Answer C), or switching brands of levothyroxine (Answer D) ignore the basic problem of malabsorption. Giving parenteral levothyroxine (Answer E) is unnecessarily aggressive.

EDUCATIONAL OBJECTIVE:
Evaluate the need for high levothyroxine requirements following bowel resection.

REFERENCE(S):
Azizi F, Belur R, Albano J. Malabsorption of thyroid hormones after jejunoileal bypass for obesity. *Ann Intern Med.* 1979;90(6):941-942.

Stone E, Leiter LA, Lambert JR, Silverberg JD, Jeejeebhoy KN, Burrow GN. L-thyroxine absorption in patients with short bowel. *J Clin Endocrinol Metab.* 1984;59(1):139-141.

Gadiraju S, Lee CJ, Cooper DS. Levothyroxine dosing following bariatric surgery. *Obes Surg.* 2016;26(10):2538-2542.

4 ANSWER: C) Thyroid lobectomy

All of the options provided could achieve euthyroidism in this patient with a toxic adenoma. However, if she opts for therapy with antithyroid medication (Answer B) she will be committed to lifelong treatment since toxic nodules do not remit. Thyroid lobectomy for toxic adenoma (Answer C) results in a high cure rate (treatment failure of <1%) with only a 2% to 3% risk for postoperative hypothyroidism. Radioactive iodine treatment for toxic adenoma (Answer A) results in a higher risk for hypothyroidism than does thyroid lobectomy, with progressively increasing rates of hypothyroidism that approach 60% at 20 years. The risk for posttreatment hypothyroidism is higher in patients with underlying thyroid autoimmunity, as is the case in this patient who is TPO antibody positive. Ethanol injection (Answer D) is not routinely recommended as a treatment for toxic adenoma because of high rates of thyroid pain and other complications. Finally, radiofrequency ablation (Answer E) is potentially appealing for this patient due to low reported complication rates and a very low risk for permanent hypothyroidism. However, this technique is relatively new and not routinely being used in the United States.

EDUCATIONAL OBJECTIVE:
Summarize factors in decision-making regarding available treatment modalities for toxic nodules.

REFERENCE(S):
Bonnema SJ, Hegedüs L. Radioiodine therapy in benign thyroid diseases: effects, side effects, and factors affecting therapeutic outcome. *Endocr Rev.* 2012;33(6):920-980.

Ross DS, Burch HB, Cooper DS, et al. 2016 American Thyroid Association Guidelines for Diagnosis and Management of Hyperthyroidism and Other Causes of Thyrotoxicosis. *Thyroid.* 2016;26(10):1343-1421.

5 ANSWER: D) Tyrosine kinase inhibitor therapy

The tyrosine kinase inhibitors are a group of drugs that affect several proteins involved in the modulation of cell growth (*see table*). Receptor kinases are involved in both normal cellular function and pathologic processes such as oncogenesis, metastasis, tumor angiogenesis, and maintenance of the tumor microenvironment. Tyrosine kinase inhibitors are small, orally active molecules that inhibit phosphorylation of tyrosine molecules at key ATP-binding sites. Affected targets include VEGF receptors 2 and 3, platelet-derived growth factor receptor, Flt-3, c-kit, and RET. On the basis of phase III trials showing beneficial effects, 2 tyrosine kinase inhibitors, vandetanib and cabozantinib, have been approved for treatment of medullary thyroid cancer in patients with extensive local disease or distant metastases. Although complete remissions are very rare with these agents, disease stabilization and prolongation of progression-free survival have been found when compared with placebo (30.5 vs 19.3 months for vandetanib; 11.2 vs 4 months for cabozantinib in phase III trials) (thus, Answer D is correct). Palliative therapy is another option in this patient, given the limited, albeit improved, response duration for tyrosine kinase inhibitors.

Radiolabeled anti-CEA antibodies (not calcitonin antibodies [Answer A]) have been evaluated in medullary thyroid cancer and certain gastrointestinal tumors, with less than impressive results. Cytotoxic chemotherapy (Answer B) has been applied to therapy for metastatic medullary thyroid cancer, with limited utility; most regimens involve dacarbazine combined with a second agent (not adriamycin and cisplatin). Focal radiotherapy (Answer C) will not delay the systemic progression of metastatic disease in this patient. There is no role for somatostatin analogue therapy (Answer E) in this case.

Table. Tyrosine Kinase Inhibitors Currently Approved for Use in Advanced Thyroid Cancer.

Tyrosine Kinase Inhibitor	Type of Thyroid Cancer	Effectiveness: Progression-Free Survival Compared With Placebo*
Vandetanib	Medullary	30.5 vs 19.3 months
Cabozantinib	Medullary	11.2 vs 4 months
Sorafanib	Differentiated	10.8 vs 5.8 months
Lenvatinib	Differentiated	18.3 vs 3.6 months

*Note: enrolled populations were different; efficacy cannot be compared directly across studies. Many other multikinase inhibitors are currently being investigated for use in advanced thyroid cancer.

EDUCATIONAL OBJECTIVE:
List indications for tyrosine kinase inhibitor therapy in advanced medullary thyroid cancer.

REFERENCE(S):
Bernet V, Smallridge R. New therapeutic options for advanced forms of thyroid cancer. *Expert Opin Emerg Drugs.* 2014;19(2):225-241.

Wells SA Jr, Asa SL, Dralle H, et al; American Thyroid Association Guidelines Task Force on Medullary Thyroid Carcinoma. Revised American Thyroid Association Guidelines for the Management of Medullary Thyroid Carcinoma. *Thyroid.* 2015;25(6):567-610.

Valerio L, Pieruzzi L, Giani C, et al. Targeted therapy in thyroid cancer: state of the art. *Clin Oncol (R Coll Radiol).* 2017;29(5):316-324.

6 ANSWER: D) Iatrogenic subclinical hyperthyroidism

In large studies, subclinical hypothyroidism has been associated with increased cardiovascular risk and subtly increased symptom scores. Adverse effects of subclinical hypothyroidism have been most clearly demonstrated when the serum TSH level is 10 mIU/L or greater. However, very large-scale trials would likely be required to demonstrate benefits, and no intervention trial to date has demonstrated a consistent improvement in sense of well-being or energy level (Answer C), weight reduction (Answer A), or improvement in cognitive function (Answer B) with treatment of subclinical hypothyroidism when the baseline TSH is less than 10 mIU/L. While some, but not all, studies have shown decreases in LDL cholesterol following initiation of levothyroxine treatment for subclinical hypothyroidism, HDL cholesterol (Answer E) is typically not altered in subclinically hypothyroid patients. Current recommendations in the absence of unequivocal evidence for treatment benefit are to treat subclinical hypothyroidism when the TSH level is consistently greater than 10 mIU/L and to individualize treatment decisions when the TSH level is between 5 and 10 mIU/L. An analysis of the NHANES-III population survey (Third National Health and Nutrition Examination Survey) has shown that normal elderly patients without goiter or serologic evidence of Hashimoto thyroiditis have a rightward shift in the upper normal limit for TSH, with the upper 95% confidence interval ranging to approximately 7.5 mIU/L in octogenarians. However, the TSH level of 8.9 mIU/L in this patient is most likely truly abnormal. Patients with positive TPO antibodies, such as this one, are at higher risk for overt hypothyroidism and may be particularly good candidates for levothyroxine therapy to prevent this progression. It is important to monitor treatment appropriately because iatrogenic subclinical hyperthyroidism (Answer D) is clearly detrimental and studies have shown that 14% to 21% of individuals taking levothyroxine are overtreated.

EDUCATIONAL OBJECTIVE:
Describe the limited evidence for benefit of levothyroxine initiation when the TSH level is less than 10 mIU/L.

REFERENCE(S):

Hennessey JV, Espaillat R. Diagnosis and management of subclinical hypothyroidism in elderly adults: a review of the literature. *J Am Geriatr Soc.* 2015;63(8):1663-1673.

Javed Z, Sathyapalan T. Levothyroxine treatment of mild subclinical hypothyroidism: a review of potential risks and benefits. *Ther Adv Endocrinol Metab.* 2016;7(1):12-23.

Baumgartner C, Blum MR, Rodondi N. Subclinical hypothyroidism: summary of evidence in 2014. *Swiss Med Wkly.* 2014;144:w14058.

Stott DJ, Rodondi N, Kearney PM, et al; TRUST Study Group. Thyroid hormone therapy for older adults with subclinical hypothyroidism. *N Engl J Med.* 2017;376(26):2534-2544.

Surks MI, Boucai L. Age- and race-based serum thyrotropin reference limits. *J Clin Endocrinol Metab.* 2010;95(2):496-502.

Pearce EN. Update in lipid alterations in subclinical hypothyroidism. *J Clin Endocrinol Metab.* 2012;97(2):326-333.

7 **ANSWER: A) 70%-90%**
The image shows a nodule with a high risk of malignancy (70%-90%, Answer A): it has classic features associated with papillary thyroid cancer, including hypoechogenicity, irregular margins, and scattered microcalcifications (*arrow*). Nodules with a very low risk for malignancy (Answer D) include spongiform nodules with clearly defined margins. Intermediate suspicion patterns associated with a 10% to 20% risk of malignancy (Answer C) include hypoechoic nodules with smooth margins but without microcalcifications, extrathyroidal extension, or a taller-than-wide shape. There is no currently defined ultrasonography pattern associated with a 20% to 40% malignancy risk (Answer B).

EDUCATIONAL OBJECTIVE:
Identify ultrasonographic features consistent with high risk for papillary thyroid carcinoma.

REFERENCE(S):

Haugen BR, Alexander EK, Bible KC, et al. 2015 American Thyroid Association Management Guidelines for Adult Patients with Thyroid Nodules and Differentiated Thyroid Cancer: the American Thyroid Association Guidelines Task Force on Thyroid Nodules and Differentiated Thyroid Cancer. *Thyroid.* 2016;26(1):1-133.

Brito JP, Gionfriddo MR, Al Nofal A, et al. The accuracy of thyroid nodule ultrasound to predict thyroid cancer: systematic review and meta-analysis. *J Clin Endocrinol Metab.* 2014;99(4):1253-1263.

8 **ANSWER: E) TSH, 0.01 mIU/L; total T$_4$, 5.0 µg/dL (64.4 nmol/L); total T$_3$, 70 ng/dL (1.1 nmol/L); free T$_4$, 2.8 ng/dL (36.0 pmol/L)**
This patient, previously euthyroid on a stable levothyroxine dosage, has recently started taking anabolic steroids. Unlike estrogens, which increase thyroxine-binding globulin values, androgens substantially decrease thyroxine-binding globulin. Euthyroid patients who are not talking levothyroxine would be expected to develop decreased serum total T$_4$ and T$_3$ levels while on high-dosage

androgens, but, due to hypothalamic-pituitary-thyroid axis feedback, would be able to maintain normal free T_4 and serum TSH values (Answer D). However, a patient taking a fixed dosage of levothyroxine has the potential to become hyperthyroid when starting high-dosage androgens. Given marked variability in the ability of different androgens to aromatize, exact changes in thyroid function values are difficult to predict. However, Answer E is the only one of the available choices that shows both a downward shift in total T_4 and T_3 values and a lack of compensation. In patients starting estrogens instead of androgens, opposite patterns might be observed: an increase in thyroxine-binding globulin driving increased total thyroid hormone values in which euthyroidism might be maintained in someone who was euthyroid at baseline (Answer B), but which might lead to hypothyroidism (Answer A) in a patient on levothyroxine. Clinically, it is important to measure TSH 6 to 8 weeks after initiating estrogen or androgen therapy in patients on thyroid hormone replacement.

EDUCATIONAL OBJECTIVE:
Diagnose androgen excess as a cause of a decrease in thyroxine-binding globulin and altered thyroid hormone requirements.

REFERENCE(S):
Tahboub R, Arafah BM. Sex steroids and the thyroid. *Best Pract Res Clin Endocrinol Metab.* 2009;23(6):769-780.

9 **ANSWER: E) Increase the levothyroxine dosage to 88 mcg daily**

This patient has central hypothyroidism due to her previous pituitary surgery. It is important to recognize that patients with central hypothyroidism may secrete a bioactive form of TSH; in this case, serum free T_4 is low and TSH is either normal or slightly elevated. In such patients, the serum TSH may drop precipitously when even low-dosage levothyroxine is initiated. The goal of therapy in central hypothyroidism is a free T_4 value in the upper half of the reference range. Discontinuing levothyroxine (Answer A) is incorrect because this patient's hypothyroidism is already undertreated. In the single study examining this to date, there was no added benefit of combination T_4/T_3 therapy

(Answer C) in patients with secondary hypothyroidism when compared with outcomes of patients treated with adequate dosages of levothyroxine alone. Methimazole (Answer B) is not indicated since the patient is hypothyroid. Continuing the current levothyroxine dosage and increasing the hydrocortisone dosage (Answer D) would not adequately treat her underlying hyperthyroidism.

EDUCATIONAL OBJECTIVE:
Use free T_4 values rather than TSH values for therapeutic targets in the management of central hypothyroidism.

REFERENCE(S):
Persani L. Clinical review: central hypothyroidism: pathogenic, diagnostic, and therapeutic challenges. *J Clin Endocrinol Metab.* 2012;97(9):3068-3078.

Chaker L, Bianco AC, Jonklaas J, Peeters RP. Hypothyroidism. *Lancet.* 2017 [Epub ahead of print]

Jonklaas J, Bianco AC, Bauer AJ; American Thyroid Association Task Force on Thyroid Hormone Replacement. Guidelines for the treatment of hypothyroidism: prepared by the American Thyroid Association Task Force on Thyroid Hormone Replacement. *Thyroid.* 2014;24(12):1670-1751.

10 **ANSWER: B) Serum thyroglobulin measurement**

The differential diagnosis for patients with thyrotoxicosis and a low radioactive iodine uptake includes painless and postpartum thyroiditis, subacute thyroiditis, struma ovarii (with low radioactive iodine uptake in the neck, but uptake in the pelvis on whole-body scan), factitious or iatrogenic thyroiditis, amiodarone use, and recent high-dose iodine exposure. In this male patient, struma ovarii and postpartum thyroiditis are not possibilities. He is not taking amiodarone. Subacute thyroiditis is unlikely given the lack of a viral prodrome, fever, or thyroid tenderness, so assessing his erythrocyte sedimentation rate (Answer C) is incorrect. The urinary iodine concentration is not consistent with recent excessive iodine exposure, so repeating the radioactive iodine uptake following a low-iodine diet (Answer A) is unlikely to change results. In this patient, the most likely diagnoses are either factitious thyrotoxicosis or painless thyroiditis. Graves disease has already been ruled out by the low radioactive iodine uptake, so thyroid-stimulating immunoglobulin measurement (Answer E) is incorrect. Thyroid ultrasonography with color Doppler (Answer D) would show absent hypervascularity with both of these entities. However, the serum thyroglobulin concentration (Answer B) in this thyroglobulin antibody–negative patient would be elevated in painless thyroiditis but low in factitious thyrotoxicosis.

EDUCATIONAL OBJECTIVE:
Construct the differential diagnosis for low radioiodine uptake thyrotoxicosis.

REFERENCE(S):
De Leo S, Lee SY, Braverman LE. Hyperthyroidism. *Lancet*. 2016;388(10047):906-918.

Ross DS, Burch HB, Cooper DS, et al. 2016 American Thyroid Association Guidelines for Diagnosis and Management of Hyperthyroidism and Other Causes of Thyrotoxicosis. *Thyroid*. 2016;26(10):1343-1421.

11 ANSWER: E) Referral for total thyroidectomy

In the Bethesda classification system for reporting thyroid cytopathology, nodules with indeterminate results, which include Bethesda class III (atypia of uncertain significance/follicular lesion of uncertain significance [AUS/FLUS]) and class IV (follicular neoplasm/suspicious for follicular neoplasm [FN/SFN]) are sometimes selected for molecular testing. Testing using a small panel of mutations known to be associated with thyroid cancer is most helpful when a mutation or rearrangement is present (higher positive predictive value) and is generally not helpful when no mutation is identified (lower negative predictive value) because many cancers do not contain the limited set of abnormalities sought in the test (*see image*). In this patient with follicular neoplasm on FNAB and a positive finding of a *RET/PTC* rearrangement, there is a high enough risk of thyroid cancer (80%-90%) that a total thyroidectomy (Answer E) is recommended. The *RET/PTC* gene rearrangement, found in 20% to 70% of papillary thyroid cancers, causes constitutive activation of transcription of the RET tyrosine-kinase domain in follicular cells, leading to uncontrolled cell proliferation.

Another form of molecular testing—a gene expression classifier (uses a microarray of a large panel of genes associated with either benign or

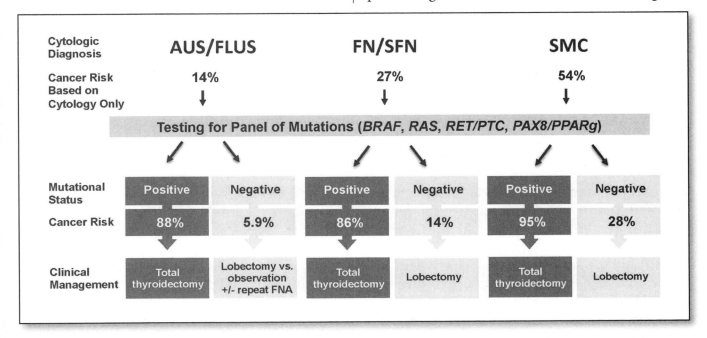

Reprinted from Nikiforov YE, Ohori NP, Hodak SP, et al. Impact of mutational testing on the diagnosis and management of patients with cytologically indeterminate thyroid nodules: a prospective analysis of 1056 FNA samples. *J Clin Endocrinol Metab*. 2011;96(11):3390-3397.

malignant thyroid nodules)—is currently only available from a single source. Limited data for this molecular classifier suggest that it is associated with a higher negative predictive value such that, in general, if negative, no surgery would be recommended. No study to date has examined the tandem use of both technologies, although the cost of this approach could be prohibitive. A lobectomy (Answer D) is inappropriate because of the high risk of malignancy, as a completion thyroidectomy would most likely be required when pathologic examination confirms a malignant nodule. Performing thyroid ultrasonography (Answer A), FNAB (Answer B), or molecular testing (Answer C) again in 6 months would incorrectly avoid thyroid surgery.

EDUCATIONAL OBJECTIVE:
Apply molecular testing to thyroid nodule evaluation.

REFERENCE(S):

Nikiforov YE, Ohori NP, Hodak SP, et al. Impact of mutational testing on the diagnosis and management of patients with cytologically indeterminate thyroid nodules: a prospective analysis of 1056 FNA samples. *J Clin Endocrinol Metab*. 2011; 96(11):3390-3397.

Alexander EK, Kennedy GC, Baloch ZW, et al. Preoperative diagnosis of benign thyroid nodules with indeterminate cytology. *N Engl J Med*. 2012;367(8):705-715.

Romei C, Elisei R. *RET*/PTC Translocations and Clinico-Pathological Features in Human Papillary Thyroid Carcinoma. *Front Endocrinol (Lausanne)*. 2012;3:54.

12 **ANSWER: E) Repeated surveillance testing in 1 year**

This patient has microscopic local invasion of tumor and positive central compartment lymph node disease. According to the AJCC-7 staging system (American Joint Committee on Cancer, 7th edition) and the newer AJCC-8 staging system, his tumor is classified as T3,N1,M0, stage I. After surgery and radioiodine therapy, the patient has persistent elevation of serum thyroglobulin, but this is down-trending over time. According to current recommendations for restratification of risk on the basis of response to initial therapy, he has had an acceptable response to therapy, with unstimulated thyroglobulin less than 1.0 ng/mL (<1.0 μg/L) and stimulated thyroglobulin less than 10 ng/mL (<10 μg/L). Numerous studies have demonstrated progressive spontaneous decreases in thyroglobulin over years after initial therapy. The best option in this patient is to continue to monitor without intervention or additional unnecessary testing (Answer E).

PET-CT (Answer B) can be considered in patients with cancer who are at high risk and have elevated serum thyroglobulin (>10 ng/mL [>10 μg/L]) and a negative whole-body scan. However, such imaging is not indicated in this patient who has low and declining serum thyroglobulin values. Noncontrast chest CT (Answer C) is the most sensitive test for small lung metastases and may be obtained in patients with cancer who are at high risk and have elevated or rising serum thyroglobulin values. Neck MRI (Answer D) is occasionally useful for visualization of metastatic disease not well visualized by ultrasonography or contrast neck CT, but this is not the case here. There is no evidence for spurious thyroglobulin measurements, and assessing serum thyroglobulin over time in the same assay is preferred due to intra-assay variability (thus, Answer A is incorrect).

EDUCATIONAL OBJECTIVE:
Recommend an appropriate surveillance strategy for differentiated thyroid cancer.

REFERENCE(S):

Yim JH, Kim WB, Kim EY, et al. The outcomes of first reoperation for locoregionally recurrent/persistent papillary thyroid carcinoma in patients who initially underwent total thyroidectomy and remnant ablation. *J Clin Endocrinol Metab*. 2011;96(7):2049-2056.

Al-Saif O, Farrar WB, Bloomston M, Porter K, Ringel MD, Kloos RT. Long-term efficacy of lymph node reoperation for persistent papillary thyroid cancer. *J Clin Endocrinol Metab*. 2010;95(5):2187-2194.

Haugen BR, Alexander EK, Bible KC, et al. 2015 American Thyroid Association Management Guidelines for Adult Patients with Thyroid Nodules and Differentiated Thyroid Cancer: The

American Thyroid Association Guidelines Task Force on Thyroid Nodules and Differentiated Thyroid Cancer. *Thyroid*. 2016;26(1):1-133.

13 ANSWER: A) Repeat thyroid function tests in 6 months

Subclinical hyperthyroidism, in which serum TSH values are low but peripheral thyroid hormone is normal, is relatively common, affecting approximately 1.5% of the US adult population. About 5% of patients progress to overt hyperthyroidism, an outcome that is more likely when TSH is fully suppressed. Up to one-third of subclinical hyperthyroid patients may spontaneously become euthyroid again; this is most common when the underlying cause of their hyperthyroidism is Graves disease and when the baseline TSH level is between 0.1 and 0.4 mIU/L. Subclinical hyperthyroidism has been associated with increased risk for all-cause and cardiovascular mortality, atrial fibrillation, osteoporosis, and fracture. However, there is currently limited evidence for treatment benefit, particularly in younger individuals, and treatment confers some risks. Current guidelines recommend observation (Answer A) rather than treatment (Answers C, D, and E) for asymptomatic patients younger than 65 years who do not have cardiac disease or osteoporosis in whom the TSH is persistently lower than normal but 0.1 mIU/L or greater. β-adrenergic blockade (Answer B) might be useful in the setting of hyperthyroid symptoms or tachycardia, but this patient has neither.

EDUCATIONAL OBJECTIVE:
List indications for treatment of subclinical hyperthyroidism.

REFERENCE(S):
Ross DS, Burch HB, Cooper DS, et al. 2016 American Thyroid Association Guidelines for Diagnosis and Management of Hyperthyroidism and Other Causes of Thyrotoxicosis. *Thyroid*. 2016;26(10):1343-1421.

Carle A, Andersen SL, Boelaert K, Laurberg P. Management of endocrine disease: subclinical thyrotoxicosis: prevalence, causes and choice of therapy. *Eur J Endocrinol*. 2017;176(6): R325-R337.

Vadiveloo T, Donnan PT, Cochrane L, Leese GP. The Thyroid Epidemiology, Audit, and Research Study (TEARS): the natural history of endogenous subclinical hyperthyroidism. *J Clin Endocrinol Metab*. 2011;96(1):E1-E8.

14 ANSWER: D) FNAB again and measurement of thyroglobulin in aspirate

Measuring thyroglobulin in the fluid obtained from FNAB aspirates of lymph nodes (Answer D) is referred to as thyroglobulin "washout" because the specimen is obtained by rinsing the hub of the needle used for lymph node FNAB with 1 cc of normal saline. FNAB alone, without thyroglobulin washout, may fail to diagnose thyroid cancer in up to 20% of cases. The utility of this technique in cases such as the one described is now well established. The higher the aspirate thyroglobulin level, the more accurate the result. Washout thyroglobulin concentrations greater than 10 ng/mL (>10 µg/L) are both sensitive and 90% specific for tumor metastatic to the sampled lymph node. Because of the risk of nonspecific PET uptake in reactive lymph nodes, "positive" PET images must generally be confirmed with tissue sampling before referring the patient for reoperation (Answer A). PET-CT uptake within the suspicious lymph node has already been demonstrated in this patient, so repeating PET-CT with recombinant human TSH stimulation (Answer B) is not required. MRI of the neck (Answer C) would not add to this case. Not treating this patient with strongly suspected persistent disease (Answer E) is inappropriate. After identifying metastatic disease to lymph nodes, the next step is generally to refer for surgical removal to include compartmental dissection in previously nonoperated compartments, as cervical lymph nodes are often relatively radioiodine resistant.

EDUCATIONAL OBJECTIVE:
Explain the limitations of PET-CT imaging in patients with persistent thyroid cancer.

REFERENCE(S):
Urken ML, Milas M, Randolph GW, et al. Management of recurrent and persistent metastatic lymph nodes in well-differentiated thyroid cancer: a multifactorial decision-making guide

for the thyroid cancer care collaborative. *Head Neck*. 2015;37(4):605-614.

Haugen BR, Alexander EK, Bible KC, et al. 2015 American Thyroid Association Management Guidelines for Adult Patients with Thyroid Nodules and Differentiated Thyroid Cancer: The American Thyroid Association Guidelines Task Force on Thyroid Nodules and Differentiated Thyroid Cancer. *Thyroid*. 2016;26(1):1-133.

15 ANSWER: C) Plasmapheresis

This patient has developed thyroid storm after discontinuing methimazole. The diagnosis of thyroid storm can be made empirically or through the use of diagnostic scoring systems. Both the Burch-Wartofsky point score (75 points) and the Japan Thyroid Association system ("Thyroid storm-1, Combination-2") would categorize this patient as having thyroid storm. Emergent thyroidectomy has been used in similar patients when other conventional medical therapies fail.

Because antithyroid drugs cannot be started in this patient, other means must be used to prepare him for thyroidectomy. Plasmapheresis (Answer C), as well as plasma exchange and charcoal perfusion, has been used successfully in this setting in the immediate preoperative period since it removes plasma-containing proteins such as immunoglobulins and thyroxine-binding globulin. Hemodialysis (Answer A) does not remove the majority of thyroid hormone, because it is bound to binding proteins. Changing from intravenous propranolol to intravenous esmolol would make sense because of the ability to rapidly titrate the latter. However, changing to atenolol (Answer B), which is even less titratable than propranolol and does not provide propranolol's beneficial effect on blocking conversion of T_4 to T_3, would be incorrect. Intravenous immunoglobulin therapy (Answer D) has not been used effectively in the treatment of thyroid storm.

EDUCATIONAL OBJECTIVE:
Manage life-threatening thyrotoxicosis and use plasmapheresis in patients unable to take antithyroid drugs.

REFERENCE(S):
Warnock AL, Cooper DS, Burch HB. Life-threatening thyrotoxicosis: thyroid storm and adverse effects of antithyroid drugs. In: Mattfin G, ed. *Endocrine Medical Emergencies*. Endocrine Press: 2014.

Ross DS, Burch HB, Cooper DS, et al. 2016 American Thyroid Association Guidelines for Diagnosis and Management of Hyperthyroidism and Other Causes of Thyrotoxicosis. *Thyroid*. 2016;26(10):1343-1421.

Akamizu T, Satch T, Isozaki O, et al; Japan Thyroid Association. Diagnostic criteria, clinical features, and incidence of thyroid storm based on nation-wide surveys. *Thyroid*. 2012;22(7):661-679.

16 ANSWER: A) External beam radiation therapy to the thyroid bed

This patient has persistent, nonresectable thyroid cancer involving the trachea and recurrent laryngeal nerve, and the tumor does not appear to be radioiodine avid. These findings are an indication for external beam radiation therapy (Answer A). Tyrosine kinase inhibitor therapy (Answer B) may be used in these patients. However, the benefit of tyrosine kinase inhibitor therapy appears to be transient, whereas external beam radiation therapy is potentially tumoricidal. Repeated radioiodine therapy (Answer C) will not be helpful in this patient with non–radioiodine-avid disease. Conventional chemotherapy (Answer D) is of limited, if any, benefit in the treatment of thyroid cancer. Not treating this patient (Answer E) is inappropriate because he has known persistent, locally invasive disease.

EDUCATIONAL OBJECTIVE:
Recommend external beam radiation therapy in a patient with persistent, nonresectable, non–radioiodine-avid thyroid cancer.

REFERENCE(S):
Haugen BR, Alexander EK, Bible KC, et al. 2015 American Thyroid Association Management Guidelines for Adult Patients with Thyroid Nodules and Differentiated Thyroid Cancer: The American Thyroid Association Guidelines Task Force on Thyroid Nodules and Differentiated Thyroid Cancer. *Thyroid*. 2016;26(1):1-133.

Powell C, Newbold K, Harrington KJ, Bhide SA, Nutting CM. External beam radiotherapy for differentiated thyroid cancer. *Clin Oncol (R Coll Radiol).* 2010;22(6):456-463.

17 ANSWER: C) Thyroid-stimulating immunoglobulin level

Overall, without considering individual risk factors, the chance of remission after 12 to 18 months of antithyroid drug therapy is 30% to 50%. Men, persons older than 40 years, individuals with large goiters, cigarette smokers, and those with higher baseline thyroid hormone levels are less likely to achieve remission (thus, Answers A, D, and E are incorrect). After 12 to 18 months of antithyroid drug treatment, thyroid-stimulating immunoglobulin levels (Answer C) can be used to refine estimates for the likelihood of remission. Patients with negative thyroid receptor antibodies after 18 months of antithyroid drug treatment are more likely to remit than those in whom thyroid receptor antibodies remain detectable. In this patient who is euthyroid on methimazole but whose thyroid-stimulating immunoglobulin level remains high, the likelihood of long-term remission is only approximately 15%. TPO antibody titers (Answer B) are not associated with the probability of remission.

EDUCATIONAL OBJECTIVE:
List predictors of remission in Graves hyperthyroidism.

REFERENCE(S):
Franklyn JA, Boelaert K. Thyrotoxicosis. *Lancet.* 2012;379(9821):1155-1166.

Barbesino G, Tomer Y. Clinical review: clinical utility of TSH receptor antibodies. *J Clin Endocrinol Metab.* 2013;98(6):2247-2255.

Carella C, Mazziotti G, Sorvillo F, et al. Serum thyrotropin receptor antibodies concentrations in patients with Graves' disease before, at the end of methimazole treatment, and after drug withdrawal: evidence that the activity of thyrotropin receptor antibody and/or thyroid response modify during the observation period. *Thyroid.* 2006;16(3):295-302.

18 ANSWER: E) Cardiac tamponade

This patient has developed a large pericardial effusion (diminished heart sounds, low voltage on electrocardiography; a chest x-ray would also show an enlarged cardiac silhouette) (Answer E). She is already being treated with corticosteroids to prevent adrenal insufficiency (Answer A). Although she is at risk for developing cardiac ischemia (Answer B) as the thyroid hormone levels are increased, nothing in the scenario points to this diagnosis. The hypothyroid heart refers to decreased contractility and decreased pulse rate—both contributing to a decreased cardiac output at a time when peripheral vascular resistance is increased. The patient is at risk for congestive heart failure (Answer D) from this mechanism, but again nothing in the scenario suggests this etiology for the decline in her cardiac function. Although the TSH remains mildly elevated 48 hours after initiating intravenous levothyroxine treatment, the free T_4 is in the reference range. Thus, inadequate thyroid hormone replacement (Answer C) is unlikely.

EDUCATIONAL OBJECTIVE:
Identify signs of cardiac tamponade in a patient with myxedema coma.

REFERENCE(S):
Savage MW. Endocrine emergencies. *Postgrad Med J.* 2004;80(947):506-515.

Karu AK, Khalife WI, Houser R, VanderWoude J. Impending cardiac tamponade as a primary presentation of hypothyroidism: case report and review of literature. *Endocr Pract.* 2005;11(4):265-271.

19 ANSWER: A) Perform FNAB

This patient presents with thyrotoxicosis and neck pain with low radioactive iodine uptake, consistent with subacute thyroiditis. He has been treated with anti-inflammatory therapy with little improvement. Over a period of only 3 weeks he has had progressive asymmetric thyroid enlargement, now accompanied by dysphagia. The diagnosis in this patient was anaplastic thyroid cancer with thyrotoxicosis due to a destructive thyroiditis. There have been numerous reports of this unusual presentation of anaplastic thyroid cancer in the medical literature, and some patients have been treated with prolonged courses of corticosteroids before a correct diagnosis has been made. These patients typically have exceptionally aggressive disease and very limited survival. Although this is an atypical presentation, very rapid thyroid enlargement in an older patient should always prompt concern for anaplastic thyroid cancer. FNAB (Answer A) will determine his underlying diagnosis.

Prednisone (Answer C) may help with the pain from his thyroid inflammation. However, switching to prednisone, starting methimazole (Answer B), or performing contrast CT of the neck (Answer D) would all fail to determine the underlying diagnosis. In addition, methimazole is generally not useful in the management of low iodine uptake inflammatory thyroiditis, since thyroid hormone synthesis is not increased. Thyroidectomy (Answer E) should not be performed in the absence of a definitive diagnosis.

EDUCATIONAL OBJECTIVE:
Recognize low radioactive iodine uptake thyrotoxicosis and neck pain with rapid thyroid growth and no response to steroids as anaplastic cancer.

REFERENCE(S):
Kumar V, Blanchon B, Gu X, et al. Anaplastic thyroid cancer and hyperthyroidism. *Endocr Pathol.* 2005;16(3):245-250.

Heymann RS, Brent GA, Hershman JM. Anaplastic thyroid carcinoma with thyrotoxicosis and hypoparathyroidism. *Endocr Pract.* 2005;11(4):281-284.

Smallridge RC, Ain KB, Asa SL, et al; American Thyroid Association Anaplastic Thyroid Cancer Guidelines Taskforce. American Thyroid Association guidelines for management of patients with anaplastic thyroid cancer. *Thyroid.* 2012;22(11):1104-1139.

20 **ANSWER: B) Repeated thyroglobulin and thyroglobulin antibody measurements in 6 weeks using the same radioimmunoassay**

This patient has an elevated serum thyroglobulin value shortly after undergoing thyroidectomy for thyroid cancer. Thyroglobulin measurement is a sensitive tool for thyroid cancer surveillance, especially in thyroglobulin antibody–negative patients such as this one, but it is important to be aware of its limitations. In this case, it is simply too soon to measure the serum thyroglobulin postoperatively; values tend to be elevated in the first few days to weeks after surgery given serum thyroglobulin elevations caused by the surgical manipulation of the thyroid gland and the serum half-life of thyroglobulin. It is generally recommended to wait 6 weeks after thyroidectomy or 3 months after radioactive iodine ablation before the initial postoperative thyroglobulin measurement. If the measurements are repeated in 6 weeks (Answer B), it is likely that the thyroglobulin level will be substantially lower.

Ideally, thyroglobulin should be measured with the same assay over time due to substantial intra-assay variability (as much as 40%-60%) between methods. Repeating the measurement immediately with a different assay (Answer A) will still most likely result in an uninterpretable value because of timing. Measuring thyroglobulin in serially diluted sera (Answer C) can determine whether thyroglobulin is artifactually elevated (or, less frequently, artifactually decreased) due to the presence of heterophile antibodies. Such antibodies can form a bridge between capture and detection antibody leading to a false thyroglobulin measurement in immunometric assays. However, heterophile antibodies are unlikely to have caused an artifactual thyroglobulin elevation in this patient, since thyroglobulin was measured by radioimmunoassay. There is no indication for PET/CT scan (Answer D) since the serum thyroglobulin may well fall within the next few weeks. The patient has a low-risk tumor based on surgical pathology, so radioactive iodine ablation (Answer E) is not indicated.

EDUCATIONAL OBJECTIVE:
Identify common pitfalls with the use of serum thyroglobulin for thyroid cancer surveillance.

REFERENCE(S):
Giovanella L, Clark PM, Chiovato L, et al. Thyroglobulin measurement using highly sensitive assays in patients with differentiated thyroid cancer: a clinical position paper. *Eur J Endocrinol.* 2014;171(2):R33-R46.

Haugen BR, Alexander EK, Bible KC, et al. 2015 American Thyroid Association Management Guidelines for Adult Patients with Thyroid Nodules and Differentiated Thyroid Cancer: The American Thyroid Association Guidelines Task Force on Thyroid Nodules and Differentiated Thyroid Cancer. *Thyroid*. 2016;26(1):1-133.

21 ANSWER: C) TSH, 0.2 mIU/L; total T₄, 2.5 µg/dL (31.2 nmol/L); total T₃, 25 ng/dL (0.4 nmol/L); free T₄, 0.5 ng/dL (6.4 pmol/L)

This patient has been admitted to the intensive care unit for sepsis and multiorgan failure and her condition is deteriorating. She would be expected to have the classic changes in thyroid hormone levels that occur as a result of an acute nonthyroidal illness of this severity. The most prevalent and pronounced change of thyroid function during nonthyroidal illness is a low T_3 level, present in 70% or more of hospitalized patients, and it may be considered, with a few notable exceptions, the sine qua non of euthyroid sick syndrome. Total T_4 is frequently low in patients with severe nonthyroidal illness and a very low T_4 portends a poor prognosis. Free T_4 generally remains in the normal range, but may be frankly low in gravely ill or moribund patients, such as the patient in this case. TSH is frequently normal early in illness, but it may also be suppressed in critical illness and then elevated during the recovery stages (generally it is <20 mIU/L). Using the process of elimination, only Answers B and C have a low T_3 value. Answer B has a slightly elevated serum TSH level, which can be seen in the recovery stage after a nonthyroidal illness, but this patient is unfortunately not recovering. Answer C, with more severe alterations in T_3, as well as depressions in both total and free T_4, is a better fit for this particular moribund patient.

EDUCATIONAL OBJECTIVE:
Identify expected thyroid function test patterns in the recovery from severe nonthyroidal illness.

REFERENCE(S):
Farwell AP. Nonthyroidal illness syndrome. *Curr Opin Endocrinol Diabetes Obes*. 2013;20(5):478-484.

Van den Berghe G. Non-thyroidal illness in the ICU: a syndrome with different faces. *Thyroid*. 2014;24(10):1456-1465.

22 ANSWER: D) Repeat thyroid function tests in 4 to 6 weeks

The primary differential in this patient is between Graves disease and gestational thyrotoxicosis. Gestational thyrotoxicosis is the most frequent cause of hyperthyroidism in the first trimester. It is typically seen in women with hyperemesis gravidarum and is caused by markedly elevated serum β-hCG levels. The concentration of β-hCG correlates with the severity of nausea, and gestational thyrotoxicosis is unusual in women without clinically significant nausea and vomiting. Gestational thyrotoxicosis resolves spontaneously as β-hCG levels fall after weeks 10 to 12 of gestation. Graves disease is far more likely to be the cause of hyperthyroidism in this case because the thyrotoxicosis has not resolved after 12 weeks' gestation, T_3 is relatively elevated compared with T_4 levels, the thyroid-stimulating immunoglobulin is positive, and she has no nausea or vomiting. However, her hyperthyroidism is subclinical: while the TSH level is low, the free T_4 and total T_3 levels are appropriate for her stage of gestation. Note that due to increasing levels of thyroxine-binding globulin, total T_3 levels increase starting at week 7 of gestation until they plateau at week 16. A reasonable estimate for a gestational age–specific upper limit for total T_3 can be derived by adding 5% to the upper limit of the non-pregnancy total T_3 reference range each week starting at week 7. The upper limit will be 150% of the nonpregnancy reference range at week 16, and subsequently will remain stable for the rest of gestation.

Free T_4 assays generally do not perform well in pregnancy due to interference from high serum levels of binding globulins and esterified fatty acids, and although the effects of pregnancy are assay-specific, most assays provide artifactually low free T_4 values in the second and third trimesters. The free T_4 index, an older method in which both total T_4 and a test of serum thyroid hormone uptake such as the thyroid hormone–binding ratio are measured in order to calculate the level of free T_4, is more robust than commercial free T_4 assays in pregnancy and is preferred for the estimation of free T_4 in pregnant women when available.

Large cohort studies suggest that there is no obstetric risk associated with subclinical hyperthyroidism in pregnancy. This patient should be monitored to watch for progression to overt hyperthyroidism (Answer D), but she does not need treatment. Both methimazole (Answer A) and propylthiouracil (Answer B) are teratogenic and should not be used in women without overt hyperthyroidism. Thyroidectomy (Answer E) can be performed safely in the second trimester of pregnancy, but it is not warranted for subclinical hyperthyroidism. While short-term use of β-adrenergic blocker in pregnancy is sometimes warranted for the reduction of hyperthyroid symptoms, atenolol (Answer C), which is a US FDA pregnancy category D drug, should not be used during gestation. Propranolol or labetalol are safer choices in pregnancy.

EDUCATIONAL OBJECTIVE:
Diagnose and manage subclinical hyperthyroidism in pregnant women.

REFERENCE(S):

Alexander EK, Pearce EN, Brent GA, et al. 2017 Guidelines of the American Thyroid Association for the Diagnosis and Management of Thyroid Disease During Pregnancy and the Postpartum. *Thyroid.* 2017;27(3):315-389.

Cooper DS, Laurberg P. Hyperthyroidism in pregnancy. *Lancet Diabetes Endocrinol.* 2013;1(3):238-249.

Lee RH, Spencer CA, Mestman JH, et al. Free T4 immunoassays are flawed during pregnancy. *Am J Obstet Gynecol.* 2009;200(3):260.e1-e6.

23 **ANSWER: D) Thyroidectomy from collar incision**

The CT shows a substernal goiter with mass effect on the trachea. The patient is symptomatic, with positional dyspnea, most likely due to the compression of his trachea by the asymmetrically enlarged thyroid when he lies on his side. More than 90% of substernal goiters can be "delivered" through a collar incision (Answer D).

The remaining therapeutic options listed are less helpful. Specifically, this euthyroid patient's thyroid mass is unlikely to respond significantly to levothyroxine suppressive therapy (Answer A). Recombinant human TSH treatment (Answer B) with radioiodine in a patient with an intact thyroid is potentially dangerous due to a release of thyroid hormone from the gland under the influence of recombinant human TSH. Thermal ablation (Answer C) would not prove useful in reducing the size of this very large substernal goiter. No intervention (Answer E) would be inappropriate given his symptomatic disease.

EDUCATIONAL OBJECTIVE:
Devise an approach to a symptomatic substernal goiter.

REFERENCE(S):

Bahn RS, Castro MR. Approach to the patient with nontoxic multinodular goiter. *J Clin Endocrinol Metab.* 2011;96(5):1202-1212.

Fast S, Nielsen VE, Bonnema SJ, Hegedüs L. Dose-dependent acute effects of recombinant human TSH (rhTSH) on thyroid size and function: comparison of 0.1, 0.3 and 0.9 mg of rhTSH. *Clin Endocrinol (Oxf).* 2010;72(3):411-416.

Bonnema SJ, Hegedüs L. Radioiodine therapy in benign thyroid diseases: effects, side effects, and factors affecting therapeutic outcome. *Endocr Rev.* 2012;33(6):920-980.

24 **ANSWER: E) 10%**

Patients with non–radioiodine-avid distant metastases from differentiated thyroid cancer have a poor prognosis. Durante et al examined disease-specific survival in patients who had differentiated thyroid cancer with and without radioiodine uptake and found 10-year survival rates of 60% in patients with uptake in the metastatic disease but only 10% survival in those without radioiodine uptake (thus, Answer E is correct). Attempts have been made to restore radioiodine uptake in these lesions. Ho et al showed that a subgroup of such patients treated with the MAPK kinase (MEK) inhibitor selumetinib had a restoration of radioiodine avidity.

EDUCATIONAL OBJECTIVE:
Predict survival in advanced dedifferentiated thyroid cancer.

REFERENCE(S):

Durante C, Haddy N, Baudin E, et al. Long-term outcome of 444 patients with distant metastases from papillary and follicular thyroid carcinoma:

benefits and limits of radioiodine therapy. *J Clin Endocrinol Metab.* 2006;91(8):2892-2899.

Ho AL, Grewal RK, Leboeuf R, et al. Selumetinib-enhanced radioiodine uptake in advanced thyroid cancer. *N Engl J Med.* 2013;368(7):623-663.

25 ANSWER: D) Thyroid ultrasonography with color Doppler

This patient developed thyrotoxicosis shortly after the discontinuation of amiodarone. Amiodarone can persist for months in tissues such as liver and lung, and amiodarone-induced thyrotoxicosis may actually occur after drug discontinuation. Among the answers provided, thyroid ultrasonography with color Doppler (Answer E) is most likely to establish whether this is type 1 amiodarone-induced thyrotoxicosis (iodine-induced hyperthyroidism) vs type 2 (inflammatory thyroiditis). Thyroidal vascularity is typically diffusely increased in type 1 amiodarone-induced thyrotoxicosis, but absent in type 2. Recent reports suggest that ^{99m}Tc-sestamibi, although not among the provided choices, would also be a reasonable option for distinguishing between the 2 entities. Radioactive iodine uptake (Answer A) is typically low in both type 1 and type 2 amiodarone-induced thyrotoxicosis due to the high levels of nonradioactive iodine present in amiodarone. An initial study in the 1990s suggested that IL-6 (Answer B), a marker for inflammation, was elevated in type 2 amiodarone-induced thyrotoxicosis and low in type 1, but this test has subsequently been shown to be of very poor utility in distinguishing between the two. Finally, TPO antibodies (Answer C) do not discriminate between the entities.

EDUCATIONAL OBJECTIVE:
Explain testing modalities for distinguishing between the 2 types of amiodarone-induced thyrotoxicosis.

REFERENCE(S):

Danzi S, Klein I. Amiodarone-induced thyroid dysfunction. *J Intensive Care Med.* 2015;30(4):179-185.

Bogazzi F, Bartalena L, Martino E. Approach to the patient with amiodarone-induced thyrotoxicosis. *J Clin Endocrinol Metab.* 2010;95(6):2529-2535.

Tomisti L, Urbani C, Rossi G, et al. The presence of anti-thyroglobulin (TgAb) and/or anti-thyroperoxidase antibodies (TPOAb) does not exclude the diagnosis of type 2 amiodarone-induced thyrotoxicosis. *J Endocrinol Invest.* 2016;39(5):585-591.

Wang J, Zhang R. Evaluation of 99mTc-MIBI in thyroid gland imaging for the diagnosis of amiodarone-induced thyrotoxicosis. *Br J Radiol.* 2017;90(1071):20160836.

26 ANSWER: C) Familial dysalbuminemic hyperthyroxinemia

Familial dysalbuminemic hyperthyroxinemia (Answer C) is the most common inherited form of hyperthyroxinemia. It is found in 0.1% to 1.8% of individuals and is most common in Hispanic populations. Patients with familial dysalbuminemic hyperthyroxinemia are frequently overlooked with the widespread measurement of TSH alone to screen for thyroid dysfunction. Although free T_4 by equilibrium dialysis yields normal values in patients with familial dysalbuminemic hyperthyroxinemia, many free T_4 assays that are more susceptible to binding-protein changes give spurious elevations in free T_4, due to the altered protein binding (*see figure*).

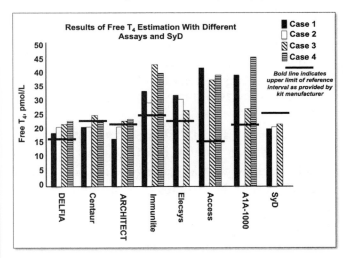

Adapted with permission of the American Association for Clinical Chemistry from Cartwright D, O'Shea P, Rajanayagam O, et al. Familial dysalbuminemic hyperthyroxinemia: a persistent diagnostic challenge. *Clin Chem.* 2009;55(5):1044-1046, permission conveyed through Copyright Clearance Center, Inc.

Familial dysalbuminemic hyperthyroxinemia is transmitted in an autosomal dominant fashion and is the result of gain-of-function mutations in the *ALB* gene encoding albumin that enhance the affinity of albumin for T_4, but generally not for T_3. As a result, reliance on total T_4 (elevated) or free T_4 index (also elevated, since this is a product of a normal T_3 resin and an elevated T_4) testing may be misleading.

A defect in 5′-monodeiodination due to selenium deficiency (Answer A) is much less common than familial dysalbuminemic hyperthyroxinemia. This patient does not have a TSH-secreting pituitary adenoma (Answer E) given that she is clinically euthyroid and T_3 levels are normal. This is not thyroid hormone resistance (Answer D) nor familial thyroxine-binding globulin excess (Answer B) because the total T_3 level is normal rather than elevated—an elevated total T_3 level would be expected in each of these disorders.

EDUCATIONAL OBJECTIVE:
Diagnose familial dysalbuminemic hyperthyroxinemia on the basis of clinical findings and thyroid function test results.

REFERENCE(S):
Pappa T, Ferrara AM, Refetoff S. Inherited defects of thyroxine-binding proteins. *Best Pract Res Clin Endocrinol Metab*. 2015;29(5):735-747.

Pannain S, Feldman M, Eiholzer U, Weiss RE, Scherberg NH, Refetoff S. Familial dysalbuminemic hyperthyroxinemia in a Swiss family caused by a mutant albumin (R218P) shows an apparent discrepancy between serum concentration and affinity for thyroxine. *J Clin Endocrinol Metab*. 2000;85(8):2786-2792.

27 **ANSWER: A) Primary hypothyroidism**
Sunitinib is a tyrosine kinase inhibitor used to treat certain malignancies such as renal cell carcinoma and gastrointestinal stromal tumors. Studies show that sunitinib can induce primary hypothyroidism (Answer A) in up to 85% of patients. Furthermore, sunitinib seems to increase the levothyroxine dosage requirement in hypothyroid patients. None of the remaining disorders (Answers B, C, D, and E) would be expected as a result of sunitinib therapy. Multiple other tyrosine kinase inhibitors, including sorafenib, cabozantinib, nilotinib, and pazopanib, are also associated with the development of hypothyroidism.

EDUCATIONAL OBJECTIVE:
Predict the most common effect that sunitinib has on thyroid function.

REFERENCE(S):
Makita N, Iiri T. Tyrosine kinase inhibitor-induced thyroid disorders: a review and hypothesis. *Thyroid*. 2013;23(2):151-159.

Desai J, Yassa L, Marqusee E, et al. Hypothyroidism after sunitinib treatment for patients with gastrointestinal stromal tumors. *Ann Intern Med*. 2006;145(9):660-664.

Illouz F, Braun D, Briet C, Schweizer U, Rodien P. Endocrine side-effects of anti-cancer drugs: thyroid effects of tyrosine kinase inhibitors. *Eur J Endocrinol*. 2014;171(3):R91-R99.

28 **ANSWER: E) Orbital decompression surgery**
This patient is at risk for permanent vision loss due to ischemic neuropathy, and high-dosage glucocorticoid therapy has already failed. He should undergo urgent orbital decompression surgery (Answer E).

Teprotumumab (Answer D) is a monoclonal antibody that inhibits the IGF-1 receptor and has recently been shown to effectively improve symptoms of active moderate-to-severe Graves ophthalmopathy, but this would not take effect rapidly enough to prevent threatened vision loss. Strabismus surgery (Answer C) may ultimately be needed, but it would be premature to perform this while the Graves eye disease is still active and evolving, and it would not reduce his risk for imminent vision loss. There are conflicting clinical trial data regarding the efficacy of rituximab (Answer B) in patients with moderate-to-severe Graves eye disease, but, even if it were effective, it would not work rapidly enough to be an appropriate choice in this clinical setting. Similarly, orbital radiotherapy (Answer A) is effective in about half of patients with moderate-to-severe eye disease, but the effects would not be rapid enough for this to be an appropriate response to sight-threatening disease.

EDUCATIONAL OBJECTIVE:
List indications for orbital decompression surgery in Graves orbitopathy.

REFERENCE(S):

Bartalena L, Tanda ML. Clinical practice. Graves' ophthalmopathy. *N Engl J Med.* 2009;360(10): 994-1001.

Wiersinga WM. Advances in treatment of active, moderate-to-severe Graves' ophthalmopathy. *Lancet Diabetes Endocrinol.* 2017;5(2):134-142.

Smith TJ, Kahaly GJ, Ezra DG, et al. Teprotumumab for thyroid-associated ophthalmopathy. *N Engl J Med.* 2017;376(18):1748-1761.

29 ANSWER: B) Screen for occult celiac disease

Celiac disease (Answer B) is a relatively common autoimmune condition that results in intolerance to dietary gluten. Malabsorption is characteristic of overt celiac disease, and refractory hypothyroidism due to levothyroxine malabsorption is well recognized. Recently, a higher-than-expected incidence of occult or previously unrecognized celiac disease has been found in patients with autoimmune thyroid disease. Similarly, unexplained vitamin D deficiency and resultant low bone mass on densitometry can occur in patients with previously unrecognized celiac disease. Several studies have shown the prevalence of celiac disease in patients with autoimmune thyroid disease to be approximately 3% to 5%, compared with approximately 1% in control populations. Similarly, a higher-than-expected prevalence of autoimmune thyroid disease has been described in patients with known celiac disease. Previously unsuspected celiac disease has been described both in patients with malabsorption of levothyroxine and in patients with vitamin D deficiency. Levothyroxine malabsorption in celiac disease is reversed with a gluten-free diet.

The remaining options are not plausible. Four hours of separation of levothyroxine from calcium supplements is generally considered sufficient (thus, Answer A is incorrect). The TSH and free T_4 assays are concordant, making antibody interference with the TSH assay unlikely (thus, Answer C is incorrect). T_3/T_4 combination therapy (Answer D) is preferred by some patients, although randomized controlled trials to date have not provided clear evidence for symptomatic improvement. However, this patient is not complaining of symptoms, and changing to combination therapy will not address the underlying problem.

EDUCATIONAL OBJECTIVE:
Diagnose celiac sprue as an etiology of uncontrolled hypothyroidism.

REFERENCE(S):

Virili C, Bassotti G, Santaguida MG, et al. Atypical celiac disease as cause of increased need for thyroxine: a systematic study. *J Clin Endocrinol Metab.* 2012;97(3):E419-E422.

Jonklaas J. Risks and safety of combination therapy for hypothyroidism. *Expert Rev Clin Pharmacol.* 2016;9(8):1057-1067.

30 ANSWER: C) The risk of future infection is 50%

This patient has a thyroglossal duct cyst present in the midline superior to the thyroid gland (denoted by arrows on the CT images). The thyroglossal duct is the tract that the developing thyroid follows in its embryologic descent from the base of the tongue to its final anatomic position in the neck. When the tract persists, it is prone to cyst formation along its length. According to the literature, these lesions are prone to bacterial infection at a lifetime rate of approximately 50% if left untreated (Answer C). The treatment is generally surgical resection together with removal of the central portion of the hyoid bone (this surgery is known as the Sistrunk procedure).

The incidence of thyroid cancer (Answer B) within a thyroglossal duct cyst is only 1%. Thyroglossal duct cysts do not respond to thyroid hormone suppressive therapy (Answer E) or radioiodine (Answer D) and are unlikely to completely resolve spontaneously (Answer A) at this stage.

EDUCATIONAL OBJECTIVE:
Summarize risks for cancer and infection in a thyroglossal duct cyst.

REFERENCE(S):

Rayess HM, Monk I, Svider PF, Gupta A, Raza SN, Lin HS. Thyroglossal duct cyst carcinoma: a systematic review of clinical features and outcomes. *Otolaryngol Head Neck Surg.* 2017;156(5):794-802.

Gioacchini FM, Alicandri-Ciufelli M, Kaleci S, Magliulo G, Presutti L, Re M. Clinical presentation and treatment outcomes of thyroglossal duct cysts: a systematic review. *Int J Oral Maxillofac Surg.* 2015;44(1):119-126.

APPENDIX A: LABORATORY REFERENCE RANGES

Reference ranges vary among laboratories. Conventional units are listed first with SI units in parentheses.

Lipid Values

High-density lipoprotein (HDL) cholesterol
Optimal.............................>60 mg/dL (>1.55 mmol/L)
Normal..................40-60 mg/dL (1.04-1.55 mmol/L)
Low....................................<40 mg/dL (<1.04 mmol/L)
Low-density lipoprotein (LDL) cholesterol
Optimal.........................<100 mg/dL (<2.59 mmol/L)
Low....................100-129 mg/dL (2.59-3.34 mmol/L)
Borderline-high...130-159 mg/dL (3.37-4.12 mmol/L)
High...................160-189 mg/dL (4.14-4.90 mmol/L)
Very high ....≥190 mg/dL (≥4.92 mmol/L)
Non-HDL cholesterol
Optimal.........................<130 mg/dL (<3.37 mmol/L)
Borderline-high...130-159 mg/dL (3.37-4.12 mmol/L)
High...............................≥240 mg/dL (≥6.22 mmol/L)
Total cholesterol
Optimal.........................<200 mg/dL (<5.18 mmol/L)
Borderline-high...200-239 mg/dL (5.18-6.19 mmol/L)
High...............................≥240 mg/dL (≥6.22 mmol/L)
Triglycerides
Optimal.........................<150 mg/dL (<3.88 mmol/L)
Borderline-high...150-199 mg/dL (3.88-5.15 mmol/L)
High.................200-499 mg/dL (5.18-12.92 mmol/L)
Very high ....≥500 mg/dL (≥12.95 mmol/L)
Lipoprotein (a).............≤30 mg/dL (≤1.07 μmol/L)
Apolipoprotein B.........50-110 mg/dL (0.5-1.1 g/L)

Hematologic Values

Erythrocyte sedimentation rate............ 0-20 mm/h
Haptoglobin ....30-200 mg/dL (300-2000 mg/L)
Hematocrit ....41%-50% (0.41-0.51) (male);
35%-45% (0.35-0.45) (female)
Hemoglobin A_{1c}......4.0%-5.6% (20-38 mmol/mol)
Hemoglobin 13.8-17.2 g/dL (138-172 g/L) (male);
12.1-15.1 g/dL (121-151 g/L) (female)
International normalized ratio 0.8-1.2
Mean corpuscular volume (MCV).......80-100 μm³
(80-100 fL)
Platelet count ...150-450 × 10³/μL (150-450 × 10⁹/L)
Protein (total)................... 6.3-7.9 g/dL (63-79 g/L)

Reticulocyte count.....0.5%-1.5% of red blood cells
(0.005-0.015)
White blood cell count....................4500-11,000/μL
(4.5-11.0 × 10⁹/L)

Thyroid Values

Thyroglobulin ....3-42 ng/mL (3-42 μg/L)
(after surgery and radioactive iodine treatment:
<1.0 ng/mL [<1.0 μg/L])
Thyroglobulin antibodies..≤4.0 IU/mL (≤4.0 kIU/L)
Thyrotropin (TSH) ....0.5-5.0 mIU/L
Thyroid-stimulating immunoglobulin ....≤120%
of basal activity
Thyroperoxidase (TPO) antibodies......<2.0 IU/mL
(<2.0 kIU/L)
Thyroxine (T_4) (free) ....0.8-1.8 ng/dL
(10.30-23.17 pmol/L)
Thyroxine (T_4) (total).......................5.5-12.5 μg/dL
(94.02-213.68 nmol/L)
Free thyroxine (T_4) index 4-12
Triiodothyronine (T_3) (free)..............2.3-4.2 pg/mL
(3.53-6.45 pmol/L)
Triiodothyronine (T_3) (total) ....70-200 ng/dL
(1.08-3.08 nmol/L)
Triiodothyronine (T_3), reverse.............10-24 ng/dL
(0.15-0.37 nmol/L)
Triiodothyronine uptake, resin.................25%-38%
Radioactive iodine uptake.........3%-16% (6 hours);
15%-30% (24 hours)

Endocrine Values

Serum

Aldosterone ....1-21 ng/dL (27.7-582.5 pmol/L)
Alkaline phosphatase ....50-120 U/L
(0.84-2.00 μkat/L)
Alkaline phosphatase (bone-specific)...... ≤20 μg/L
(adult male); ≤14 μg/L (premenopausal female);
≤22 μg/L (postmenopausal female)
Androstenedione ....65-210 ng/dL
(2.27-7.33 nmol/L) (adult male); 80-240 ng/dL
(2.79-8.38 nmol/L) (adult female)

Antimullerian hormone .... 0.7-19.0 ng/mL
(5.0-135.7 pmol/L) (male, >12 years);
0.9-9.5 ng/mL (6.4-67.9 pmol/L) (female,
13-45 years); <1.0 ng/mL (<7.1 pmol/L)
(female, >45 years)

Calcitonin .... <16 pg/mL (<4.67 pmol/L)
(basal, male); <8 pg/mL (<2.34 pmol/L)
(basal, female); ≤130 pg/mL (≤37.96 pmol/L)
(peak calcium infusion, male); ≤90 pg/mL
(≤26.28 pmol/L) (peak calcium infusion, female)

Carcinoembryonic antigen .... <2.5 ng/mL
(<2.5 μg/L)

Chromogranin A .... <93 ng/mL (<93 μg/L)

Corticosterone .... 53-1560 ng/dL
(1.53-45.08 nmol/L) (>18 years)

Corticotropin (ACTH) .... 10-60 pg/mL
(2.2-13.2 pmol/L)

Cortisol (8 AM)... 5-25 μg/dL (137.9-689.7 nmol/L)

Cortisol (4 PM).... 2-14 μg/dL (55.2-386.2 nmol/L)

C-peptide .... 0.9-4.3 ng/mL (0.30-1.42 nmol/L)

C-reactive protein.. 0.8-3.1 mg/L (7.62-29.52 nmol/L)

Cross-linked N-telopeptide of type 1 collagen ....
5.4-24.2 nmol BCE/mmol creat (male);
6.2-19.0 nmol BCE/mmol creat (female)

Dehydroepiandrosterone sulfate (DHEA-S)

Patient Age	Female	Male
18-29 years	44-332 μg/dL (1.19-9.00 μmol/L)	89-457 μg/dL (2.41-12.38 μmol/L)
30-39 years	31-228 μg/dL (0.84-6.78 μmol/L)	65-334 μg/dL (1.76-9.05 μmol/L)
40-49 years	18-244 μg/dL (0.49-6.61 μmol/L)	48-244 μg/dL (1.30-6.61 μmol/L)
50-59 years	15-200 μg/dL (0.41-5.42 μmol/L)	35-179 μg/dL (0.95-4.85 μmol/L)
≥60 years	15-157 μg/dL (0.41-4.25 μmol/L)	25-131 μg/dL (0.68-3.55 μmol/L)

Deoxycorticosterone .... <10 ng/dL (<0.30 nmol/L)
(>18 years)

1,25-Dihydroxyvitamin D_3 .... 16-65 pg/mL
(41.6-169.0 pmol/L)

Estradiol .... 10-40 pg/mL (36.7-146.8 pmol/L)
(male); 10-180 pg/mL (36.7-660.8 pmol/L)
(follicular, female); 100-300 pg/mL
(367.1-1101.3 pmol/L) (midcycle, female);
40-200 pg/mL (146.8-734.2 pmol/L) (luteal,
female); <20 pg/mL (<73.4 pmol/L)
(postmenopausal, female)

Estrone .... 10-60 pg/mL (37.0-221.9 pmol/L)
(male); 17-200 pg/mL (62.9-739.6 pmol/L)

(premenopausal female); 7-40 pg/mL
(25.9-147.9 pmol/L) (postmenopausal female)

α-Fetoprotein .... <6 ng/mL (<6 μg/L)

Follicle-stimulating hormone (FSH) ....
1.0-13.0 mIU/mL (1.0-13.0 IU/L) (male);
<3.0 mIU/mL (<3.0 IU/L) (prepuberty, female);
2.0-12.0 mIU/mL (2.0-12.0 IU/L) (follicular,
female); 4.0-36.0 mIU/mL (4.0-36.0 IU/L)
(midcycle, female); 1.0-9.0 mIU/mL (1.0-9.0 IU/L)
(luteal, female); >30 mIU/mL (>30 IU/L)
(postmenopausal, female)

Free fatty acids .... 10.6-18.0 mg/dL (0.4-0.7 nmol/L)

Gastrin .... <100 pg/mL (<100 ng/L)

Growth hormone (GH) .... 0.01-0.97 ng/mL
(0.01-0.97 μg/L) (male); 0.01-3.61 ng/mL
(0.01-3.61 μg/L) (female)

Homocysteine .... ≤1.76 mg/L (≤13 μmol/L)

β-Human chorionic gonadotropin (β-hCG) ....
<3.0 mIU/mL (<3.0 IU/L) (nonpregnant female);
>25 mIU/mL (>25 IU/L) indicates a positive
pregnancy test

β-Hydroxybutyrate ...... <3.0 mg/dL (<300 μmol/L)

17-Hydroxypregnenolone .... 29-189 ng/dL
(0.87-5.69 nmol/L)

17α-Hydroxyprogesterone .... <220 ng/dL
(<6.67 nmol/L) (adult male); <80 ng/dL
(<2.42 nmol/L) (follicular, female); <285 ng/dL
(<8.64 nmol/L) (luteal, female); <51 ng/dL
(1.55 nmol/L) (postmenopausal, female)

25-Hydroxyvitamin D... <10 ng/mL (<25.0 nmol/L)
(severe deficiency); 10-24 ng/mL (25.0-59.9 nmol/L)
(mild to moderate deficiency); 25-80 ng/mL
(62.4-199.7 nmol/L) (optimum levels);
>80 ng/mL (>199.7 nmol/L) (toxicity possible)

Inhibin B .... 15-300 pg/mL (15-300 ng/L)

Insulinlike growth factor 1 (IGF-1)

Patient Age	Female	Male
18 years	162-541 ng/mL (21.2-70.9 nmol/L)	170-640 ng/mL (22.3-83.8 nmol/L)
19 years	138-442 ng/mL (18.1-57.9 nmol/L)	147-527 ng/mL (19.3-69.0 nmol/L)
20 years	122-384 ng/mL (16.0-50.3 nmol/L)	132-457 ng/mL (17.3-59.9 nmol/L)
21-25 years	116-341 ng/mL (15.2-44.7 nmol/L)	116-341 ng/mL (15.2-44.7 nmol/L)
26-30 years	117-321 ng/mL (15.3-42.1 nmol/L)	117-321 ng/mL (15.3-42.1 nmol/L)
31-35 years	113-297 ng/mL (14.8-38.9 nmol/L)	113-297 ng/mL (14.8-38.9 nmol/L)

Patient Age	Female	Male
36-40 years	106-277 ng/mL (13.9-36.3 nmol/L)	106-277 ng/mL (13.9-36.3 nmol/L)
41-45 years	98-261 ng/mL (12.8-34.2 nmol/L)	98-261 ng/mL (12.8-34.2 nmol/L)
46-50 years	91-246 ng/mL (11.9-32.2 nmol/L)	91-246 ng/mL (11.9-32.2 nmol/L)
51-55 years	84-233 ng/mL (11.0-30.5 nmol/L)	84-233 ng/mL (11.0-30.5 nmol/L)
56-60 years	78-220 ng/mL (10.2-28.8 nmol/L)	78-220 ng/mL (10.2-28.8 nmol/L)
61-65 years	72-207 ng/mL (9.4-27.1 nmol/L)	72-207 ng/mL (9.4-27.1 nmol/L)
66-70 years	67-195 ng/mL (8.8-25.5 nmol/L)	67-195 ng/mL (8.8-25.5 nmol/L)
71-75 years	62-184 ng/mL (8.1-24.1 nmol/L)	62-184 ng/mL (8.1-24.1 nmol/L)
76-80 years	57-172 ng/mL (7.5-22.5 nmol/L)	57-172 ng/mL (7.5-22.5 nmol/L)
≥80 years	53-162 ng/mL (6.9-21.2 nmol/L)	53-162 ng/mL (6.9-21.2 nmol/L)

Insulinlike growth factor binding ......2.5-4.8 mg/L protein 3

Insulin ....1.4-14.0 µIU/mL (9.7-97.2 pmol/L)

Islet-cell antibody assay ....0 Juvenile Diabetes Foundation units

Luteinizing hormone (LH)............1.0-9.0 mIU/mL (1.0-9.0 IU/L) (male); <1.0 mIU/mL (<1.0 IU/L) (prepuberty, female); 1.0-18.0 mIU/mL (1.0-18.0 IU/L) (follicular, female); 20.0-80.0 mIU/mL (20.0-80.0 IU/L) (midcycle, female); 0.5-18.0 mIU/mL (0.5-18.0 IU/L) (luteal, female); >30 mIU/mL (>30 IU/L) (postmenopausal, female)

Metanephrines (plasma fractionated)
   Metanephrine....................<57 pg/mL (<289 pmol/L)
   Normetanephrine...........<148 pg/mL (<808 pmol/L)

75-g oral glucose tolerance test
   Blood glucose values ....60-100 mg/dL (3.3-5.6 mmol/L) (fasting); <200 mg/dL (<11.1 mmol/L) (1 hour); <140 mg/dL (<7.8 mmol/L) (2 hour)
   Between 140-200 mg/dL (7.8-11.1 mmol/L) is considered impaired glucose tolerance or prediabetes. Greater than 200 mg/dL (11.1 mmol/L) is a sign of diabetes mellitus.

50-g oral glucose tolerance test for gestational diabetes ....<140 mg/dL (<7.8 mmol/L) (1 hour)

100-g oral glucose tolerance test for gestational diabetes .....<95 mg/dL (<5.3 mmol/L) (fasting);

<180 mg/dL (<10.0 mmol/L) (1 hour); <155 mg/dL (<8.6 mmol/L) (2 hour); <140 mg/dL (<7.8 mmol/L) (3 hour)

Osteocalcin............9.0-42.0 ng/mL (9.0-42.0 µg/L)

Parathyroid hormone, intact (PTH) ..10-65 pg/mL (10-65 ng/L)

Parathyroid hormone–related protein (PTHrP) ....14-27 pg/mL (14-27 ng/L)

Progesterone.... ≤1.2 ng/mL (≤3.8 nmol/L) (male); ≤1.0 ng/mL (≤3.2 nmol/L) (follicular, female); 2.0-20.0 ng/mL (6.4-63.6 nmol/L) (luteal, female); ≤1.1 ng/mL (≤3.5 nmol/L) (postmenopausal, female); >10.0 ng/mL (>31.8 nmol/L) (evidence of ovulatory adequacy)

Proinsulin .....26.5-176.4 pg/mL (3.0-20.0 pmol/L)

Prolactin ...4-23 ng/mL (0.17-1.00 nmol/L) (male); 4-30 ng/mL (0.17-1.30 nmol/L) (nonlactating female); 10-200 ng/mL (0.43-8.70 nmol/L) (lactating female)

Prostate-specific antigen... <2.0 ng/mL (<2.0 µg/L) (≤40 years); <2.8 ng/mL (<2.8 µg/L) (≤50 years); <3.8 ng/mL (<3.8 µg/L) (≤60 years); <5.3 ng/mL (<5.3 µg/L) (≤70 years); <7.0 ng/mL (<7.0 µg/L) (≤79 years); <7.2 ng/mL (<7.2 µg/L) (≥80 years)

Renin activity, plasma, sodium replete, ambulatory ....0.6-4.3 ng/mL per h

Renin, direct concentration ....30-40 pg/mL (0.7-1.0 pmol/L)

Sex hormone–binding globulin........1.1-6.7 µg/mL (10-60 nmol/L) (male); 2.2-14.6 µg/mL (20-130 nmol/L) (female)

α-Subunit of pituitary glycoprotein hormones.......<1.2 ng/mL (<1.2 µg/L)

Testosterone (bioavailable) ....0.8-4.0 ng/dL (0.03-0.14 nmol/L) (20-50 years, female on oral estrogen); 0.8-10.0 ng/dL (0.03-0.35 nmol/L) (20-50 years, female not on oral estrogen); 83.0-257.0 ng/dL (2.88-8.92 nmol/L) (male 20-29 years); 72.0-235.0 ng/dL (2.50-8.15 nmol/L) (male 30-39 years); 61.0-213.0 ng/dL (2.12-7.39 nmol/L) (male 40-49 years); 50.0-190.0 ng/dL (1.74-6.59 nmol/L) (male 50-59 years); 40.0-168.0 ng/dL (1.39-5.83 nmol/L) (male 60-69 years)

Testosterone (free)............................9.0-30.0 ng/dL (0.31-1.04 nmol/L) (male); 0.3-1.9 ng/dL (0.01-0.07 nmol/L) (female)

Testosterone (total)............................300-900 ng/dL
   (10.4-31.2 nmol/L) (male); 8-60 ng/dL
   (0.3-2.1 nmol/L) (female)
Vitamin B$_{12}$............ 180-914 pg/mL (180-914 ng/L)

Chemistry Values

Alanine aminotransferase .... 10-40 U/L
   (0.17-0.67 µkat/L)
Albumin............................ 3.5-5.0 g/dL (35-50 g/L)
Amylase ....26-102 U/L (0.43-1.70 µkat/L)
Aspartate aminotransferase .... 20-48 U/L
   (0.33-0.80 µkat/L)
Bicarbonate..............21-28 mEq/L (21-28 mmol/L)
Bilirubin (total)....0.3-1.2 mg/dL (5.1-20.5 µmol/L)
Blood gases
   Po_2, arterial blood..... 80-100 mm Hg (10.6-13.3 kPa)
   Pco_2, arterial blood .... 35-45 mm Hg (4.7-6.0 kPa)
Blood pH 7.35-7.45
Calcium.............. 8.2-10.2 mg/dL (2.1-2.6 mmol/L)
Calcium (ionized)......................... 4.60-5.08 mg/dL
   (1.2-1.3 mmol/L)
Carbon dioxide ....22-28 mEq/L (22-28 mmol/L)
CD$_4$ cell count .... 500-1400/µL (0.5-1.4 × 10^9/L)
Chloride...............96-106 mEq/L (96-106 mmol/L)
Creatine kinase ....50-200 U/L (0.84-3.34 µkat/L)
Creatinine .... 0.7-1.3 mg/dL (61.9-114.9 µmol/L)
   (male); 0.6-1.1 mg/dL (53.0-97.2 µmol/L) (female)
Ferritin .... 15-200 ng/mL (33.7-449.4 pmol/L)
Folate ....≥4.0 ng/mL (≥4.0 µg/L)
Glucose .... 70-99 mg/dL (3.9-5.5 mmol/L)
γ-Glutamyltransferase....2-30 U/L (0.03-0.50 µkat/L)
Iron .... 50-150 µg/dL (9.0-26.8 µmol/L) (male);
   35-145 µg/dL (6.3-26.0 µmol/L) (female)
Lactate dehydrogenase......................... 100-200 U/L
   (1.7-3.3 µkat/L)
Lactic acid.......... 5.4-20.7 mg/dL (0.6-2.3 mmol/L)
Lipase ....10-73 U/L (0.17-1.22 µkat/L)
Magnesium.......... 1.5-2.3 mg/dL (0.6-0.9 mmol/L)
Osmolality ...275-295 mOsm/kg (275-295 mmol/kg)
Phosphorus.......... 2.3-4.7 mg/dL (0.7-1.5 mmol/L)
Potassium.................3.5-5.0 mEq/L (3.5-5.0 mmol/L)
Prothrombin time....................................8.3-10.8 s
Serum urea nitrogen ....8-23 mg/dL
   (2.9-8.2 mmol/L)
Sodium............ 136-142 mEq/L (136-142 mmol/L)
Transferrin saturation 14%-50%
Troponin I .... <0.6 ng/mL (<0.6 µg/L)
Tryptase ....<11.5 ng/mL (<11.5 µg/L)
Uric acid........ 3.5-7.0 mg/dL (208.2-416.4 µmol/L)

Urine

Albumin.................................... 30-300 µg/mg creat
   (3.4-33.9 µg/mol creat)
Albumin-to-creatinine ratio .... <30 mg/g creat
Aldosterone ....3-20 µg/24 h (8.3-55.4 nmol/d)
   (should be <12 µg/24 h [<33.2 nmol/d] with
   oral sodium loading—confirmed with 24-hour
   urinary sodium >200 mEq)
Calcium........... 100-300 mg/24 h (2.5-7.5 mmol/d)
Catecholamine fractionation
   Normotensive normal ranges:
      Dopamine .... <700 µg/24 h (<4567 nmol/d)
      Epinephrine .... <35 µg/24 h (<191 nmol/d)
      Norepinephrine..... <170 µg/24 h (<1005 nmol/d)
Cortisol....................4-50 µg/24 h (11-138 nmol/d)
Dexamethasone suppression test
   (low-dose: 2 day, 2 mg daily), urinary free
   cortisol ....<10 µg/24 h (<27.6 nmol/d)
Creatinine ....1.0-2.0 g/24 h (8.8-17.7 mmol/d)
Glomerular filtration rate (estimated) ... >60 mL/min
   per 1.73 m^2
5-Hydroxyindole acetic acid ....2-9 mg/24 h
   (10.5-47.1 µmol/d)
Iodine (random) .... >100 µg/L
17-Ketosteroids.........................6.0-21.0 mg/24 h
   (20.8-72.9 µmol/d) (male); 4.0-17.0 mg/24 h
   (13.9-59.0 µmol/d) (female)
Metanephrine fractionation
   Metanephrine.............. <400 µg/24 h (<2028 nmol/d)
   Normetanephrine....... <900 µg/24 h (<4914 nmol/d)
   Total metanephrine .. <1000 µg/24 h (<5260 nmol/d)
Osmolality .... 150-1150 mOsm/kg
   (150-1150 mmol/kg)
Oxalate ....<40 mg/24 h (<456 mmol/d)
Phosphate ....0.9-1.3 g/24 h (29.1-42.0 mmol/d)
Potassium...........17-77 mEq/24 h (17-77 mmol/d)
Sodium........... 40-217 mEq/24 h (40-217 mmol/d)
Uric acid................... <800 mg/24 h (<4.7 mmol/d)

Saliva

Cortisol (salivary), midnight .... <0.13 µg/dL
   (<3.6 nmol/L)

Semen

Semen analysis .... >20 million sperm/mL;
   >50% motility

ACTH = corticotropin
ACE inhibitor = angiotensin-converting enzyme inhibitor
ALT = alanine aminotransferase
AST = aspartate aminotransferase
BMI = body mass index
CNS = central nervous system
CT = computed tomography
DHEA = dehydroepiandrosterone
DHEA-S = dehydroepiandrosterone sulfate
DNA = deoxyribonucleic acid
DXA = dual-energy x-ray absorptiometry
FDA = Food and Drug Administration
FNAB = fine-needle aspiration biopsy
FSH = follicle-stimulating hormone
GH = growth hormone
GHRH = growth hormone–releasing hormone
GnRH = gonadotropin-releasing hormone
hCG = human chorionic gonadotropin
HDL = high-density lipoprotein

HIV = human immunodeficiency virus
HMG-CoA reductase inhibitor = 3-hydroxy-3-methylglutaryl coenzyme A reductase inhibitor
IGF-1 = insulinlike growth factor 1
LDL = low-density lipoprotein
LH = luteinizing hormone
MCV = mean corpuscular volume
MRI = magnetic resonance imaging
NPH insulin = neutral protamine Hagedorn insulin
PET = positron emission tomography
PTH = parathyroid hormone
PTHrP = parathyroid hormone–related protein
T_3 = triiodothyronine
T_4 = thyroxine
TPO antibodies = thyroperoxidase antibodies
TRH = thyrotropin-releasing hormone
TSH = thyrotropin
VLDL = very low-density lipoprotein